The Plague Files

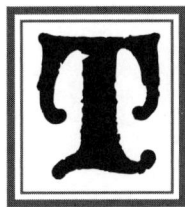

The Plague Files

CRISIS MANAGEMENT IN SIXTEENTH-CENTURY SEVILLE

ALEXANDRA PARMA COOK AND NOBLE DAVID COOK

LOUISIANA STATE UNIVERSITY PRESS ✳ BATON ROUGE

This publication was made possible in part by a grant from the Program for Cultural Cooperation between Spain's Ministry of Culture and United States Universities.

Published by Louisiana State University Press
Copyright © 2009 by Louisiana State University Press
All rights reserved
Manufactured in the United States of America
First printing

Designer: AMANDA MCDONALD SCALLAN
Typefaces: MINION, DISPLAY BLACKMOOR
Typesetter: J. JARRETT ENGINEERING, INC.
Printer and binder: THOMSON-SHORE, INC.

Library of Congress Cataloging-in-Publication Data

Cook, Alexandra Parma.
    The plague files : crisis management in sixteenth-century Seville / Alexandra Parma Cook and Noble David Cook.
        p. ; cm.
    Includes bibliographical references and index.
    ISBN 978-0-8071-3404-7 (cloth : alk. paper) 1. Plague—Spain—Seville—History—16th century. I. Cook, Noble David. II. Title.
    [DNLM: 1. Plague—history—Spain. 2. History, 16th Century—Spain. WC 350 C773p 2009]
    RC178.S72S48 2009
    614.5'73209468609031—dc22

                                                                        2008038037

For the Sevillanos of today, and yesterday

CONTENTS

ACKNOWLEDGMENTS

This project began, as often others do, by a chance "discovery" in 1990 of a cache of documents while we were engaged in another investigation, in this case a preliminary study of the social and economic history of Triana, the maritime district of Seville.[1] We were working in Seville's Municipal Archive, looking through hundreds of sixteenth- and seventeenth-century documents, and came across a special volume of bound papers that dealt with a suspected outbreak of the bubonic plague. The information was rich and fascinating, and given our long-standing interest in epidemic disease, it immediately fired up our imagination. We began collecting data not only on our original Triana project but on the plague as well. Unfortunately, owing to other endeavors, the actual writing dragged on for many years, with frequent interruptions.

Friends and colleagues have been subjected over the years to our enthusiastic recounting of the progress of "the plague book," and we thank them for their indulgence and apologize for not naming them all. Our special gratitude for their friendship and support goes to Mari Luz Peña and José Hernández Palomo, Enriqueta Vila Vilar, George Lovell, Graciela and Nicolás Sánchez Albornoz, the late Franklin Pease and Mariana Pease, Margarita Suárez, Rafael Varón, Miguel Costa, and Karoline Cook. Consuelo Varela and Juan Gil have given of their time and expertise, and we have shared many happy hours together on both sides of the Atlantic. We are especially indebted to James Boyden, Juan Gil, Richard Kagan, and two anonymous readers for their magnanimous and valuable comments. Maps were prepared by Joseph Stoll of the Syracuse University Cartographic Lab under the direction of David Robinson. We also want to thank our Sevillian friends outside the profession whose generosity has been boundless: Emilia Morón and Luis Sánchez and their (and our) extended

1. These documents have been consulted by various historians; see, for example, José Velázquez y Sánchez, *Anales epidémicos: Reseña histórica de las enfermedades contagiosas en Sevilla desde la reconquista cristiana hasta nuestros días (1866)* (Seville: Colección Clásicos Sevillanos, Ayuntamiento de Sevilla, 1996); and, more recently, Juan Ignacio Carmona García, *La peste en Sevilla* (Seville: Ayuntamiento de Sevilla, 2004).

family. We thank our friends and neighbors, Rosa Muñiz and Manuel Parejo, for alerting us to and loaning us their copy of *Melchor y la señora del Robledo*. We appreciate Margit and Graeme Dutton-Forshaw's hospitality during our brief research trip to Britain, and we have many fond memories of pub hopping.

Original support for the study that began in 1990–91 came from the joint Spanish-U.S. Committee for Cultural and Educational Cooperation. In subsequent years we have been fortunate to spend several summers continuing research in Seville's archives. There were two longer periods. In 1998–99 a generous grant from the American Council of Learned Societies provided a full year of concentrated research. A sabbatical from Florida International University in 2001–02 allowed us to fine-tune the plague account as well as continue research on Triana.

Without helpful and knowledgeable archivists and librarians, historians would find it difficult to carry out their work. We wish to thank the wonderful staffs of the Archivo Municipal de Sevilla (and its then-director, Doña Eulalia de la Cruz Bugallal); the Sala de Manuscritos of the Biblioteca Nacional in Madrid; the Archivo General de Indias in Seville; the British Library in London; the Library of Congress in Washington, D.C.; and the interlibrary loan librarians at Florida International University. We also thank Doña Isabel Simó, past director of the Archivo Histórico Provincial of Seville and current director of the Archivo General de Indias. Our special gratitude goes to Don Agustín Pinto Pabón, head of the Sala de Investigaciones, and the entire staff of the Archivo Histórico Provincial of Seville that over the years has become our second home. We not only appreciate all their assistance but, more important, we cherish their friendship and conversation. For help with the illustrations we thank Consuelo Varela and J. Carlos Martínez of the Escuela de Estudios Hispanoamericanos in Seville, and at Florida International University, Ivan E. Santiago and Rocío González of the Educational Technology Resource Center. Katherine Kimball's professionalism as a copyeditor is evident throughout the text. Last but not least, our special thanks go to our editor, Alisa Plant, who became as excited as we are about the events and lives that we attempt to recreate in this small history.

ABBREVIATIONS

Unless otherwise indicated, all translations are our own.
Archival works have been cited using the following abbreviations:

AGI	Archivo General de Indias
AHPS	Archivo Histórico Provincial de Sevilla
AMS	Archivo Municipal de Sevilla
BL	British Library
BNM	Biblioteca Nacional, Madrid

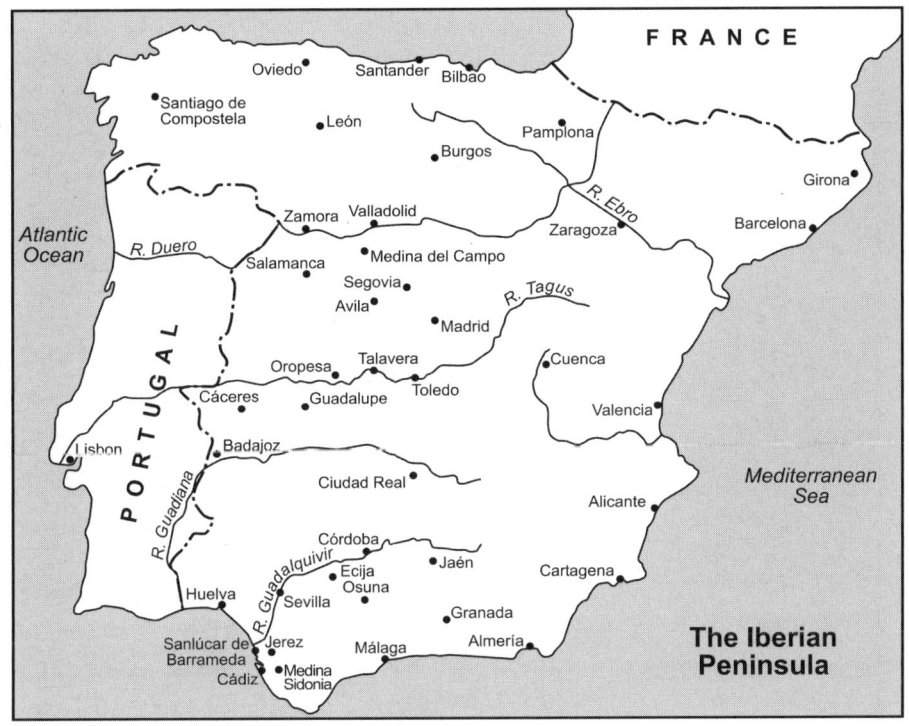

The Iberian Peninsula

David Robinson

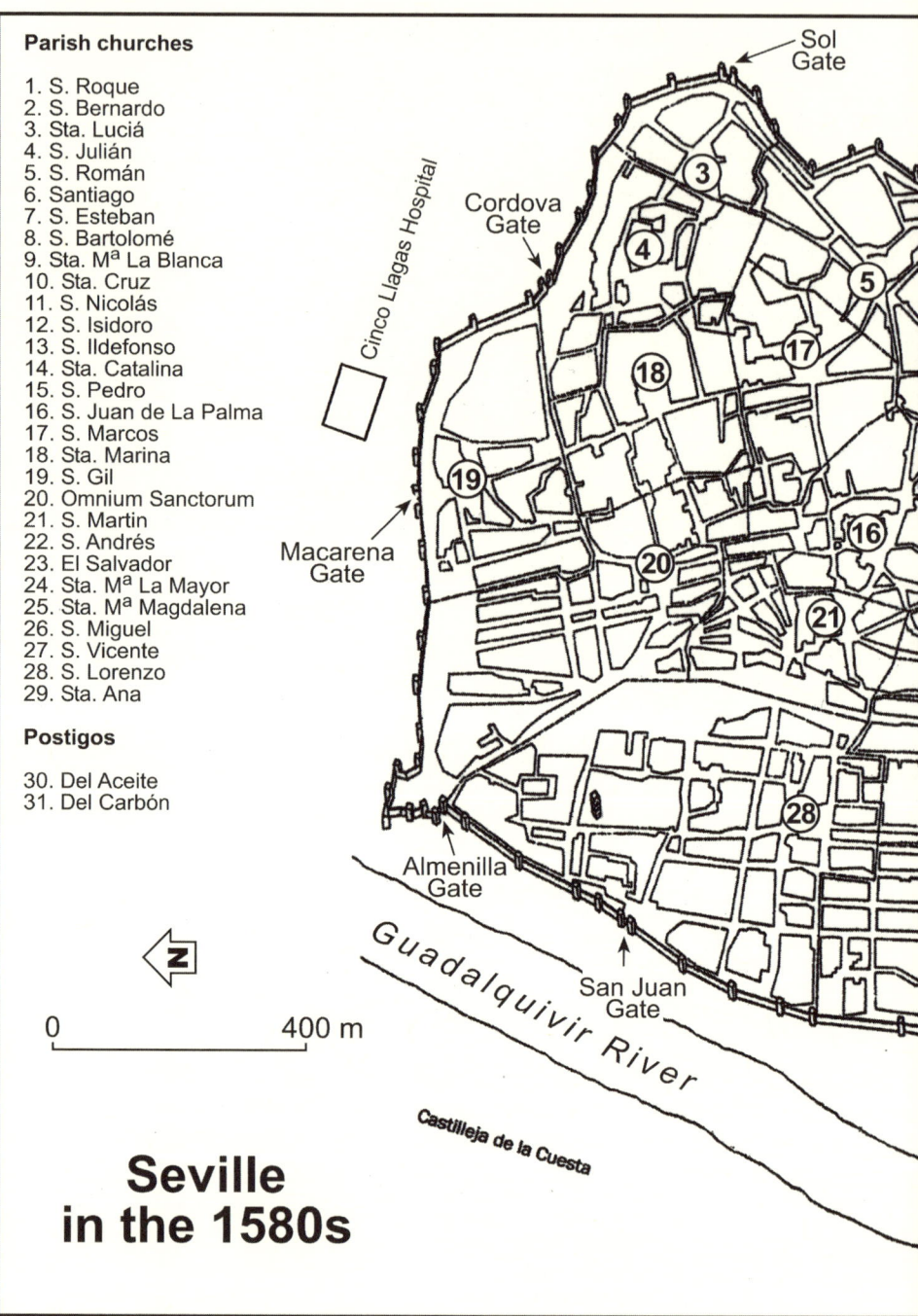

Parish churches

1. S. Roque
2. S. Bernardo
3. Sta. Luciá
4. S. Julián
5. S. Román
6. Santiago
7. S. Esteban
8. S. Bartolomé
9. Sta. Mª La Blanca
10. Sta. Cruz
11. S. Nicolás
12. S. Isidoro
13. S. Ildefonso
14. Sta. Catalina
15. S. Pedro
16. S. Juan de La Palma
17. S. Marcos
18. Sta. Marina
19. S. Gil
20. Omnium Sanctorum
21. S. Martin
22. S. Andrés
23. El Salvador
24. Sta. Mª La Mayor
25. Sta. Mª Magdalena
26. S. Miguel
27. S. Vicente
28. S. Lorenzo
29. Sta. Ana

Postigos

30. Del Aceite
31. Del Carbón

Cinco Llagas Hospital

Sol Gate

Cordova Gate

Macarena Gate

Almenilla Gate

San Juan Gate

Guadalquivir River

Castilleja de la Cuesta

N

0   400 m

Seville
in the 1580s

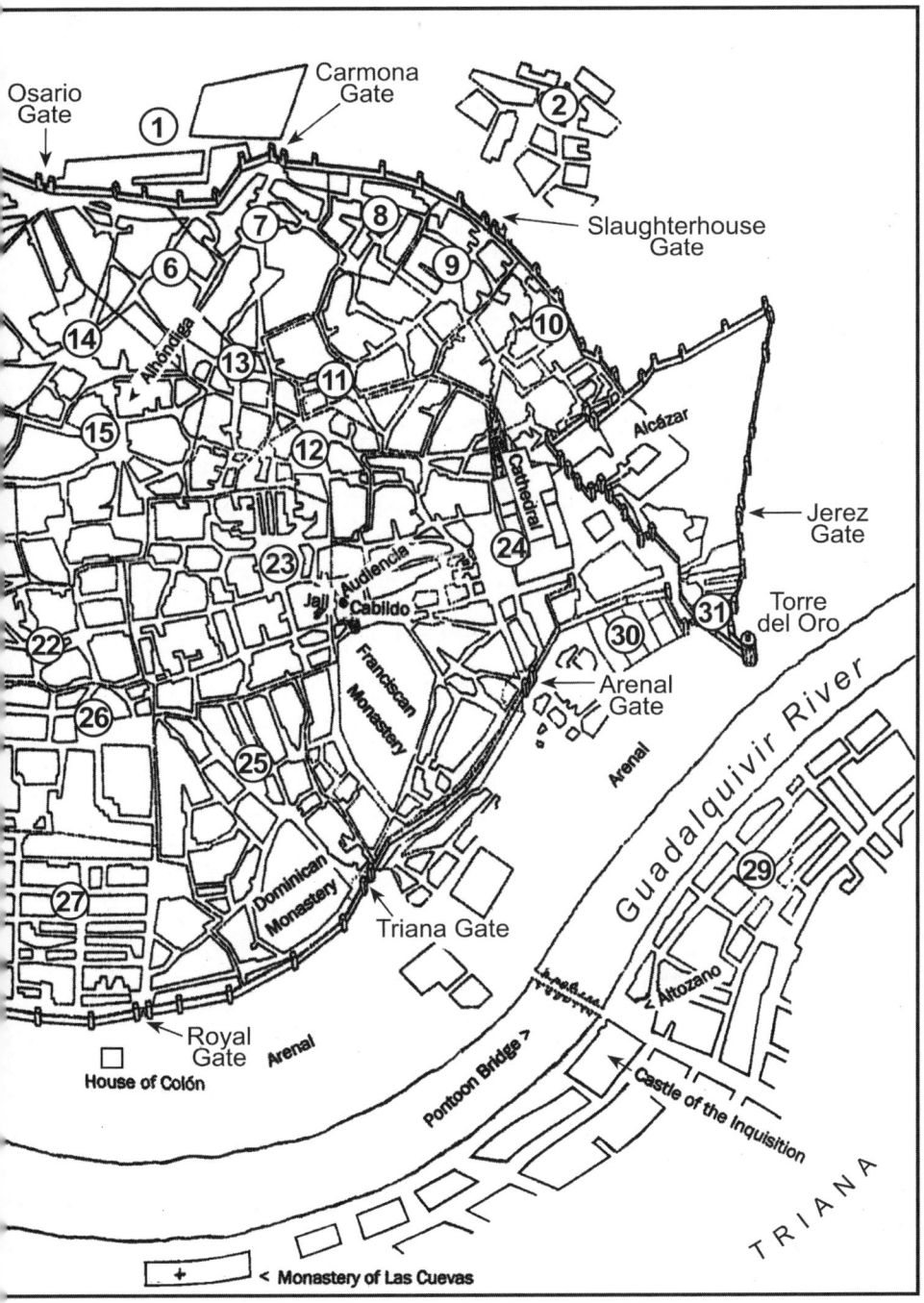

Osario
Gate

Carmona
Gate

① 1

② 2

Slaughterhouse
Gate

⑦ 7

⑧ 8

⑥ 6

⑨ 9

⑭ 14

Alhóndiga

⑬ 13

⑪ 11

⑩ 10

⑮ 15

⑫ 12

Alcázar

Jerez
Gate

Cathedral

⑳ 24

Jail Audiencia

⑳ 23

Cabildo

⑳ 30

③① 31

Torre
del Oro

㉒ 22

Franciscan
Monastery

Arenal
Gate

㉖ 26

Arenal

Guadalquivir River

㉕ 25

⑳ 29

㉗ 27

Dominican
Monastery

Altozano

Triana Gate

Royal
Gate   Arenal

House of Colón

Pontoon Bridge ›

Castle of the Inquisition

T R I A N A

+   ‹ Monastery of Las Cuevas

David Robinson

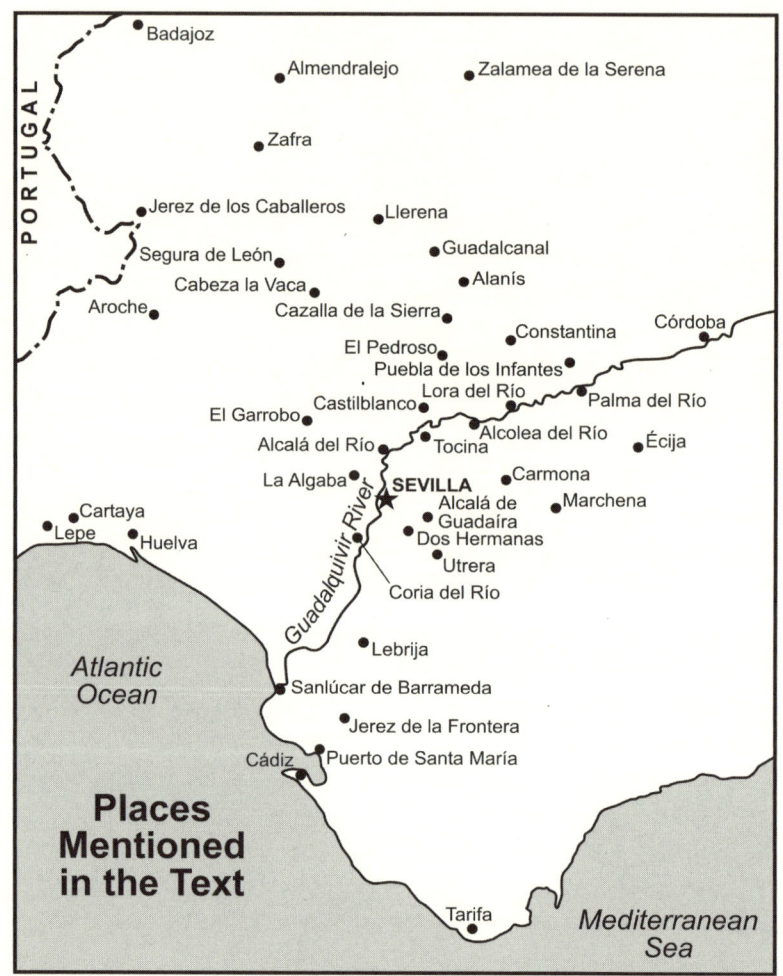

Places
Mentioned
in the Text

David Robinson

INTRODUCTION

Seville was one of Europe's largest Atlantic port cities in the late sixteenth century, comparable in size to Lisbon, London, and Antwerp. Only Paris and Venice had more inhabitants than Seville.[1] The urban complex was a vibrant, cosmopolitan place that attracted migrants from nearby towns and other areas of Andalusia as well as Extremadura and further afield. The population included traders and merchants from Castilian cities such as Medina del Campo, León, and Burgos, and many Basques, Galicians, and Catalans lived in Seville. There were numerous residents from the Kingdom of Naples and Sicily, the commercial and banking cities of Genoa and Venice, and some from Greece. There were people from Flanders, France, and Germany as well as England, but there was an especially large community of Portuguese, given the proximity of their homeland to Seville. Slave ownership bestowed status, and many Sevillians had not just African slaves but also an occasional Amerindian captive.

From a vantage point near the crest of the bluff of Castilleja de la Cuesta overlooking the Guadalquivir River basin, the spectator could discern to the east the elegant Muslim prayer tower, the Giralda, capped by the Christian belfry with its magnificent weathervane, towering above the cathedral and the nearby Alcázar. Elements of Islamic Spain were still visible, determinedly standing even three centuries after the 1248 Christian *reconquista* (reconquest). The Triana plain spread across the foreground, its vineyards producing palatable wines as well as vinegar and its many vegetable gardens and olive and fruit trees supplying Seville's hungry population and the export trade. Even from a distance one could easily trace the mighty river and note the imposing castle housing the tribunal of the Inquisition. The fearsome fortress sat on the west bank of the Guadalquivir, dominating the maritime district of Triana, and near the centuries-old pontoon bridge linking the western suburb to the city proper on

1. Estimates of Seville's population in the 1580s range from 120,000 to 150,000; see Ruth Pike, *Aristocrats and Traders: Sevillian Society in the Sixteenth Century* (Ithaca, N.Y.: Cornell University Press, 1972), 12–13; and Antonio Domínguez Ortiz, *La sociedad española en el siglo XVII* (Madrid: Consejo Superior de Investigaciones Científicas, 1964), 140–41.

the east side of the river. The massive wall surrounding Seville, dotted with towers and gates, was clearly visible. A prolonged look would reveal the outlines of the narrow winding streets of the older sections of the city and the dozens of church towers as well as numerous monasteries and convents. Gazing in a northeasterly direction toward Cordova, the observer might pick out on the far side of the river the house built by Hernando Colón and, on the nearer side, the Carthusian Monastery of Santa María de las Cuevas.[2]

All this supposes our observer was surveying the scene on a clear day. Often the basin was blanketed by the thick smoke of hundreds of ovens and furnaces baking tiles and all types of pottery. Triana was the major center for the production not only of these articles but also of soap, bread, and hardtack and gunpowder to supply the demands of the army and navy. The heavy air was further contaminated by the steaming pots of the caulkers sealing the hulls of the ships careened on the riverbank. Early modern Seville was polluted, and its streets were filthy. Offal and human and animal excrement tended to be tossed into the street, and garbage often piled up to the point that passage became difficult. City officials periodically passed measures to clean the city, but such cleaning was a sporadic operation. The streets would be cleared of garbage, but it would soon start accumulating again; and when the filth and stench reached a certain point, or the plague threatened, the councilors would issue new directives for waste removal.

The best water came from the nearby Archbishop's Spring (Fuente del Arzobispo) or was piped in by the Carmona aqueduct from another spring near Alcalá de Guadaíra and then distributed throughout the city. But water was expensive, and many residents used the river or relied on water of questionable quality from shallow wells. The river carried not only Seville's refuse but also the waste of every other settlement upriver.[3] Furthermore, it flooded regularly. The *marismas*, the alluvial floodplain of the lower Guadalquivir, made an ideal breeding ground for mosquitoes, and with them came mosquito-borne diseases, especially during the rainy season.

The Guadalquivir River was cluttered with vessels of all kinds, from skiffs

2. We have used Spanish names for people and places except when they are particularly well known by an English equivalent. Although we would refer to Cristóbal Colón as Christopher Columbus, we have kept his son as Hernando Colón.

3. Juan Ignacio Carmona, *Crónica urbana del malvivir (s. XIV–XVII): Insalubridad, desamparo y hambre en Sevilla* (Seville: Universidad de Sevilla, 2000), 21–23.

ferrying people across to a variety of fishing boats, some equipped with nets for taking mullet or smaller fish. At the upper end of the scale were the large ships employed in the transatlantic trade, with their sails furled, some careened, others anchored downstream. In addition, one could see a myriad of other vessels, some transporting wheat from Sicily and North Africa, others used for trade in the eastern Mediterranean, dozens of boats employed by coastal fishermen, and other barks trading with Lisbon, Galicia, and the far away ports of the Low Countries.[4]

Seville witnessed the first fleets arriving from the New World, and quickly the city and its river became Spain's gateway for transatlantic commerce, controlled by the House of Trade (Casa de la Contratación) founded at the outset of the sixteenth century. Seville is an inland port connected to the sea by the Guadalquivir River, which empties into the Atlantic Ocean at Sanlúcar de Barrameda. The journey up or down the river was not without peril, particularly as ships became larger and heavier, and many were unable to cross the treacherous sandbar at Sanlúcar or to undertake the trip between Seville and the mouth of the Guadalquivir. By the mid-seventeenth century, Cádiz, in spite of being more vulnerable to enemy attacks, supplanted Seville as the primary port for the Indies trade.[5] During the course of the sixteenth century, as Seville's role in the transatlantic trade expanded, its population exploded, and its inhabitants benefitted to varying degrees from profits reaped in the Americas. Some

4. There is as yet no comprehensive urban history of early modern Seville in English. There are several useful works about Seville in Spanish; see Antonio José Albardonedo Freire, *El urbanismo de Sevilla durante el reinado de Felipe II* (Seville: Ediciones Guadalquivir, 2002); Francisco Morales Padrón, *Historia de Sevilla: La ciudad del quinientos* (Seville: Universidad de Sevilla, 1983); and Antonio Domínguez Ortiz, *La Sevilla del siglo XVII* (Seville: Universidad de Sevilla, 1986). Numerous studies in English address specific aspects of life in the city; see Pike, *Aristocrats and Traders,* and the same author's *Enterprise and Adventure: The Genoese in Seville and the Opening of the New World* (Ithaca, N.Y.: Cornell University Press, 1966); Mary Elizabeth Perry, *Crime and Society in Early Modern Seville* (Hanover, N.H.: University Press of New England, 1980), and the same author's *Gender and Disorder in Early Modern Seville* (Princeton, N.J.: Princeton University Press, 1990). For Seville's sailors, see Pablo E. Pérez-Mallaína, *Spain's Men of the Sea: Daily Life in the Indies Fleets in the Sixteenth Century,* trans. Carla Rahn Phillips (Baltimore: Johns Hopkins University Press, 1998). Seville receives ample coverage in Richard L. Kagan, ed., *Spanish Cities of the Golden Age: The Views of Anton van den Wyngaerde* (Berkeley and Los Angeles: University of California Press, 1989), 327–33.

5. For a discussion of the ports and the river route, see Pérez-Mallaína, *Spain's Men of the Sea,* 1–9.

merchants became fabulously wealthy, while small artisans or innkeepers may have seen more modest gains. At the same time, as in any large city, poverty and crime coexisted with riches.

This was the city that Don Fernando de Torres y Portugal, the Count of Villar, faced when he began his duties as chief administrative officer. The count, who had served earlier as *corregidor* (royal governor) of Salamanca, was named royal governor (*asistente,* Seville's term for a corregidor) of Seville by King Philip II in 1579, and almost from the start epidemics combined with food shortages were among his major concerns. A nobleman from Jaén, the count was a capable administrator not easily intimidated by challenges, whether posed by natural disasters or the Inquisition. He faced both and on both sides of the Atlantic. Shortly after his tenure in Seville ended, Fernando de Torres y Portugal was named viceroy of Peru. Governing Seville provided valuable preparation for a future viceroy, and the Count of Villar was not the only governor of this booming Andalusian commercial center to become a viceroy in Spanish America.[6]

The duties of Seville's royal governor were multifold and similar to those of a corregidor elsewhere in Castile. As Marvin Lunenfeld aptly phrases, an early modern governor was "the omnicompetent servant." He acted as judge, military commander, and chief executive as well as the presiding officer in the meetings of the municipal council. The powers of the official varied from one jurisdiction to another and were based on the nature of the royal appointment and past privileges that may have been granted to localities. The general tendency under the Catholic Monarchs (Ferdinand and Isabel) and the first Habsburgs was toward increasing centralization and the extension of royal authority over both municipalities and local powerful lords.[7]

The authority of the royal governor of Seville extended far beyond the urban core and the bustling seaport. It encompassed numerous places (*lugares*), hamlets, villages, and towns, extending as far distant as Fregenal to the north, on the edge of Extremadura; Utrera to the east; Lebrija near the Atlantic port

6. Miguel Molina Martínez, "Los Torres y Portugal: Del señorío de Jaén al virreinato peruano," in *Andalucía y América en el siglo XVI: Actas de las II jornadas de Andalucía y América,* ed. Bibiano Torres Ramírez and José Hernández Palomo (Seville: Escuela de Estudios Hispano-Americanos, 1983), 2:35–66.

7. Marvin Lunenfeld, *Keepers of the City: the Corregidores of Isabella I of Castile (1474–1504)* (Cambridge: Cambridge University Press, 1987), chap. 1, 1–9.

of Sanlúcar de Barrameda in the south; and the mountaintop fortress town of Aroche, near the border with Portugal, to Seville's west. The city's jurisdiction encompassed a total of sixty-eight towns, not counting the many small hamlets and places that were subject to Seville's control, which included the power to approve local elections, name commanders of fortresses, collect certain taxes, and demand services in time of emergencies. Some places had special *fueros* (charters), granted by previous rulers, that protected many local privileges. Others were under the domination of the greater nobility, who held authority by generations-old royal grants. The authority of the city of Seville and its municipal council, as well as its governor, was often challenged by the lesser political entities, with complaints going to the royal council and monarch.[8]

The administration of Seville was similar to that of other Castilian centers of the time. The city council normally met three times a week, on Monday, Wednesday, and Friday. During the meetings, presided over by the governor or his deputy, the councilors sat in their assigned seats according to rank, starting with the chief constable (*alguacil mayor*), who was on the governor's right. The royal governor of Seville, always a nobleman, was a direct representative of the king, and his duties included not only governing the city and its territory but also the administration of justice, something that often put the governor in conflict with the Royal Appellate Court (Audiencia). His appointment normally lasted three years, and he usually resided in apartments of Seville's Alcázar, the fortress palace constructed by the Muslims and modified by successive Christian rulers.

Don Fernando de Torres y Portugal, the Count of Villar, certainly possessed the requisite status of "titled nobility" to serve as royal governor of Seville. The seat of the family's fortune was tied to an estate in the modest village of Villardompardo, only thirty kilometers distant from the city of Jaén, where the family maintained its urban palace. The origins of the *mayorazgo* (entailed estate) of the Torres y Portugal lineage are rooted in the Christian reconquista of Andalusia from Muslim domination. Among Don Fernando's ancestors were a Portuguese *infante* (prince) as well as a daughter of King Enrique II of Castile. In 1576 Philip II bestowed the title of count on Don Fernando and confirmed certain past privileges. Among others, the Count of Villar was hereditary standard-bearer of Jaén and the keeper of the keys of the city, and he had

<hr>

8. Morales Padrón, *La ciudad del quinientos,* 209.

the privilege of entering meetings of the municipal council with his sword un-sheathed. Don Fernando inherited the income from the tax revenue owed by various occupational groups in Jaén and Villardompardo—carpenters, black-smiths, shoemakers, dyers, silk workers, and others—and throughout his life-time he would often be in court defending these rights.

Nobility was also a prerequisite for other members of the municipal council (*cabildo*), such as the *caballeros veinticuatros* (aldermen), and by the sixteenth century even the *jurados* (councilmen), though in Seville many wealthy mer-chants, often of *converso* origin (that is, Jewish converts to Christianity), inter-married with the old Christian elite. The definition of *nobility* is inexact, and in the context of this work it follows the outline established by Lunenfeld. With a few exceptions among the veinticuatros, the nobility ranked beneath the titled greater aristocracy and ranged from an *hidalgo,* a person who was able by birth to claim exemption from payment of taxes, to the knight (*caballero*). The men holding municipal office were required to be native Sevillians, with the excep-tion of the chief constable, who, after 1556, had to be an outsider; and although these were royal appointments, those with adequate pedigree and cash could buy the position and often did.

Many offices, including the alguacil mayor, the six *alcaldes mayores* (chief justices), and the *alférez mayor* (chief standard-bearer), were held by prominent families and passed from father to son. During the late sixteenth century, the office of chief constable was linked to the family of the Duke of Alcalá, and the six chief justices persisted under the control of the families of the Duke of Me-dina Sidonia, the Duke of Béjar, the Duke of Arcos, the Marquis of Villanueva, the Marquis of Tarifa, and Martín Cerón. In spite of the name, by the sixteenth century the number of the veinticuatros was not fixed at twenty-four but fluc-tuated widely.

Each of Seville's parishes was represented by two jurados, who were ex-pected to reside in their district and were responsible for implementing the de-cisions of the city council in their jurisdiction. Unlike the veinticuatros, the jurados did not have a vote but only a voice during council meetings. They also met in their own council, the *cabildo de jurados,* and they were expected to in-form the king of any mismanagement of the city, which they often did. The governor was aided by two deputies, and many of the other council members also relied on lieutenants. There were lesser offices, for example, the *fieles ejecu-*

tores, who controlled weights and measures and also inspected the jail, the condition of the protective city wall and gates, and the bridge, as well as the city's sanitation.

Seville's politics of the period were dominated by two antagonistic factions: the Guzmanes, headed by the Duke of Medina Sidonia, and the Ponces de León, under the umbrella of the Duke of Arcos. Most councilors in Seville belonged to one or the other faction, and there were numerous and shifting alliances between individuals and groups. Although the Count of Villar was often frustrated by efforts of the veinticuatros to promote their own positions at the expense of the Crown's interests, he handled factionalism with remarkable skill. He worked by quiet persuasion, even acting "as alderman at times and ceasing to be governor," navigating "sometimes with much softness and at other times not so much," to secure their support.[9] The issues treated by the cabildo varied, and the discussions were often heated; the threat of plague produced some of the more lively exchanges.

The plague periodically appeared in Andalusia during the course of the sixteenth century. There was a particularly nasty bout in Seville in 1568, when "from April until August, more than 8,000 people died of the plague."[10] The next decade saw the city relatively free of contagion. But the calm was broken as the 1570s approached their close. Contemporaries viewed the plague as God's punishment, and they considered mass contrition an important deterrent. When Saint Teresa of Avila abandoned the city in 1576, she condemned its immorality. But in the meantime the church had done its part to enhance Seville's moral standing as the remains of San Fernando, the king who had recaptured the city for Christianity three centuries earlier, his son, Alfonso X, the

9. Quoted in José Ignacio Fortea Pérez, "Sevilla y las Cortes de Castilla en el reinado de Felipe II," in *Sevilla, Felipe II y la Monarquía Hispánica*, ed. Carlos Alberto González Sánchez (Seville: Ayuntamiento de Sevilla, 1999), 64–65; Morales Padrón, *La ciudad del quinientos*, 209–19; Antonio Domínguez Ortiz, "Salarios y atribuciones de los asistentes de Sevilla," *Archivo hispalense* 7, no. 20 (1946): 207–13. For a general study of the foundations of municipal government in early modern Spain, see Lunenfeld, *Keepers of the City*. Regarding the Count of Villar, see Luis Miguel Costa, "Patronage and Bribery in Sixteenth-Century Colonial Peru: The Government of Viceroy Conde del Villar and the Visita of Licentiate Alonso Fernández de Bonilla" (Ph.D. diss., Florida International University, 2005); and Molina Martínez, "Los Torres y Portugal," 2:36–37, 54–55.

10. Archivo Municipal de Sevilla (AMS), sec. 11 (Archivo-Biblioteca del Conde del Águila), vol. 20.

Wise, and their queens were transferred to the stately royal chapel in the cathedral in June of 1579. The Count of Villar and the members of the city government took a prominent part in the solemn ceremonies and processions.

But relics, important as they seemed to contemporaries, could not protect the city from periodic outbreaks of sickness or other dangers. Epidemic disease often brought with it food shortages and economic hardships. Nor was the populace immune from natural disasters such as droughts or floods, locust devastation and crop failures. There were other stresses on Seville's populace. Not long after the Count of Villar arrived at city hall, the gunpowder factory, which stood in Triana, the district across the river from the Torre del Oro, exploded. The contemporary historian, Alonso de Morgado, who lived at the other end of the city, remembered eating his midday meal on Monday, 18 May 1579, when he "felt that the whole house shook"; "there was no house, nor church in all of Seville," he added, "where the same was not felt."[11] A large part of Triana was destroyed, and more than 150 people were killed; "some of them flying through the air fell into the river and drowned." The powerful explosion shattered windows of the cathedral and roused the city council into action. The authorities agreed that gunpowder should not be produced or even stored in large quantities in populated areas. Unfortunately, it took more than a year and another explosion, though a much less damaging one, before gunpowder production was moved further outside of Triana.[12]

Seville's population was a heterogeneous mix of local residents and transients. People came from the nearby countryside to conduct their business in the city or to visit relatives, arriving from all points of the peninsula and further afield. Most important, the fleets from the Indies or those leaving for the overseas colonies generated incessant human traffic. The congestion, the climate, inadequate diet, and poor hygiene, along with the constant movement in and out of the city, provided fertile ground for disease, and it was not uncommon that epidemics flared up and carried away large numbers of victims.

In the sixteenth century the understanding of sickness, both symptoms and cure, was incomplete. Even today new threats to public health crop up to confound medical specialists, who by painstaking investigation peel away uncertainty until they understand the nature, the cause, and ultimately the cure of

11. Alonso de Morgado, *Historia de Sevilla* [1587] (Seville: J. M. Ariza, 1887), 178–79.

12. AMS, sec. 11, vol. 20 (18 May 1579); AMS, sec. 10 (Actas Capitulares), 1579 [2] (20 May) and 1580 [1] (18 May).

the disease. The modern scourges of HIV (human immunodeficiency virus), the Ebola virus, SARS (severe acute respiratory syndrome), and avian flu all come frighteningly to mind, and drug-resistant strains of diseases once thought to be under control again threaten. The sixteenth-century approach to sickness was far from scientific. We are reasonably certain that Seville, like other southern European cities of the time, faced periodic episodes of smallpox, measles, mumps, typhus, typhoid, lockjaw, influenza, bubonic plague, tuberculosis, syphilis, malaria, and perhaps yellow fever as well as other afflictions.

Few of these ailments could have been diagnosed accurately by the early modern physician. After all, most began with a fever, body aches, drowsiness or lethargy, vomiting and diarrhea, and coughs, followed by one type or another of skin eruption. Only if certain patterns were evident was the doctor able to point with some certainty to a specific "disease," such as smallpox or measles, correctly identified by the Persian physician Rhazes in the ninth century and studied by Spanish doctors who regularly saw them among children. The distinction between these two was easily recognizable in the differing nature of the manifestations on the epidermis. Typhus was first recognized and described as it ravaged armies in the Spanish reconquista of Granada in the 1480s and then continued killing troops and defenders during Spanish warfare on the Italian peninsula. The very name the Spanish gave it, *tabardillo*, was associated with the reddish-brown spots on the skin, largely on the trunk of the body, the area covered by the vest, or *tabardo*. Leprosy was also well known by its symptoms, and a vast literature including methods of control was published. Early modern Spanish doctors also studied and described epidemic syphilis, associated with the return of Christopher Columbus's men from the Indies.

The scourge that received greatest attention was the bubonic plague, introduced in modern form into Europe in the 1340s. Although heated debate continues over the massive mortality of the fourteenth century and over the correct identification of the disease, the mere idea of the plague was enough to frighten early modern men and women, as continued outbreaks of disease with plague-like symptoms occurred. Treatise after treatise on the plague and other diseases was published by sixteenth-century physicians in Spain and elsewhere. Many doctors provided their own specific "cures," and some even set out in search of new medications, in the Americas, in the Philippines, and elsewhere. Nevertheless, until the nineteenth century when *Yersinia pestis*, the bacteria that causes the plague, was identified, the transmission of the disease was a mystery. When doctors and local authorities combating the spread of the plague ordered the burning of victims' clothing and bedding, they may have unwittingly destroyed some of the actual culprits in disease transmission, the ubiquitous fleas, whose infected bite sickened the victim. But they did not understand the etiology of the plague or the role of rodents and their parasites in its transmission.[13]

The physicians of the Iberian peninsula were among the best at the time, as they borrowed from and maintained the healing traditions of Islamic and Jewish medical practitioners. Some students training for the profession traveled abroad to Bologna or other famous medical schools, while a larger number studied at the medical faculties of the Universities of Alcalá de Henares, Salamanca, Seville, and Granada as well as other venerable peninsular institutions. To avoid quackery and malpractice, doctors were examined and licensed by a government oversight board, the Protomedicato, before they could practice in the realm. This control over the profession set Castile off from most of the rest of Europe.

The basic education of university-trained doctors was rooted in the classic works of medicine composed by Hellenistic authorities and in the paradigm of the humors. In this view, illness was caused by an imbalance of the four basic bodily humors or fluids: blood, phlegm, choler, and black bile (or melancholy). If doctors had been able to identify the sickness, application of a correct cure was just as problematic. The most commonly accepted ways to restore the imbalance in the bodily fluids were purging and bleeding, although sweating or cooling of the body might be prescribed in appropriate cases, often coupled with the first two treatments. Patients with weakened constitutions might not survive the shock of the cure, further contributing to elevated mortality caused by the infection. The apothecary had a host of potential concoctions to assist the patient fighting off sickness. The pharmacists were also controlled by the Protomedicato, and they were tested and licensed before they could open up a

13. For a useful modern compendium of these and other diseases, see Kenneth F. Kiple, ed., *The Cambridge World History of Human Disease* (Cambridge: Cambridge University Press, 1993), especially Ann G. Carmichael, "Bubonic Plague," 628–31. Regarding the controversy over identification of medieval plague, see, for example, David Herlihy, *The Black Death and the Transformation of the West* (Cambridge, Mass.: Harvard University Press, 1997), posthumously edited by Samuel Cohn, who rejects the bubonic or pneumonic plague as the "Black Death" of the fourteenth century. For a survey of the epidemic chronology of Seville, see Velázquez y Sánchez, *Anales epidémicos*. See also Kristy Sue Wilson Bowers, "Plague, Politics, and Municipal Relations in Sixteenth-Century Seville" (Ph.D. diss., Indiana University, 2001).

botica (pharmacy). Some of the medications, both chemical and organic, did help relieve symptoms, and numerous books on the subject were published during the period.[14]

Labeling of health care givers in the sixteenth century is quite distinct from today's more precise terminology, and we have attempted to be consistent. When referring to a "doctor" we imply that he held the university title of doctor. We use the term "physician" generically to refer to both doctor and surgeon or to a licentiate who was licensed to practice medicine but did not have the full university degree of doctor. In the sources, witnesses at times called someone doctor even though he held no degree. The oft-used term "barber surgeon" (*barbero cirujano*) can be confusing, because some are simple barbers, while others are actually surgeons with more formal training and are just labeled *barberos*.

In spite of its title, this brief book is not only about the plague. Numerous excellent studies of the disease exist already; they focus on various cities, with detailed analyses of the nature and preferred treatments for the disease and the training and quality of the health providers. Historians of medicine have done fine work on London, various cities and provinces in the Low Countries, France, Germany, Scandinavia, Italy, and even Greece, covering the sixteenth through eighteenth centuries. Spain has also received substantial though less well known attention, by largely Spanish historians.[15]

14. Francisco Guerra, *Historia de la medicina* (2 vols., Madrid: Ediciones Norma, 1982–89) and the same author's *Epidemiología americana y filipina, 1492–1898* (Madrid: Ministerio de Sanidad y Consumo, 1999) are basic references and provide important bibliographical information. Although there is no study in English of early modern Spain's medical profession comparable to Richard L. Kagan's *Lawsuits and Litigants in Castile, 1500–1700* (Chapel Hill: University of North Carolina Press, 1981) for the legal profession, there has been an explosion of books and articles in Spanish on health and all aspects of the medical field. These are discussed later in the text. For a general survey, see Nancy G. Siraisi, *Medieval and Early Renaissance Medicine: An Introduction to Knowledge and Practice* (Chicago: University of Chicago Press, 1990).

15. The list of available titles includes Ann G. Carmichael, *Plague and the Poor in Renaissance Florence* (Cambridge: Cambridge University Press, 1986); Carlo M. Cipolla, *Cristofano and the Plague: A Study of the History of Public Health in the Age of Galileo* (London: Collins, 1973), and *Fighting the Plague in Seventeenth-Century Italy* (Madison: University of Wisconsin Press, 1981); Giulia Calvi, *Histories of a Plague Year: The Social and the Imaginary in Baroque Florence* (Berkeley and Los Angeles: University of California Press, 1989); Jean-Noël Biraben, *Les hommes et la peste en France et dans les pays européens et méditerranéens* (2 vols., Paris: Mouton, 1975–76); Klaus Schwarz, *Die Pest in Bremen: Epidemien und freier Handel in einer deutschen Hafenstadt, 1350–1713* (Bremen, Germany: Selbstverlag des Staatsarchivs Bremen, 1996); Paul Slack, *The Impact of Plague in Tudor and Stuart England* (Oxford: Oxford University Press, 1990); John Aberth, *From the Brink of the*

Our intention is to examine a much broader topic, generally not as well studied by historians: how did city officials in a large early modern urban complex deal with crises that arose —not as a single epidemic or natural disaster but rather in a series of waves, none great enough in itself to break down the system but several combined, sufficient to challenge the social and economic order? In this case, over a period of less than thirty months, Seville and its hinterland faced crop failures brought on by climatic variations and locust infestations, spoilage of imported grains with consequent famine and starvation, unrest as a result of the billeting of foreign troops associated with a projected invasion of a neighboring country, the threatened uprising of a sizable ethnic-religious minority, poverty and pollution, the explosion of a major gunpowder factory, and, of course, disease in many forms.

The crises facing the councilors seemed unending. Reading through the municipal council records reminds one of some present-day proceedings of deliberative bodies, be they city councils, state or provincial legislatures, or even national congresses. There was plenty of debate, and dissent was not uncommon. Decisions were voted on, and although the royal governor's authority was great, council members attempted to sway the opinion of their fellow officers. The municipal authorities received a stream of petitions, dealing with both community issues and personal matters. The governor or his deputies handled some of these requests, others were presented to the entire cabildo, and many were referred to commissions established to contend with a given problem.

We have chosen in this narrative to let the protagonists' voices be heard as much as possible as we follow them on their daily routines. Although the detailed records of the sessions of Seville's city council provide the documentary foundation of our reconstruction, they are only a part of the material we use. Seville's municipal archive is a rich depository of documents detailing the city's long history, and this work has benefitted from many relating to the present topic. We have also found much additional information in the notarial records. They are especially challenging because of the difficult paleography and the te-

---

Apocalypse: Confronting Famine, War, Plague, and Death in the Later Middle Ages (New York: Routledge Press, 2000); Mavis E. Mate, *Daughters, Wives, and Widows after the Black Death: Women in Sussex, 1350–1535* (Woodbridge, U.K.: Boydell and Brewer, 1998); and José Luis Betrán, *La peste en la Barcelona de los Austrias* (Lleida, Spain: Milenio, 1996).

dium associated with the sheer mass of information included by the notaries. But they provide contracts that are directly relevant: payments for medicines, rentals, salaries for nurses, and wills. The words and observations of some of our key figures, for example, the governor of Seville, appear in official state correspondence. Whenever it is relevant to the narrative, we incorporate medical treatises, some written by our key figures, including Bartolomé Hidalgo's *Thesoro de la verdadera cirugía* and Nicolás Monardes's *Historia medicinal.* Furthermore, we have used the descriptions of contemporaries who lived and wrote in Seville during the early modern period, such as Rodrigo Caro's *Antigüedades,* Cristóbal de Chaves's *Relación de la Cárcel de Sevilla,* Alonso de Morgado's *Historia de Sevilla,* and Francisco Pacheco's *Retratos,* as well as the later chronicle of Diego Ortiz de Zúñiga, *Anales eclesiásticos,* among others.

Our hope is that by staying close to the words of the protagonists, carefully recorded by town scribes, and the writing of other contemporaries, today's reader can enter, if only briefly, into their world and face with them the challenges they confronted daily as they went about their work. The book is populated by councilmen, physicians, pharmacists, merchants, farmers, even slaves and children. There appear frequent and often intimate glimpses of women, not only as wives but also as nurses, shopkeepers, innkeepers, bakers, and small-scale merchants. Through the voices of health care givers, and of those able to tell their own story, we see and at times can almost feel the excruciating pain of those stricken down by sickness. We interject only when we believe it necessary to fill in details, at times in footnotes, to assist the reader in better understanding the background and setting and the protagonists' actions.

This microhistory focuses on a city and its citizens and outside administrators battling seemingly successive crises during a narrow three-year period encompassing the tenure of its governor, Don Fernando de Torres y Portugal, the Count of Villar. The threat of a deadly and feared disease always took center stage for the authorities, but the municipal council records indicate that the aldermen and a host of lesser city officials, along with the governor, did not neglect other more routine matters. What is ultimately noteworthy is that in spite of numerous emergencies, Seville's bureaucracy functioned with relative normality to provide the basic services necessary for the survival of her citizens.

1

PLAGUE IN LISBON

It is taken for certain that there is plague in Lisbon.
—DIEGO MEXÍA

SEVILLE'S MASSIVE STONE CITY HALL, completed in 1564, shared the principal public plaza with a large Franciscan monastery as well as the Audiencia and the Royal Jail. The Plaza of San Francisco itself was the favorite site for both religious and secular spectacles. Bull-fights and horse games, autos-da-fé and processions from the nearby cathedral were common. Visits of important dignitaries to the city and major events, be they births, deaths, and marriages of royalty or military victories, all were celebrated in the city's principal square. An enthusiastic city booster in the early seventeenth century, Rodrigo Caro, marveled at the beauty of the city hall as the "envy of all the nations." He added up the number of greater and lesser officials who served in it, finding there were 147, "which makes it in both numbers and in quality, one of the most illustrious senates in all of Christendom."[1]

On the morning of 21 October 1579 the city council of Seville met for its usual Wednesday gathering, presided over by the royal governor, the Count of Villar. Following other items of business, the veinticuatro Diego Mexía announced, "It is taken for certain that there is plague in Lisbon." Furthermore, according to a letter dispatched from Lisbon on 8 October, "the situation is worsening in the city." Mexía lamented that "the Portuguese have come fleeing into this city with their wives and children, and continue to do so." He urged the city council to verify this alarming news and demanded immediate action, should it prove to be true. The Count of Villar concurred; after a short discussion, the cabildo members designated Diego Mexía and another veinticuatro, Bartolomé López de Mesa, to collect more information and to confer with the

1. Rodrigo Caro, *Antigvedades, y principado de la ilvstrissima civdad de Sevilla. Y chorographia de sv convento ivridico, o antigva chancilleria* [1634] (Seville: Ediciones Alfar, 1998), 62r–v.

appropriate people on what measures to take to protect the city. They were to give a full report to the governor so that the council could move quickly to avert the impending crisis.[2]

One of the councilors, Bartolomé de Hoces, suggested that several members, including Diego Mexía, should meet that same afternoon in the Count of Villar's lodgings at the Alcázar to continue the discussion regarding "what would be expedient to do for the security and protection of this city and its land." He also proposed that Don Diego de Portugal join Diego Mexía and Bartolomé López de Mesa as one of the commissioners of the plague. Most agreed, and in the end the officials added three more deputies to the commission: the veinticuatros Don Pedro Ponce, el Primero, Gaspar Ruiz de Montoya, and Don Andrés de Monsalve. The council asked the men to pay attention to the various issues related to the question and to inquire directly from those persons who had communication with the infected areas. The council members also agreed that anyone coming from Lisbon should be prevented from entering Seville and that the river approach should be guarded, because they assumed that the infection would arrive by ship. Before the meeting was adjourned, the Count of Villar named two additional deputies, the Marquis of Villamanrique and Melchor del Alcázar, and consented to meet the plague commission in his residence the following afternoon, giving the deputies time to gather more information.[3]

The measures to stop the plague from spreading differed little from those adopted in the fourteenth century when the Black Death reappeared in Europe after centuries of calm. In the wake of that horrendous calamity, Italian city-states established commissions consisting of respected citizens and physicians to deal with sanitation and disposal of the dead, as well as combating the disease itself. Florence, Venice, Lucca, and Perugia, for example, all took steps to keep foreigners outside the city walls. Pistoia issued some of the most stringent ordinances, including those designed to prevent travelers from infected areas from entering or bringing in old clothes. The authorities ordered meat markets to be inspected to ensure the food was fresh. They also prohibited large numbers of people from gathering at funerals and regulated the depths of graves. The city adopted new measures, some annulling earlier ones, to accommodate

2. AMS, sec. 10, 1579 [3].
3. Ibid.

changing situations as the disease progressed.[4] By the sixteenth century, many of these steps had become routine whenever the plague threatened, not only in Italy but in the rest of Europe, including Seville.

The plague commission reported back to the full council on 23 October, two days after the initial announcement by Diego Mexía. It was clear that the city needed to act. Don Gerónimo de Montalvo urged the Count of Villar to name a trustworthy individual to travel immediately to the areas in Portugal where the plague had been reported to gather information on the nature of the disease. He recommended that the city's steward (*mayordomo*), Diego del Postigo, be authorized to cover the travel expenses out of the city coffers. Following a short discussion, the councilors approved Don Gerónimo's recommendations.[5]

The first question of quarantining a ship came to the cabildo's notice on Wednesday, 4 November. The shipmaster Salvador González had just arrived on the vessel *Nuestra Señora de Ayuda* and requested permission to unload his merchandise. He had been detained by officials who told him that because there was plague in Portugal, he could not proceed. *Maestre* González protested that their information was untrue and insisted that he should be allowed to unload the goods, but to no avail; he had to wait until reports came back from Portugal.

Five days later, on 9 November, a letter arrived from Don Pedro Girón, the Duke of Osuna, confirming that plague had broken out in Portugal. After it was read to the assembled cabildo, the Marquis of Villamanrique, one of the chief justices, spoke.[6] He contended that this letter, along with the testimony provided by Bartolomé López de Mesa, was convincing. The marquis argued that the plague commission, armed with this information, should act and if necessary issue orders that Seville and the places within her jurisdiction should

4. Anna Montgomery Campbell, *The Black Death and the Men of Learning* (New York: Columbia University Press, 1931), 112–17. For Pistoia's ordinances, see Rosemary Horrox, trans. and ed., *The Black Death* (Manchester, U.K.: Manchester University Press, 1994), 194–203. See also Cipolla, *Fighting the Plague in Italy*.

5. AMS, sec. 10, 1579 [3].

6. Don Alvaro Manrique de Zúñiga, the Marquis of Villamanrique, was the uncle of the Duke of Medina Sidonia; in 1585 he became viceroy of New Spain. See Peter Pierson, *Commander of the Armada: The Seventh Duke of Medina Sidonia* (New Haven, Conn.: Yale University Press, 1989), 53.

set up a quarantine against anyone arriving from Portugal. All of those present at this meeting agreed and decided to thank the Duke of Osuna for his efforts.

Eleven days later, on Friday, 20 November 1579, the cabildo received a petition from Andrés Gutiérrez, the owner of a caravel loaded with fish that had arrived from Portugal. He requested permission to enter the port of Seville. The council decided to investigate. There was also a slave ship held up in the river, presumably because its cargo came from Portugal. One of the more outspoken veinticuatros, Diego Ortiz Melgarejo, argued that since the ship had already been anchored in the river for more than twenty days, they should issue license to unload the cloth and slaves. The councilors discussed the matter, and in the end caution prevailed. The governor supported the notion that the ship and its cargo should be carefully inspected and that a physician, Dr. Rodrigo de León, should go along and examine the slaves on board. If Dr. León found them to be healthy, they could disembark.

The city council continued to receive disconcerting news. There was plague in the North African port of Ceuta, and local officials suspected that the disease had been introduced by a woman from Portugal. The cabildo, faced with an imminent threat of contagion, decided to send representatives to meet with the archbishop of Seville, Don Cristóbal de Rojas y Sandoval, as well as the members of the Cathedral Chapter to inform church authorities on the course of action the city was taking. In keeping with the prevailing belief that plague was a sign of God's ire, the deputies were to request that all the monasteries and churches in Seville begin prayers to ward off the pestilence.

Seville was protected on all sides by a centuries-old stone wall, but one part of the city, the district of Triana, which lay across the Guadalquivir River, had no wall and was more vulnerable to outside influences. Triana, with its principal church of Santa Ana, was the largest parish in the city. Because of its maritime connections, Triana has traditionally been described as the "sailor's barrio." Although it was populated by wealthy ship captains, as well as lowly sailors, Triana's residents were no less diverse than the rest of Seville. Numerous merchants, doctors, artisans, tavern keepers, and day laborers resided there. The inquisitors, secretaries, and many familiars of the Inquisition lived in Triana. Clergymen attached to the parish of Santa Ana made Triana their home, and members of various religious orders occupied several monasteries and convents in the barrio. There were judges, lawyers, notaries, tax collectors, poor and wealthy widows, Moriscos (Muslim converts to Christianity), Gypsies, and slaves, as well as free blacks. Most residents proclaimed to be *vecinos* (citizens) of Triana rather than just of Seville. As in the rest of the city, there was a large transient population. Triana was connected to the main part of the city by a massive pontoon bridge, a busy artery bustling with both residents and countless travelers. There were also boats that ferried people back and forth between Triana and the rest of Seville.

Triana, proudly declaring itself the guard of Seville, could nevertheless be a conduit for an epidemic, allowing sickness to pass into the main part of the city. When the cabildo met on Monday, 7 December, the Count of Villar told those assembled that it now seemed expedient to block the streets of Triana with temporary walls, as had been done in the past whenever the city was threatened by the plague, and that guards be placed there, as well as on all the roads entering the city. The city paid the guards for their services. For example, Cristóbal Donayre, a "guard of the plague," received on 21 May 1580 a payment of 3,978 *maravedís* (almost 11 ducats) for his work.[7]

During the same meeting, the governor informed the council that he had received reports of plague not only in Portugal and Ceuta but in Genoa, as well.[8] Two days later a royal provision arrived from Madrid officially authorizing Seville to set up a plague commission.[9] Although the city council ostensibly needed the central government's permission to form a special commission, the governor and the councilors could not afford to remain idle while waiting for it to be granted, and they took the necessary steps to protect the city even before the royal license reached them.

A number of people suggested that it would be wise to stop the sale of *carne mortezina*—meat from animals who died of natural causes rather than by slaughter. The members of the plague commission discussed the question of selling and eating carrion, which they believed could carry infection, and on 8 January 1580 Gaspar Ruiz de Montoya reported to the council. The commissioners had agreed that carrion should be banned and proposed that the *arrendador* (tax farmer) of the tax on this type of meat be asked to relinquish his share of the *alcabala* (sales tax) for the current year and be compensated by the

7. Archivo Histórico Provincial de Sevilla (AHPS), Protocolos notariales, leg. 2365, fol. 1043r–v.

8. AMS, sec. 10, 1579 [3].

9. AMS, sec. 10, 1580 [3], misbound.

city with twelve thousand maravedís (thirty-two ducats). The cabildo readily authorized this course of action.

Seville's city council was not only battling a potential plague outbreak; it faced another more immediate danger: locusts. In the era before modern chemical pesticides were developed, people competed with insect and animal pests, which frequently consumed crops in the fields before they matured for harvest. In good years, the agriculturalist's output was sufficient to absorb the loss owing to insects, birds, and rodents, leaving a surplus for human consumption. But there were natural cycles over which the early modern farmer had no control, and one of the more destructive ones involved locusts. It is now known that the locust is nothing more than one of several types of grasshoppers. Normally, grasshoppers lead a relatively solitary life, and natural predators keep their numbers in check. But under certain not well understood conditions they become more active and gregarious. They suddenly eat more, grow larger, change color, and mate more frequently. Clusters, then swarms, and finally millions of insects explode into clouds of ravenous creatures devouring every piece of vegetation in their path. In their devastating march the locusts could denude hundreds of miles of croplands.

The cabildo had been receiving numerous petitions from towns and villages within its jurisdiction asking for help to kill the locusts. The city council discussed the threat during the meeting of 9 December, and its members agreed to send a representative to investigate the seriousness of the infestation. The Count of Villar chose Rodrigo Sánchez to survey the damage.[10] The jurado returned on 5 March 1580 with disconcerting news. He had been "inspecting the district of Seville to find the locusts and their eggs, and had discovered large tracts of land where they were."

The city acted quickly, ordering a public proclamation to recruit people to kill the locusts and to offer them payment of one *real* for "each *almud* of the [locusts'] egg sacks and eggs."[11] Gaspar Ruiz pointed out that one real might not be quite enough and suggested that an additional quarter or half real might make the people more willing to participate in the eradication of the vermin. The "locust killers" were to bring their find to the Slaughterhouse Gate (Puerta

10. AMS, sec. 10, 1579 [4].

11. *Canuto* is the Spanish term, indicating the tube that is formed by the earth adhering to the eggs deposited by the female locust. The *almud* was approximately 27.75 liters, though the measure varied according to time and region.

del Matadero) of the city, where Rodrigo Sánchez, along with a notary, would record the amounts collected and then burn the insects and their eggs.[12] Each person was to be paid as soon as the share was measured. In addition, the members of the cabildo decided that if there were no volunteers then the count should order each parish to contribute a certain number of people who also would be paid per almud.

Ten days later, the jurado came back lamenting that he went out with "142 men, women, and youngsters to remove the seed and eggs of the locust," but in spite of all their efforts, they "were unable to take more than four *fanegas*, more or less."[13] Rodrigo Sánchez warned that the infestation was serious; nevertheless, many in the council complained about the expenditure.

The ever-blunt veinticuatro, Diego Ortiz Melgarejo, declared that they should not be hiring day workers but should instead order the parishes to provide people "to go out and kill the locusts" and pay the workers, at the end of each day, four reales from the *propios*.[14] Following a heated discussion, Ortiz Melgarejo's proposal passed. By the middle of April the plan was in place, although trouble developed when three dishonest overseers were found to be underpaying workers and pocketing the difference. The jurado Juan de Avendaño had alerted the city council to the scam and demanded that these overseers be punished and removed from their posts.

Along with the practical measures adopted to kill the locusts, the councilors thought it prudent to ask church authorities for help. They proposed a general procession the following Sunday, with prayers to rid the land of the insects.[15] Furthermore, when "a man from this city" offered his services "to very easily kill all the locusts in this city and its districts" for a thousand ducats, a large sum, the councilors were disposed to look into it, though all concurred that the man would not be paid until he had successfully performed the task.[16] The city council did not leave any method untested, because the fear of locusts almost matched the fear of the plague.

12. Slaughterhouse Gate was also known as the Meat Gate (Puerta de la Carne).

13. The exact capacity of the fanega (approximately a bushel or 55.5 liters) varied according to time and region. There were two almudes in a fanega.

14. *Propios* constituted the city's income-earning properties. The income could be in the form of rents or fees.

15. AMS, sec. 10, 1580 [1] (15 April).

16. Ibid. (29 April).

Early in the next century, for example, Seville's city council in desperation sent Father Alonso Yáñez del Castillo "to conjure the said locusts." He was to go to all the afflicted places, and wherever he went he was to receive "lodging and food necessary for his person and one servant and a mule . . . in order to make the said exorcisms." Each of the communities that benefitted from Father Yáñez del Castillo's services was to pay his servant six reales a day or face a fine. When the priest finished his mission, he reported to Seville's cabildo that he had spent thirty-two days going to all the affected communities, including Coria, Dos Hermanas, Las Cabezas, Utrera, Villafranca de la Marisma, Alcalá de Guadaíra, and many more, "and I said the masses and the fields were blessed and the said locusts were exorcized and with God Our Lord's mercy the few that remain do not cause damage anymore." It was not uncommon in sixteenth-century Spain, if all else failed, to conduct exorcisms or trials, sometimes presided over by an image of the Virgin Mary, to excommunicate the locusts and thus protect the crops.[17]

At the end of January 1580, Seville was still free of disease, and people were grumbling about the strict regulations of quarantine. On 29 January the residents living near the Osario Gate unsuccessfully petitioned the cabildo to lift the restrictions on their gate and to permit free entrance. A few months later they were complaining about garbage and offal being dumped outside the gate, warning that it "engenders pestilence." The measures to protect Seville from the plague were creating difficulties for many of her citizens as well as visitors. Certainly the disruption of commerce was becoming a problem, especially for the large number of Sevillians whose livelihood depended on trade. Moreover, although Seville remained free of plague, there was concern elsewhere in Spain that the city had already been infected. On 24 April 1580 the city council of Medina del Campo discussed the threat of plague entering its community as a result of commerce with Seville.[18] Yet in spite of numerous complaints and the rising costs of quarantine, the Count of Villar and the council refused to lift the orders and did not open the city gates.

17. AMS, Escribanía de Cabildo, sec. 4, vol. 21, doc. 2 (1617). For locust trials and exorcisms, see William A. Christian, Jr., *Local Religion in Sixteenth-Century Spain* (Princeton, N.J.: Princeton University Press, 1989), 28–31. See also Jodi Bilinkoff, *The Avila of Saint Teresa: Religious Reform in a Sixteenth-Century City* (Ithaca, N.Y.: Cornell University Press, 1989), 154.

18. AMS, sec. 10, 1580 [1] (22 March). Gerardo Moraleja Pinilla, *Historia de Medina del Campo* (Medina del Campo, Spain: Mateo Alaguero, 1971), 240.

2

CARING FOR SICK SOLDIERS

They could cause by their death some contagious disease.
—GASPAR RUIZ DE MONTOYA

I N NATIONAL EMERGENCIES, the Crown secured the funds necessary to carry forward the effort by a series of measures: forced loans, new or sharply increased taxes, conscription of men to serve in the armies, obligatory quartering of soldiers, and requests for special donations. These actions took a greater toll on communities with more resources at hand, such as Seville, whose role in the transatlantic trade made it a favorite target. The annexation of Portugal by Philip II was a costly enterprise, and the Crown expected Seville and other cities to contribute. King Philip claimed the Portuguese throne as the most legitimate of all the contenders left following the death of the childless Portuguese monarch. There was some resistance in Portugal to a union with Spain, and in February 1580 Philip enlisted the Duke of Alba to assemble and lead an army to secure the king's claim. The cost of the war, which only lasted a few months, was high, and Seville was called upon to provide her share.[1]

On Monday, 30 May 1580, as the first business of the session, the Count of Villar reported that the royal agent Francisco Duarte had notified him that a contingent of four hundred German soldiers, "many of them sick," had arrived, along with their wives, in "certain caravels" and were anchored in the river. The Marquis of Santa Cruz, one of King Philip's great naval commanders, ordered the Germans to the city "to be cured and refreshed so they can be incorporated into His Majesty's army." The fleet commanded by the Marquis of Santa Cruz played a crucial part in defeating the Portuguese a few months later.[2]

1. John Lynch, *Spain under the Habsburgs, vol. 1, Empire and Absolutism, 1516–1598* (New York: Oxford University Press, 1965), 304–11, deals in detail with the annexation of Portugal.

2. Ibid., 309; AMS, sec. 10, 1580 [1] (30 May).

The Count of Villar was touching on issues that were of utmost interest to the council. The cabildo, always mindful of the danger of epidemics, was also concerned about the potential financial burden the city would face in caring for foreign troops. The count proposed to place the Germans in a hospital or in houses outside the city, "where they can be cured and fed." He believed this would be a just solution to the problem, because "if the soldiers had indeed brought contagious disease it would be very dangerous and disadvantageous for the health of the city to house them within." The count admonished the councilors that, although the city would assume the cost of housing, feeding, and curing the soldiers, they should keep in mind as they debated the question both the benefit to the Crown and "the conservation of the health of the city." The council agreed to discuss the governor's proposal and to choose several members to study the issue and decide what would be best "for the service of His Majesty and the good of this republic."[3]

Diego Ortiz Melgarejo recommended giving the royal agent, Francisco Duarte, an account of the proposal and, more important, urged the council to send physicians to examine the soldiers to determine whether they "carried contagious disease." The outspoken alderman firmly stated that if they were sick they should not be allowed to disembark at all and stressed that "it is expedient for this city and the entire kingdom that this city is healthy." He did concede that if the Germans did not pose a health threat, they should be housed and provided for outside the city. Yet he complained about the cost of the "physician and barber" because the city was facing such a serious deficit that there was no money even "to pave the streets." The veinticuatro Diego Caballero agreed, adding that Francisco Duarte had to understand that the city would quarter the soldiers for this one time only, and he emphasized that the customs and privileges of the city should not be breached.

Gaspar Ruiz de Montoya concurred that Francisco Duarte should receive a full account of the proposal and be told that the city wanted to help but faced considerable difficulties. Ruiz de Montoya pointed out that the soldiers were paid by His Majesty and their salaries should suffice to cover the costs of being quartered outside the city. He also stressed that if "the sickness they have is contagious," they should not be allowed to disembark. He conceded that the council should send a physician and a barber to examine the soldiers' condition at

3. AMS, sec. 10, 1580 [1].

the city's expense. Furthermore, the cabildo should negotiate with Duarte regarding the best place to house them.

Melchor del Alcázar, one of the more distinguished aldermen, urged the Count of Villar that immediately and "above all things" he should have the city "name knowledgeable and conscientious doctors to go and examine these sick soldiers." He declared that should the physicians find them "infected with some contagious disease," the soldiers should be forced to leave Seville and "be accommodated in places so removed that they could not inflict damage on this land." At the same time, both Melchor del Alcázar and Gaspar Ruiz de Montoya allowed that if the soldiers were not sick then they could disembark.

Telling of the importance of the debate and the complexity of the issues being raised is the response of Bartolomé López de Mesa, who reminded his colleagues of royal privileges granted to the city by past rulers and confirmed by Philip II, that "no soldiers can be housed, nor given lodging within the city or its outskirts" because it would be detrimental to the city's economy and commerce. He added that if the soldiers had to be accommodated, then the quartering should be at the cost of the Crown, not the city, and that in any case they should be stationed outside Seville. Other members spoke, and many agreed with López de Mesa's position, which protected the rights as well as the coffers of the city.

At this point the Count of Villar voiced his own stand, supporting Melchor del Alcázar's position to house the soldiers outside the city walls if they did not have a contagious disease. He also advocated that they be lodged "with the hospitality given to them as sick and poor foreigners, who have come to serve His Majesty." The session ended with a vote accepting Melchor del Alcázar's proposal first to determine the condition of the Germans and then to act accordingly.[4]

The count's explicit agreement with Melchor del Alcázar confirms the laudatory comments by the contemporary Sevillian painter and humanist, Francisco Pacheco. Pacheco extolled Melchor del Alcázar's wisdom and eloquence, noting that "his capacity and prudence were so great, that His Majesty instructed the governors he was sending to be governed by him, and he ordered him to assist them." The Count of Villar's regard for Melchor del Alcázar was mutual, as shown in the veinticuatro's defense of the governor's conduct in a letter to the

---

4. Ibid.

queen's steward written on 15 August 1580. Apparently not everyone in the city hall was satisfied with the governor, and some murmured that "in our cabildo there is no other vote than his." Melchor del Alcázar did not entirely disagree, but he pointed out that "I know well the humors of these gentlemen my companions," and he was certain that if the councilors made all the inquiries and decisions, there "would be more harm than good." He declared his loyalty to the Count of Villar and offered that "if the governor should wish to take my advice, I will try to give good counsel."

The veinticuatro was about sixty years old during this time and would die ten years later in 1590, "the same day he reached 70 years." He was not only an alderman but also a treasurer of Seville's Royal Mint and the deputy warden of the Alcázar. He belonged to one of Seville's most prominent and wealthy converso families, traditionally allied with the Duke of Medina Sidonia. Pacheco's portrait of a serious and inquisitive man lends credence to the painter's assertion of the respect Melchor del Alcázar commanded.[5]

One of the seediest neighborhoods of Seville was known as the Arenal (sandy ground), a term that aptly describes the terrain. The Arenal comprised the long strip of land between the city and the river. It was also the place where the ships traveling to or from the Indies loaded and unloaded their passengers and merchandise, which were promptly registered by the officials of the House of Trade, located just inside the city walls. The Arenal contained the shipyard (*atarazanas*), and the city wall was littered with numerous dwellings built into it. The open space bustled with a mix of artisans, merchants, travelers, sailors, beggars, thieves, and prostitutes. The rich and the poor, respectable citizens and undesirables, all mingled in the Arenal. The city's brothel, known as La Mancebía, operated there, under the auspices of the municipality and the church, as did numerous inns and taverns. The infamous *malbaratillo*, a market where stolen goods and defective merchandise were sold to unsuspecting travelers,

5. Francisco Pacheco, *Libro de descripción de verdaderos retratos de ilustres y memorables varones* [1599], ed. and intr. Pedro M. Piñero and Rogelio Reyes Cano (Seville: Diputación Provincial de Sevilla, 1985), 283–88; British Library (BL), Add. Mss. 28369, fols. 51r–52v. See also Pike, *Aristocrats and Traders*, 47–49; Juan Gil, *Los conversos y la Inquisición sevillana* (Seville: Universidad de Sevilla, 2001), 3:201–203; Ruth Pike, *Linajudos and Conversos in Seville: Greed and Prejudice in Sixteenth- and Seventeenth-Century Spain* (New York: Peter Lang, 2000), 125–27; and Ruth Pike, "The Converso Family of Baltasar del Alcázar," *Kentucky Romance Quarterly* 14 (1967): 349–65. The poet Baltasar del Alcázar was Melchor's brother.

functioned daily near the Arenal Gate. The Arenal was a notoriously dangerous place, particularly at night.[6]

There was therefore a sense of urgency when, on 1 June, the Count of Villar informed the cabildo that the sick German soldiers were "in the Arenal exposed to the sun and nightly dew" except those whom some charitable individuals had taken into their houses. The governor added that most of the Germans had been examined by two physicians who testified that the soldiers "do not carry infectious disease, rather they are ordinary and common sicknesses caused by hardship and need that they had gone through, and at present it is so great that they are dying of hunger, some in the Arenal and in other places." The count pointed out that although the sickness was not contagious, the Germans and especially the corpses of those who had died "could cause harm to the health of the city."

The governor also announced that Martín Gutiérrez Cerón and Baltasar de Aguilar thought it would be "such a just and pious thing to remedy this" that they had contacted him and the factor Francisco Duarte the previous afternoon in order "to shelter the sick in the Cinco Llagas Hospital and so last night they took there as many as they could."[7] The count and the deputies asked the hospital's administrator to take charge of the sick soldiers, but he agreed only to assist them as long as there was no cost to him. The Count of Villar exhorted the cabildo "that it would be a worthy thing for the city to see to their relief." He added that if the city did not assume the financial responsibility, then he would do it himself. The governor also alerted the councilors that there were some Italians in the city in a similar situation and suggested that they should be assisted as well.[8]

Chief Justice Martín Gutiérrez Cerón, who had been instrumental in plac-

6. Pike, *Aristocrats and Traders,* 203–11; María Dolores Pérez Murillo and others, "Aspectos urbanísticos y sociales del Arenal de Sevilla en el siglo XVI," in *Andalucía y América en el siglo XVI: Actas de las II jornadas de Andalucía y América,* ed. Bibiano Torres Ramírez and José Hernández Palomo (Seville: Escuela de Estudios Hispano-Americanos, 1983), 2:273–302. For the operation of the *mancebía,* see Francisco Vázquez García and Andrés Moreno Mengíbar, *Poder y prostitución en Sevilla* (Seville: Universidad de Sevilla, 1995).

7. In the original it often appears as hospital de la Sangre, but it was also called hospital de las Cinco Llagas. To be consistent we call it the Cinco Llagas Hospital.

8. AMS, sec. 10, 1580 [1]. At the end of his term as governor, the Count of Villar claimed to have used his own money on several occasions to help the city. It is unclear whether this was one such time; see BL, Mss. Add. 28343, fols. 345r–46v.

ing the sick soldiers in the hospital, proposed that the city give the king an account of the deplorable condition in which "these Tudescan [lower Saxony] soldiers" arrived. Revealing that his pious act was not entirely altruistic, he noted that the letter should emphasize all that was being done for them, including the charitable works. He believed the city should be able to spend up to 100,000 maravedís (267 ducats) to implement the remedies recommended by the physicians, given the importance for His Majesty's service.

The count's charitable offer to assist the sick Germans himself if the city was unable to care for them inspired another council member. Veinticuatro Ortiz Melgarejo, in his usual candid manner, declared that he would go that very day "to the hospital and select two Tudescans and order them taken to his house and he would cure them at his own cost, until they were able to make their journey."

Diego Caballero de Cabrera, conscious of the need to protect the city's privileges, made several recommendations.[9] He proposed that the Count of Villar call to his residence all the administrators of Seville's hospitals and ask them on behalf of the city to accommodate as many sick soldiers as they could. He also advised the count to question the captain of the soldiers about the eight thousand ducats that he had received in the town of Jerez de la Frontera and see whether any of the money could be distributed among the hospitals caring for the soldiers. Diego Caballero stated unequivocally that because of its ordinances the city "cannot pay the said alms . . . and cannot help in anything."

Although several members murmured in agreement, Gaspar Ruiz de Montoya observed that the city needed to remember that if these ailing soldiers were not helped "they could cause by their death some contagious disease, which could be very difficult to deal with." He exhorted his reluctant colleagues that "the city has an obligation to remedy it in time." To cover the costs, the municipality should take the money from its propios and "spend it for no more or less than in guarding the gates and roads so that those coming from a place where there is plague cannot enter." Ruiz de Montoya argued that if they were willing to spend money on killing locusts, then how could they justify not using city

9. Diego Caballero de Cabrera was the son of Diego Caballero, a wealthy and powerful merchant of converso origins, whose chapel graces Seville's cathedral near the sacristy. Above the tomb is Pedro de Campaña's painting, "Purification of the Virgin," which includes portraits of the merchant and his brother Alonso and their families. Pike, *Aristocrats and Traders,* 43–45; Gil, *Los conversos y la Inquisición,* 3:398–401.

funds "to cure and care for the sick who had been taken and will be taken to the Cinco Llagas Hospital, providing them with the necessary food and medicine." He further proposed that the council name deputies to oversee the process and to ensure that no one "who appears healthy is admitted" in the hospital.

Melchor del Alcázar and several members supported Ruiz de Montoya's position, but others in the room voiced their agreement with Diego Caballero's proposal. In the end, Ruiz de Montoya's motion passed with the proviso that if the soldiers could not be comfortably provided for in the Cinco Llagas Hospital, then other hospitals in the city should be used as well. The councilors chose the jurado Ruy Gómez to supervise the operation and allocated fifty thousand maravedís (133 ducats) to accommodate the sick soldiers.

Seville's numerous hospitals performed a double function, care of the poor as well as cure of the sick. Many hospitals had been founded by churches, Christian confraternities, or individuals as charitable institutions to take care of the less fortunate in the city. These hospitals varied in size and mission; some were established by confraternities to provide food and shelter for the poor in the city or poor travelers, others funded alms or provided dowries for poor girls, a few were charged with liberating Christian captives in North Africa or burying the poor, while yet others were entrusted with caring for orphans and abandoned children. Several hospitals were founded to cure disease, and they too were specialized. There were more than a hundred hospitals in Seville before Archbishop Rodrigo de Castro reduced their number to eighteen in 1587. Temporary hospitals, usually outside the city walls, were established in times of epidemics to care for the inordinate number of sick.

Seville's major sanitary hospitals included the Hospital of San Cosme and San Damián, popularly known as the Hospital of Las Bubas (Pox Hospital) because it treated both men and women who had contracted venereal disease. The oldest hospital, San Lázaro, was founded in 1272 to care for lepers. The Hospital of San Hermenegildo, also known as Cardenal Hospital because it had been founded by Cardinal Juan de Cervantes in the mid-fifteenth century, specialized in treating all types of injuries regardless of sex or age and employed some of the best doctors and surgeons. The Amor de Dios Hospital cured men afflicted with "fevers." The Cinco Llagas, or Sangre, Hospital had been founded in 1500 by a prominent Sevillian noblewoman, Doña Catalina de Ribera y Mendoza, to treat sick women. One of the newest centers, the Paz Hospital, founded in 1543, was dedicated to caring for the incurable poor. The Bubas Hospital was under the direct auspices of the city council, though most Sevillian sanitary hospitals were under the patronage of the church, usually the religious orders. The patrons designated administrators to run the respective institutions. The hospitals enjoyed certain endowments, which were often augmented by individual charitable gifts of widely disparate value. A significant portion of hospital funding came from bequests of agricultural land or urban properties that were rented out. Various types of bonds and mortgages, as well as incomes generated by the sale or rental of city receipts, also played a role in financing beneficent corporations.[10]

Ruy Gómez reported back to the assembled cabildo two days later, on Friday, 3 June. He related that the German soldiers in the Cinco Llagas Hospital had just been examined by a physician, "who says that sixty of them were in express need of a cure." The doctor had emphasized that in order to care for the soldiers, they needed hospital beds. Therefore, the jurado had spoken with Dr. Rodrigo de León, the administrator of the Amor de Dios Hospital, "where he knew that some of the sick had already been received." In negotiations between the two, Dr. León "replied that he would happily accept all who would fit in the available beds." Not stopping there, the diligent councilman approached several other hospitals: the Desamparados, the Padre de León, and the Cardenal Hospital, "where the sick could be taken in and cured more comfortably." Ruy Gómez pleaded with the cabildo to authorize this distribution.

Martín Gutiérrez Cerón suggested that this proposal be submitted to the count, and all except Diego Caballero agreed. Melchor del Alcázar added that "Jurado Gómez on behalf of the city should profess to the administrators that the city receives much contentment for this hospitality and that their trouble and cost will be recompensed in other things that will present themselves in the future."[11]

---

10. Juan Ignacio Carmona García, *El sistema de la hospitalidad pública en la Sevilla del antiguo régimen* (Seville: Diputación Provincial, 1979), 39–88; Eloy Domínguez-Rodiño y Domínguez-Adame, "El Hospital de las Cinco Llagas," in *Los hospitales de Sevilla*, by Fernando Chueca Goitia and others (Seville: Real Academia Sevillana de Buenas Letras, 1989), 93–96; Morales Padrón, *La ciudad del quinientos*, 115–17.

11. AMS, sec. 10, 1580 [1].

3

AVERTING A MORISCO CRISIS

Many Moriscos were taken by force to the galleys.
—DIEGO ORTIZ MELGAREJO

DURING THE MONTH OF JUNE, another matter occupied the Count of Villar and the cabildo. Seville was home to about six thousand Moriscos, Muslim converts to Christianity.[1] After the fall of Granada in 1492, Muslims were allowed to continue to practice their religion, but they faced much discrimination. By the end of the century, resentment against these policies among the Mudéjares (Muslims living in Christian lands) culminated in several rebellions both in Granada and other parts of eastern Andalusia. The authorities decided to resolve the problem by forcing Muslims throughout Castile to either convert to Christianity or leave. Most chose to remain, hoping that by ostensibly accepting Christianity they could continue to practice Islam clandestinely. Because Moriscos seemed to have been resisting integration they were always suspect and a target of the Inquisition. The frequent raids by North African corsairs along the Spanish coast, coupled with the Ottoman empire's expansion during the sixteenth century and its foothold in North Africa, contributed to fears of a Muslim invasion. In such a climate, Moriscos were viewed as Ottoman sympathizers at best and more often as active agents helping the enemy. Local authorities reacted to the threat by keeping a closer watch on the Moriscos, as did the Inquisition. They were spied on, subjected to frequent inspections in their homes, their activities scrutinized; and infractions, whether for nonpayment of taxes or any indication of old customs in dress or culture, were punishable by fines, service in the galleys, or confiscation of land and property.

On Christmas eve of 1568 Moriscos began a bloody rebellion in the Alpujar-

1. Morales Padrón, *La ciudad del quinientos,* 93, based on a census in AMS, sec. 16 (Diversos), 334.

ras Mountains of Granada, and for the next two years there was fierce fighting in the region. After the rebels were finally defeated in 1570, most Moriscos were expelled from Granada and resettled throughout Castile, including Extremadura and western Andalusia. The few who were allowed to remain in Granada appeared well integrated into the dominant Christian society. Many of the exiled Moriscos settled in Seville. Some had been enslaved as rebels, but most were free and made their living in various occupations, seemingly interacting with the rest of the populace. Yet authorities were uneasy, given the large number of Moriscos from Granada who now lived in Seville, and periodically rumors flared up that the converts were plotting an uprising.[2] In the late spring of 1580 the city council was once again concerned about the concentration of Moriscos in certain parishes and the possibility of unrest. Indeed, during a council meeting discussing the problem, the jurado Cristóbal Suárez argued that there were too many Moriscos in the city and advocated that all should be expelled.[3]

The Count of Villar informed the cabildo on Monday, 20 June, that after having made "certain inquiries," he had concluded that the Moriscos "want to rise up" and had set the date for "the eve of San Pedro" (28 June). The threat seemed serious and involved Moriscos not just in Seville but in other parts of Andalusia as well. The leader of the rebellion was thought to be Don Fernando Muley, a Morisco also known as Don Fernando Henríquez. The city council acted quickly. First, the councilors agreed to apprise the inquisitors and church authorities of the situation and ask them to conduct their own investigation and then share their findings with city officials. At the same time, the count and several council members who had formed a commission to deal with the Morisco affair met with the president and judges of the Audiencia to discuss the best course of action to protect the city from strife.

The officials decided to proclaim several orders in various parts of the city.

2. Antonio Domínguez Ortiz and Bernard Vincent, *Historia de los moriscos: Vida y tragedia de una minoría* (Madrid: Alianza Universidad, 1997), 17–56. See also Ruth Pike, "An Urban Minority: The Moriscos of Seville," *International Journal of Middle East Studies* 2 (1971): 368–77; Pike, *Aristocrats and Traders*, 154–70; David Coleman, *Creating Christian Granada: Society and Religious Culture in an Old-World Frontier City, 1492–1600* (Ithaca, N.Y.: Cornell University Press, 2003), 180–85; and Morales Padrón, *La ciudad del quinientos*, 93–94. For analysis of the relationship between the Ottoman Turks and the Moriscos, see Andrew C. Hess, "The Moriscos: An Ottoman Fifth Column in Sixteenth-Century Spain," *American Historical Review* 74, no. 1 (1968): 1–25.

3. AMS, sec. 10, 1580 [1] (20 May).

First, they warned residents not to mistreat Moriscos "physically or verbally, nor forcibly enter their houses, or take their property." Those who had looted anything from Moriscos were to "return and restitute it, under pain of being declared robbers." It is unclear whether this particular ordinance was passed before or after many Moriscos were attacked and robbed throughout the city that same day. Second, the civil and judicial authorities ordered all guards at city gates to prevent Moriscos from leaving or entering the city. Furthermore, each parish was to designate a plaza where citizens, armed if necessary, were to congregate; the magistrates, constables, veinticuatros, and jurados, along with as many residents as needed, were to make nightly rounds in their respective parishes.

The commissioners agreed also to warn cities such as Cordova, Écija, Jerez de la Frontera, Jaén, and Carmona. They believed that Don Fernando Henríquez Muley, who by then had fled Seville, could have gone either to Cordova or Écija, and therefore they provided local officials with a physical description of the fugitive and asked them to search for him. The authorities ordered border patrols not to let any Moriscos cross between Spain and Portugal. This time the reason was not fear of the plague but fear that reinforcements might enter or that Moriscos might escape justice. According to letters that the Count of Villar sent to various towns, warning of the plot, some Moriscos had already been arrested, but other suspects had fled Seville, and the authorities wanted to prevent their escape to Portugal.

To contain the perceived threat, officials issued proclamations throughout Seville: no Morisco, whether free or enslaved, was to "leave his house night or day" under pain of death; and the sentence for infraction was "irremissible." Moriscas were allowed to leave their dwellings "from sunrise to sunset to provision their husbands and homes," but at night the women were subject to the same curfew as the men and with the same punishment for noncompliance The authorities admonished owners of Morisco slaves to ensure that their slaves obeyed these orders.

In the afternoon the council members again met at the city hall to review the measures adopted so far. At this point they designated various plazas throughout the city as well as in Triana where armed citizens ready to defend their community could congregate at the sound of the alarm: the parish church bells would give the signal. Each councilor, as well as the governor, was assigned command of a particular plaza, where citizens were expected to report. The councilors also worked out the details of the night watch. Each parish would be responsible for providing forty citizens nightly to accompany a constable and patrol their neighborhood. To inform Philip II of the situation, the city sent a messenger to Badajoz, near the Portuguese border, where the king was directing the military campaign to secure his succession.[4]

While the commissioners were debating how to stop a potentially disastrous uprising, there was unrest in the city, particularly in Triana, and Moriscos were the principal victims. Their houses were plundered, and some were kidnapped from their homes and dragged to the galleys. Complaints came the next day. On Tuesday, 21 June, several Moriscas denounced their neighbors to the commission, lamenting that the previous day "many residents near their houses took and sacked their property and money." After hearing the women's petition, Veinticuatro Ortiz Melgarejo reported that he had learned that "many Moriscos were taken by force to the galleys that are presently in the river of this city." The Moriscos were prisoners on the ships, and the alderman was concerned because the galleys were scheduled to leave the following day; if the Moriscos were not extricated, they would be enslaved. He urged the commissioners to secure their release. The officials sent the city's chief constable, Lope Zapata Ponce de León, to talk to Don Alonso de Leyva, the general of "the galleys of Sicily," and demand that he liberate the Moriscos, whom his soldiers had abducted and at the time "have in chains." Moreover, the general should order his people to return all the goods and money that they had looted from Moriscos "in Triana and San Bernardo and other parts of this city."[5]

It is difficult to assess how much of the property stolen by soldiers or other residents was recovered, but there are indications that some victims managed to be repaid. For example, on 18 August 1580 a Morisco couple reached an agreement with another couple, their neighbors, whom they had asked to hide some things for them at the height of the confusion during the galley soldiers' raid on Triana. The Moriscos, Hernando de Baena and his wife Leonor de Aguilar, feared the looters, and in desperation they hastily "threw certain goods" into their neighbors' courtyard for safekeeping. Unfortunately, when calm returned and the couple asked for their belongings, the neighbors refused to give them back. The Moriscos sued them, and in order to avoid imprisonment the "help-

---

4. AMS, sec. 13 (Papeles importantes), siglo XVI, vol. 9, doc. 55; sec. 10, 1580 [1].

5. Ibid. For Don Alonso de Leyva's participation and death during the Spanish Armada expedition, see Pierson, *Commander of the Armada*.

ful" neighbors paid the Morisco couple 170 reales (about 15 ducats) in restitution. As late as December 1583, a group of Moriscos collected money in compensation for property stolen by the soldiers.[6]

The Count of Villar and the commissioners were trying to protect the Morisco population, but at the same time they continued to take measures designed to thwart any plot. Once they dispatched the chief constable to complain to the general of the galleys, they turned back to the rumored uprising. They decided to alert authorities throughout the district that "some Moriscos roam together, causing harm," and ordered the offenders apprehended and sent to Seville to the count. Furthermore, if the local constables came across any Moriscos who had left Seville to work, they should not bother them but should order them to return within four days, because after that they would be taken "for rebellious and they will be proceeded against with full rigor."

Three days later, on 24 June, a letter arrived from the corregidor of Cordova with excellent news: Don Fernando Henríquez Muley, the Morisco leader sought by the authorities in Seville, had been captured in Cordova. The corregidor described the fugitive as "a man of medium build, dark and slightly bald, who has a small mole on his forehead above his left eyebrow." He apparently was well spoken, seemed to be "a capable" individual, and did not possess the distinct accent in Castilian that characterized many of his compatriots because "in his language he does not show to be a Morisco." His son Alvaro Henríquez was also arrested. Cordovan officials searched their belongings, including a "chest with papers," but nothing incriminating was found. The governor of Cordova asked for guidance regarding the two prisoners: since officials could not make an easy case against Don Fernando and his son, the governor was willing to let them go unless the Count of Villar advised otherwise.[7]

The prize would not escape. The Count of Villar was convinced that Don Fernando Henríquez Muley was the ringleader of a conspiracy, and apparently the king believed it also. Soon the city received a letter from King Philip, written in Badajoz on 25 June, which reached Seville two days later. The king was still unaware of Don Fernando's arrest, and he urged the count to find and imprison the rebel leader, "take his confession," and determine who else was in-

6. AHPS, Protocolos notariales, leg. 2366, fols. 295v–97r; leg. 2375, fols. 950v–51r.

7. AMS, sec. 13, siglo XVI, vol. 9, doc. 55.

volved in the plot and arrest them as well. The tone of the letter betrays deep concern on the part of the monarch, as the details of the plot were emerging. The king believed that the Moriscos who had been dispersed ten years earlier to prevent another rebellion were planning to return to the mountains of Granada and unite. The possibility that such a large armed body could aid North African enemy ships to invade seemed frighteningly real, and the king was mobilizing all his governors in the region to act swiftly. In the letter to the governor of Seville, the hotbed of the insurgency, the king exhorted the Count of Villar to inspect Morisco houses to "see if they have any arms" and to make sure they do not leave their houses or "deal or communicate with each other nor congregate."

Earlier, the count had also informed the king of the looting and abductions of the Moriscos. King Philip related to the governor that he had already written to General Don Alonso de Leyva, reprimanding him that "if he had been present on the galleys as he was supposed to be, this would not have happened" and ordering him to find and punish the culprits. In addition, the general was to make certain that everything his soldiers had robbed from the Moriscos "whether money, jewelry, clothing and any other things . . . all should be restituted to them." If not the actual items, then at least "the value in money" of what had been taken should be paid in compensation. To ensure that the guilty would be castigated, the king asked the Count of Villar to make his own inquiries and provide appropriate punishment. In closing, he instructed the governor to determine "how many Moriscos there are in this city and its lands and Triana who can take up arms and in particular if any of them have them hidden."[8]

The letter from Cordova and the one from the king were both read during the council meeting on Monday, 27 June. As first item of business, the councilors decided to "immediately make the arms inspection and the list of Moriscos." To accomplish the task, the count assigned to each parish a veinticuatro and a jurado, who would be accompanied by a constable and a scribe. The census would include "men and women and youngsters stating their age and which ones are free and captive."[9] The councilors agreed that the inspectors were to "take care to inquire with great urgency what weapons the said Moriscos have."

8. Ibid.

9. Ibid. The census is found in AMS, sec. 16, 334. See also Pike, *Aristocrats and Traders,* 154–70; and Morales Padrón, *La ciudad del quinientos,* 93.

If arms were found they were to be confiscated, and the scribes were instructed to note carefully "whose possession they were in."

While the Moriscos were being disarmed, the rest of the citizenry were told that until further notice they could carry weapons, "which are understood to be a sword and dagger, at any time of the night." Indeed, the jurados and veinticuatros who had been assigned to conduct the census of the Moriscos in all the parishes were the same ones who were in charge of the night watch and of informing residents which plazas they were to come to with their arms in the event the alarm were sounded.

During the meeting the councilors also decided to report to the king, telling him all that was being done in the city regarding the Morisco crisis. At the same time, the officials thought it opportune to "indicate to His Majesty the inconveniences" caused by some of the measures, particularly the one prohibiting Morisco men from leaving their houses, rendering them unable to work and earn their living, and to stress how disruptive it would be "if this should last many days." Many Moriscos were involved in agriculture, and not being able to carry on their work, particularly during the harvest, could be detrimental not only to the Moriscos themselves but for the overall economy as well. Seville's wheat and barley harvest was poor that year, and a labor shortage only exacerbated the problem of decreasing grain supplies.[10]

The king's reply, addressed to the Count of Villar, came days later, and the councilors heard it during their meeting in the Royal Audiencia on Wednesday, 6 July. Philip II, still in Badajoz, congratulated the governor on his handling of the Morisco crisis and expressed satisfaction that he was "apprehending the culprits." The king ordered that the rebel leader Don Fernando Henríquez Muley and his son be sent from Cordova to Seville and incarcerated there in order "to verify this business." King Philip acknowledged the councilors' concern regarding the Morisco house arrest and agreed that, since most of them appeared to be quiet, they could be permitted to work outside their homes.

The royal clearance led the councilors to issue new orders, which were announced that same day. The city criers proclaimed in all the pertinent places that Moriscos "can freely leave their houses to work and gain sustenance from sunrise to sunset," but until further notice they were still not allowed to leave the city. Morisco slaves, on the other hand, as long as they were accompanied

10. See Chapter 7 of this volume.

by their masters, could be out in the streets "at any hour . . . night and day."[11] These new rules affected not only Moriscos living in Seville but those in the other communities of the district as well. The proclamation once again reiterated that no harm should be done to the Moriscos.[12]

The crisis passed. Interestingly, on the following day, a Thursday, the cabildo met for an extraordinary meeting. The Inquisition was planning to stage an auto-da-fé on Sunday, 17 July, on the Plaza of San Francisco. The penitents who had been sentenced by the Inquisition, dressed in their distinctive garb, the *sanbenito,* would be conducted in procession from the Inquisition's prison in Triana's castle, across the pontoon bridge, through the Arenal into the city, and there to the plaza. As was customary, the cabildo led by the governor would participate, but first the plaza needed to be prepared for the spectacle, and the bridge required quick repair. On the appointed day, following a Mass and the reading of the individual sentences, sixty people were reconciled, acknowledging their waywardness and promising to mend their ways. One hapless person was relinquished to secular authorities, taken outside the city walls, and burned at the stake.[13] The Inquisition's exquisite timing of this auto-da-fé, just days after a serious Morisco crisis was averted, served as a powerful warning to the local populace.

11. Most Morisco slaves in Seville at this time were enslaved during the Alpujarras rebellion. As Christians they should have been immune from slavery, but as renegades were subject to it.

12. AMS, sec. 13, siglo XVI, vol. 9, doc. 55. Don Fernando Henríquez Muley and other leaders were executed; see Henry Kamen, *Philip of Spain* (New Haven, Conn.: Yale University Press, 1997), 176, 343, n. 214. A few more rumors of Morisco uprisings surfaced before the end of the century, though they seem to have been just that. By 1609 the Spanish Crown, frustrated by the perceived Morisco inability to fully assimilate and influenced by external political developments, ordered their expulsion from Spain.

13. AMS, sec. 10, 1580 [1]; sec. 11, vol. 20; Antonio Domínguez Ortiz, *Autos de la Inquisición de Sevilla (siglo XVII)* (Seville: Biblioteca de Temas Sevillanos, 1994), 59–62, describes a typical auto-da-fé on the Plaza of San Francisco.

4

SICKNESS IN THE JAIL

An incurable ailment . . . can indeed
come from this jail and infect the whole city.
—ROYAL JAIL DEPUTIES

THE GOVERNOR AND THE SEVILLE council relied on the services of numerous physicians, particularly in times of crisis. The city had no shortage of medical professionals, though their training and level of expertise varied widely. At the highest level were university-trained doctors, who had devoted years to the study of medicine and had spent large amounts of money to earn their degrees. Although they might have enjoyed certain prestige, most earned meager incomes. Furthermore, when these learned men were called in they would diagnose an illness and prescribe treatment, but often it was the barbers and surgeons who actually performed much of the curing. Because of the time and cost involved many so-called doctors possessed only the lesser degree of licentiate. Some of the better surgeons had lower-level university training, though many did not. Most surgeons and barbers learned their profession as apprentices, working with a surgeon or barber until they were ready to pass an examination and obtain a license to practice from the Protomedicato, a central institution consolidated during the reign of Ferdinand and Isabel and designed to regulate public health and medical practitioners, from pharmacists to doctors. At the bottom of the medical profession, and outside the establishment, were the *curanderos,* healers who often traveled from village to village or town to town peddling their special skills and potions.[1]

The income derived from practicing medicine was relatively small, and many medical professionals in Seville supplemented their salaries by trade.

1. Anastasio Rojo Vega, *Enfermos y sanadores en la Castilla del siglo XVI* (Valladolid, Spain: Universidad de Valladolid, 1993), 18–38.

Whether they were doctors, surgeons, or lowly barbers, they actively participated in commerce, including the Indies trade. One of the more versatile and ingenious merchant-doctors, Dr. Melchor de la Plaza, in only one year contracted a water seller to supply fresh water for two years during theater performances in the popular Corral de Doña Elvira and sold large quantities of velvet, silver, gold, emeralds, cameos, silk doublets, and silk stockings.[2]

The medical specialist on whom the Count of Villar regularly called, Dr. Nicolás Monardes, was already in his seventies and perhaps Seville's most famous physician. Dr. Monardes was the son of a Genoese bookseller who had settled in Seville and married the daughter of a local surgeon. He was born around 1508 and in the early 1530s received his degrees in arts and in medicine at the University of Alcalá de Henares. Licentiate Nicolás Monardes then returned to Seville and did a form of internship with the Sevillian doctor Garci Pérez Morales. At that point the young physician met, and in 1537 married, his mentor's daughter, Doña Catalina de Morales. It was not until ten years later, in 1547, that Monardes finished his doctorate at the University of Seville. In addition to his book on New World medicinal plants, he was the author of several short treatises; one of his earliest was a synthesis of opinions regarding where best to bleed patients suffering from pleurisy.

Dr. Monardes also became involved in trade. He formed a commercial partnership with the merchant Juan Núñez de Herrera, selling merchandise and slaves in the New World. After the death of his associate, Dr. Monardes entered into partnership with his son-in-law, which proved disastrous. Following some bad investments his business suffered serious setbacks, and in 1567 Dr. Monardes declared bankruptcy. To avoid imprisonment in the Royal Jail, Monardes hid briefly in the Monastery of Regina Coeli until he was able to satisfy his creditors. By 1580 the doctor was back on more solid financial ground. His wife had died in 1577, and some of his children were dispersed as far away as the Indies. During the health crisis of the 1580s, Dr. Monardes continued in spite of his advanced age to assist the city by advising officials and visiting the sick. Some time before his death, Dr. Monardes was ordained a priest. When he died in 1588 he was buried in the Convent of San Leandro, next to his wife.

Nicolás Monardes tried to grow in his garden many of the medicinal plants that his agents and other travelers brought to him from the New World. He col-

2. Dr. Melchor de la Plaza's contracts can be found in AHPS, Protocolos notariales, leg. 16136.

lected information on how these plants were used in the Indies and conducted experiments himself. The outcome of this investigation resulted in his most famous work, *Historia medicinal de las cosas que se traen de nuestras Indias occidentales que sirven en medicina,* first published in 1565. Dr. Monardes provided one of the earliest descriptions of a wide variety of American plants and their medicinal properties and use. Nine years later, the doctor published a final and expanded version of his work, which also included treatises on poisons and the bezoar stone, considered the best antidote to both poisons and the plague.[3]

One of the plants that most impressed Dr. Monardes was sassafras. A Frenchman, recently arrived from Florida, had given the inquisitive physician a piece of the tree along with an explanation of its use among native Americans. According to Monardes, sassafras "water," particularly if made from the root, was an excellent remedy for a wide variety of maladies, ranging from stomach ache, constipation, diarrhea, and headache to contagious diseases. "During this past time of the plague," the doctor remarked, "many have used it to drink to preserve themselves from this sickness, and we see that none of those who used it was infected by the disease." He also recommended smelling a small piece of sassafras, "because the infected air is cleared with its pleasant scent."

Dr. Monardes used sassafras himself to ward off the plague: "I carried a piece for a long time, and have found it, in my judgment, very beneficial." He also chewed on little bits of citron or lemon rind, which he believed to be a forceful deterrent to contagion. Dr. Monardes's remedies reflected the belief that plague was caused by poisonous vapors, or miasmas, and that the best way to avoid the dreaded disease was by purifying the air, usually with aromatic woods or plants. Carrying smelling apples or just some simple herbs was essential. This solution, repeated in countless plague treatises, differed little from those suggested in the fourteenth century during the first outbreak of the Black Death. The eminent physician was convinced that by smelling a sassafras stick and chewing on citrus, "with God's help, I escaped the fire that we doctors find ourselves in."[4]

3. Francisco Rodríguez Marín, *La verdadera biografía del doctor Nicolás Monardes* [1913] (Seville: Padilla Libros, 1988), 18–33; Francisco Guerra, *Nicolás Bautista Monardes: Su vida y su obra (ca. 1493–1588)* (Mexico City: Compañía Fundidora de Fierro y Acero de Monterrey, S.A., 1961), 5–8, 32–33; regarding Monardes's age, see Chapter 31, note 2, in this volume.

4. Nicolás Monardes, *Historia medicinal de las cosas que se traen de nuestras Indias occidentales que sirven en medicina. . . .* [1574] (Seville: Padilla Libros, 1988), 51v–64r; Campbell, *Men of Learning,* 65–73.

The city council also employed physicians, barbers, and nurses to supervise health conditions and treat the sick and wounded in the two infirmaries of the Royal Jail, one for men and one for women. The city administered the Royal Jail, a large compound not far from the city hall. According to Seville's sixteenth-century historian Alonso de Morgado, "Rarely do the imprisoned men drop below 500 . . . and often they pass 1,000 and reach 1,500."[5] The prisoners, who were accommodated in separate sections for men and women, came from all walks of life and were incarcerated for minor offenses, including debt, as well as major crimes such as murder. Those with money could purchase better treatment, but for the majority it was hardly a pleasant experience. For those who could afford it, there were taverns serving food and "jail warden's wine," and "two shops with vegetables, fruits, paper and ink, oil, and vinegar" were operated directly on the premises.[6]

The jail was open and the prisoners received visitors day and night, leading to a "confluence of innumerable people who incessantly come and go . . . at all hours of the day."[7] Most of the prisoners were not shackled and were able to move about freely. Fights erupted frequently, and the injured were treated in the prison infirmary. The clergy and various confraternities attempted to alleviate some of the suffering of the inmates, especially those condemned to death. The overcrowding and the "stench, confusion and screams" led Morgado to compare the prison to "a true representation of hell on earth."[8] In such miserable conditions, disease flourished, and whenever the plague visited Seville, the inmates were among its first victims.

The deputies in charge of the Royal Jail wrote a long letter to Philip II at the beginning of May 1579 lamenting the overcrowding and the difficulties they faced in administering the prison. They confirmed Morgado's figures on the number of prisoners, stating that "every day almost one hundred people enter and leave and normally the number is 1,000 and at some times it reaches 1,300 between males and females," both locals and foreigners. They complained that in spite of the charitable nature of many citizens, their alms were insuf-

---

5. Morgado, *Historia de Sevilla*, 191–92. For a vivid contemporary description of life in Seville's jail (written between 1585 and 1597), see Cristóbal de Chaves, *Relación de la cárcel de Sevilla* (Madrid: Clásicos El Arbol, 1983). One of the more famous inmates was Miguel de Cervantes, imprisoned in the Royal Jail for debts in 1597. There were other, smaller jails in Seville.

6. Chaves, *Relación de la cárcel*, 14.

7. Morgado, *Historia de Sevilla*, 191.

8. Ibid., 192.

ficient to operate the prison, primarily because of expenses owing to "the ailments, wounds and deaths that are very common in this jail." The two infirmaries were usually filled beyond capacity, forcing "two or three ill with different sicknesses to occupy one straw bed." The officials warned that the combination of contagion could engender "an incurable ailment, which can cause the pestilence that we live in great fear of here, and it can indeed come from this jail and infect the whole city."

The officials asked the king for funds to help remedy the problem, suggesting that he could assign for "this jail and its infirmaries of men and women" half of the fines that had recently been levied on the Royal Audiencia during the latest inspection of Seville's court of justice. The fines were to be divided between the royal treasury and pious works, and the jail deputies contended that if His Majesty assigned a portion to the jail it would constitute "a great charity and alms." They did not stop there. They asked for more money from the royal treasury so that "this jail could have some property," the income from which could "help and give food to more than 300 people every day," including galley slaves.[9]

Regardless of the outcome of this petition, the financial burden on the city led the governor to reduce some expenses, including physicians' salaries. One of the prison doctors, Dr. Juan Bautista Vides, was leaving for the Indies and needed to be replaced in early June 1580. The Count of Villar recommended that the jail's administrators consult Dr. Nicolás Monardes in order to create a list of instructions for the incoming doctor. The governor proposed that they "be written on a plaque which should be placed in the infirmary." The count stated that the salary for the new doctor should not be released until he was in place and working. The governor nominated Juan Sánchez as Dr. Vides's replacement; with little discussion, the cabildo passed the count's set of proposals.

The Count of Villar's attempts to improve conditions in the prison were motivated both by a desire to provide better medical service and by the pressing need to cut the city's expenses. Later in the session the count complained about "a surgeon who earns 100 ducats a year" to "cure all those [in the jail] ill with stones." But this surgeon had not been doing the job the city was paying him to do, and the governor advised the council to discuss whether it would "be expedient to name another surgeon with a smaller salary."

9. BL, Add. Mss. 28341, fol. 341r.

Don Gerónimo de Montalvo suggested that they turn the issue over to the jail's administrators, who should find out from the *enfermero* (male nurse) how this surgeon performed the cures and his rate of success. Don Gerónimo agreed with the count that the council should attempt to hire another surgeon for less money. Veinticuatro Ortiz Melgarejo, one of the deputies of the Royal Jail who had earlier written to the king regarding the conditions in the prison, supported the notion and proposed that in the meantime they should cancel the salary of the current surgeon.[10]

On 6 July the Count of Villar informed the cabildo that the jail's surgeon, Licentiate Suárez Montero, "had been let go." The governor reiterated that although Licentiate Suárez's annual salary had been one hundred ducats, the new surgeon should be paid less, and proposed 20,000 maravedís (about 53 ducats). Two weeks later the authorities named a new surgeon, Licentiate Bustos, to treat the wounded in the jail, at the substantially reduced salary. At the same time, the prison chaplain, who also earned 100 ducats a year, received a raise. The city council decided to pay the well-connected cleric 55,000 maravedís (almost 147 ducats) to say three weekly masses during the course of the year.

The issues of sanitation and health were frequent items on the cabildo's agenda. The Guadalquivir River often flooded, causing the drains to plug, creating pools of filthy stagnant water. Shallow graves and garbage constituted another health hazard with which the council continuously grappled. Unauthorized burials were also a source of complaint. At the end of September 1579, the count prohibited burials outside the cemetery in the Plaza of San Salvador when he learned that "the priests of the church of San Salvador are burying dead bodies in the entire plaza, which is very detrimental."[11] ·

The petition of the priests of the Church of San Andrés is representative of many similar complaints. The parish as well as the nearby Amor de Dios Hospital buried their dead in the church's cemetery, and according to the petitioners about eight hundred burials were conducted each year. "We have found and seen many times," the priests lamented, "dogs removing body parts from the graves and eating them." Furthermore, they fumed, "local residents, without respect for the decency of the place, throw out at night a lot of filth and garbage from their houses into the said cemetery." The clerics asked the city to build a

10. AMS, sec. 10, 1580 [1].

11. AMS, sec. 10, 1579 [3] (25 September). Carmona García, in the first part of his book, *Crónica del malvivir,* vividly describes the filth and stench of early modern Seville and its causes.

fence around the graveyard, and they warned that quick action was needed before "the bad odor causes infection."[12]

The "filth and garbage" included everything from food scraps to excrement,
and the dumping was not confined to burial places. People often threw their
garbage, dirty water, the contents of chamber pots, indeed anything that they
needed to dispose of, right out the window, to the peril of passersby. In spite
of repeated ordinances prohibiting this practice, particularly in the daytime,
when some unlucky souls could be walking by, it continued. Outside the city
wall there were designated places, marked with wooden posts, where all the
refuse from people and animals was to be deposited, but not everyone complied. City officials mandated that citizens were responsible for maintaining the
cleanliness of their districts, and they sometimes required them to cover the expenses of the cleanup, particularly when municipal funds were running low.
The cabildo regularly grappled with the issue of cleanliness, but a health crisis
injected urgency into the debates. When city officials received a complaint related to sanitation and health, they usually sent a physician to inspect the situation before taking any steps to remedy the problem. In times of the plague or
any other outbreak of contagious disease, the councilors solicited the services
and advice of the medical community more frequently.[13]

12. AMS, sec. 13, siglo XVI, vol. 3, doc. 26.

13. Carmona García, *Crónica del malvivir*, 48–58, outlines the difficulties facing citizens and city
officials in dealing with sanitation issues throughout the sixteenth century.

5

THIS SICKNESS OF CATARRH

Receive the sick poor who wander
the city unassisted, with this sickness of catarrh.
—RUY GÓMEZ

THE GUARD AGAINST THE PLAGUE had continued during the Morisco crisis and seemed effective, though disgruntled city residents complained about the restrictions. During the cabildo meeting of Friday, 5 August, chief constable Lope Zapata Ponce de León stated that the residents of the city "receive much vexation by being sent to guard" against the plague. Furthermore, it had been expensive for the city. Lope Zapata argued that "this business has no effect, and no other place in the kingdom is guarded except Seville." Indeed, Seville was free of the plague but not free of deadly disease.

Later in the day a new warning of serious sickness in the city emerged. The council sent three veinticuatros, Diego Caballero de Cabrera, Gaspar Ruiz, and Don Diego de Portugal, as well as the jurado Diego del Postigo, to ask the hospital administrators, and especially those of the Cinco Llagas and Cardenal Hospitals, to admit the poor who were suffering with "fevers." They were to stress the importance of the sick being accommodated and treated, given "the harm that could result."[1] Three days later, the council's first item of business was a petition presented by Dr. Rodrigo de León, the administrator of the Amor de Dios Hospital, who asked that something be done about the way the sick were collected and cured because there was no more space in the hospitals. A crisis had begun, but it was not the plague that caused city officials and hospital administrators to scurry around searching for solutions. Seville, along with most of the Iberian Peninsula, found itself in the midst of a deadly influenza

---

1. AMS, sec. 10, 1580 [2].

outbreak. The sickness did not spare the king and queen. On 14 September the cabildo received news from Badajoz that Philip II, while engaged in his Portuguese campaign, had become "indisposed," though the Sevillians soon learned that he had improved. The queen, Anna of Austria, however, succumbed the following month.[2]

When the council met on Friday, 23 September, the meeting was presided over by the deputy governor, Licentiate Juan de Aguilera. He reported what everyone feared, "that the sickness of catarrh and fevers is so universal in this city that it is believed that two-thirds of all the people are sick, and more are becoming sick every day." He recommended that city officials and the Count of Villar form a commission with physicians and "with their advice provide some remedies in this city and other expedient things for the health of the people."

Bartolomé de Hoces recommended that the veinticuatros García de León, Don Gonzalo de Saavedra, and Diego de Almansa, along with jurados García de Bustamante and Bernaldino Ramírez, should meet at three o'clock that afternoon in the count's apartments at the Alcázar to discuss the issue. All agreed, and the chief constable, Lope Zapata Ponce de León, urged that they should also send these deputies to the Cathedral Chapter to "plead on behalf of the city that general processions and prayers be ordered in all the churches, appealing to Our Lord for general health, because the sickness of catarrh is intensifying and there have been some sudden deaths." He suggested that after the deputies visited the cathedral they should attempt to bring together in the School of Maese Rodrigo "the best and most efficient doctors" available in the city to discuss possible remedies "to purify the air, which appears to be spoilt and causes all these sicknesses."[3] Lope Zapata exhorted his colleagues to heed the physicians' recommendations and implement them.

The reaction of city officials to this serious epidemic, even though it was not

2. Ibid.; Vicente Pérez Moreda, *Las crisis de mortalidad en la España interior, siglos XVI–XIX* (Madrid: Siglo XXI, 1980), 252–53, notes great mortality throughout Spain from "*catarro contagioso*" in 1580, beginning in August. See also Betrán, *La peste en Barcelona*, 93–94.

3. AMS, sec. 10, 1580 [2]. The Colegio de Maese Rodrigo was founded in 1505 by Master Rodrigo de Santaella, Queen Isabel's canon priest, who wanted to establish a university in Seville. In 1508 the canon obtained papal permission to create a medical school with the same rights and privileges as the University of Salamanca. By the 1580s the university had grown both in size and prestige. See Morales Padrón, *La ciudad del quinientos,* 286–88.

the plague, was based on standard practices and beliefs of the time, repeated in various medical treatises throughout Europe. Contagious disease raging in the city was a sign of God's wrath, and to stop it petitionary processions as well as personal acts of contrition were vital. It was God's will that began the sickness, and God's will would end it. At the same time, there were practical steps, based on doctors' advice as well as the accepted notion that the elimination of miasmas would halt infectious disease. Another important measure believed to alleviate sickness was a good diet of meat, poultry, dried fruit, and nuts rather than fresh fruit, which spoiled easily and could aggravate the disease.[4]

Meat consumption in Seville was always high, and in times of epidemics the need escalated. The meat of the *carnero,* the ram, was one of the most prized for this purpose, and the wether (castrated ram) was the best of all.[5] During normal times, prices for ram's meat averaged about fourteen maravedís a pound, the meat of a wether was worth about twenty-two, and the most expensive meat, from merino rams, cost more than twenty-five maravedís. Veal cost fourteen and a half maravedís, beef ten and a half, and pork approximately thirteen. In times of shortages prices could quadruple. The animals destined for slaughter grazed outside the city in the Tablada and Tabladilla pasturelands near the slaughterhouse. The city controlled the prices of meat by sending a veinticuatro and a jurado as well as an inspector (fiel ejecutor) to the slaughterhouse every afternoon to witness the slaughter and set the price of the meat. The slaughterhouse, a large compound that included not only the animal facilities but also housing for some of the personnel and a chapel, was located not far from the Slaughterhouse Gate. Ironically, the Quemadero, the spot where heretics were burned, was also nearby.[6]

In the meeting of 23 September, the cabildo agreed to send constables to the Isla Mayor and Isla Menor, islands downriver, to bring to Seville "2,000 of the best merino and castrated rams they could find." Later in the session, the deputy governor, Juan de Aguilera, observed that "the city knows about the

---

4. Betrán, *La peste en Barcelona,* 407–13.

5. Sheep were primarily prized for their wool; only inferior, old, or sick animals were sold for meat. See Carla Rahn Phillips and William D. Phillips, *Spain's Golden Fleece: Wool Production and the Wool Trade from the Middle Ages to the Nineteenth Century* (Baltimore: Johns Hopkins University Press, 1997), 116–23.

6. Morales Padrón, *La ciudad del quinientos,* 142–43.

great shortage of poultry and game and pippins and dried fruit and nuts," and he blamed the widespread sickness for this scarcity.[7] Licentiate Aguilera recommended that to "alleviate the present need," the town criers should proclaim in the city and all the villages for the next ten or fifteen days that "all who want to bring and sell hens, chickens, fowl, game, and dried apples and nuts" can sell at the price they want, without bidding, during this period of crisis. One councilor objected to allowing unregulated prices, but in the end the motion passed. There was also concern that some constables might be sick, and the councilors decided to name temporary replacements if that proved to be the case.

Three days later the council followed up on the question of meat supply for the city. The deputy governor declared that they were all aware of "the great need for sheep that there is and the many sick that there are," and he informed the councilors that in spite of "having made inquiries on Isla Mayor and Isla Menor to get them," no animals could be located. This unwelcome news provoked a lively discussion on how to address this emergency. Diego Caballero proposed a meeting that afternoon, in the Count of Villar's residence, with the deputy of the slaughterhouse and the meat inspector to determine how many sheep were available in the nearby Tablada and Tabladilla, as well as on the islands in the Guadalquivir south of the city. Don Gonzalo de Saavedra urged the councilors to send the procurador mayor (chief solicitor), Bartolomé de Hoces, to secure as many merino rams as he could; after all, the need was great. Veinticuatro López de Mesa agreed and suggested that as an incentive to the animal dealers, "let us give them recompense and payment the day that they weigh [the meat]." Moreover, the alderman stressed that the meat should be given to the poor and warned that "the meat that appears to be spoiled should be burned and should not be weighed." Following further discussion, the measure passed.[8]

The city council faced another problem. The jail administrator was petitioning to release the prisoners "because there is great sickness." Diego Caballero de Cabrera recommended that several members review the situation and also speak to the Count of Villar before reporting back to the cabildo about "the urgency to release the prisoners from jail, because of the great risk and danger that could result if it were not done." He furthermore suggested that those who

7. Pippin is a variety of apple.

8. AMS, sec. 10, 1580 [2].

were about to serve their terms in the galleys should be included in the investigation. The councilors chose Don Gonzalo de Saavedra and Diego Caballero to make the necessary inquiries.

The next issue was also related to the current influenza outbreak: the question of the city's hospitals that were treating the poor. Jurado Gómez informed the cabildo that the Count of Villar had charged him with negotiating with the hospital administrators regarding "their disposition to receive the sick poor, who wander the city unassisted, with this sickness of catarrh." After all, the council had decided to send him to collect the poor and take them to the hospitals with the understanding that the city would cover their costs. Indeed, there was a precedent, when the hospitals recently had admitted sick soldiers. Ruy Gómez told his colleagues that he went to speak with the administrator of the Amor de Dios Hospital and conducted a tour of other hospitals. What he found was disconcerting: "All the said hospitals are so full of the sick poor that most of them are on the floor, because there are no beds to accommodate them."

The jurado stated that given this overcrowding it was impossible to carry out the city's mandates; some administrators and others who were involved, he added, suggested that the aid for the poor sick should be organized by the parishes. The city should order the respective jurados to distribute, with the help of priests, "meat and bread and medicines from the pharmacy to anyone they find poor and sick in each parish." Ruy Gómez believed that this would be the least costly and most effective way to solve the crisis. He had broached the subject with the Count of Villar the day before, and the governor had suggested he bring it before the cabildo that day. One of the chief justices, Martín Gutiérrez Cerón, was first to speak. He disagreed with the governor, pointing out that this business did not need to be discussed in the council. He believed that the problem should be handled by the health commission; as far as funding was concerned, it should be provided as necessary.

After detailed discussion, Jurado Gómez spoke again. He told the councilors that in addition to the other administrators he had talked to, he had approached Dr. Gerónimo de Herrera in the Bubas Hospital. Dr. Herrera was busy preparing to administer treatment to syphilis patients, which occurred twice a year. The standard medicine for venereal disease at this time consisted of water that had been boiled with small pieces of guaiacum, or holy wood. According to Dr. Monardes, the Spanish learned about the beneficial properties of the tree from an indigenous doctor on Hispaniola when the Europeans there first became infected with the pox. For best results, the patients were to lie in bed in a warm room and drink ten ounces of the guaiacum water "quite hot"; then they should be tightly covered, "in order to sweat well," for at least two hours. After that the patients were to be cleaned and dried and given fresh clothing. The process was to be repeated every eight hours for at least two weeks.[9] Dr. Herrera, alluding to the city's patronage of the hospital, bluntly told the jurado that "that house and his person belong to the city," and therefore he was at the cabildo's disposal. But he warned that "he was at the point of administering the waters that are normally given at this time to the sick, and that the clothing that he has there is sweaty from the sick with the pox." Under these circumstances, the doctor pointed out, treating those stricken with the flu "would hurt them" rather than help them. When the jurado finished, the deputy governor agreed with Martín Gutiérrez Cerón that these issues should be decided by the health commission, and the motion then passed.[10]

The city council's preoccupation with the sick poor followed a long tradition of helping the needy. As good Christians, the council members as well as ordinary citizens were expected to provide charitable assistance to the poor. At the same time, there were the practical concerns of "the inconvenience" to the community that would result from inaction in the face of contagious disease.[11]

9. Ibid.; Monardes, *Historia medicinal,* 12v–16r.

10. AMS, sec. 10, 1580 [2]; Carmona García, *El sistema de la hospitalidad,* 53; Jon Arrizabalaga, John Henderson, and Roger French, in *The Great Pox: The French Disease in Renaissance Europe* (New Haven, Conn.: Yale University Press, 1997), 185–88, point out how quickly guaiacum spread from Spain to the rest of Europe and supplanted painful mercury treatments.

11. Regarding charity, see, for example, Richard C. Trexler, *Public Life in Renaissance Florence* (Ithaca, N.Y.: Cornell University Press, 1991), 350–52; and Michel Mollat, *The Poor in the Middle Ages: An Essay in Social History,* trans. Arthur Goldhammer (New Haven, Conn.: Yale University Press, 1986), 104–107.

6

SANITATION IN THE CITY

The city is very dirty and has a terrible odor.
—COUNT OF VILLAR

HE MEETING OF WEDNESDAY, 28 September 1580, once again presided over by the Count of Villar, began on a positive note. The cabildo rejoiced at the good news from Badajoz that "His Majesty is well and without fever." The council members decided to show the letter to church officials along with a renewed request to hold a general procession in the city to thank "Our Lord for the health of His Majesty" and to pray "for the general health of the community." A few days later the councilors posted a letter addressed to the king expressing their satisfaction at the restoration of his health.

But in Seville there were continuing signs of sickness. Two days after learning of the king's recovery, the city council received a petition from the administrator of the Amor de Dios Hospital requesting five fanegas of wheat from the public granary each week for the hospital "because the number of sick has grown." The cabildo acted quickly and passed a unanimous resolution granting the hospital the necessary wheat during the entire month of October to provide food for the extra patients treated there.[1] The following Wednesday, 5 October, the cabildo decided to send several members to inspect the city's hospitals and the treatment being administered to the sick. The councilors were particularly concerned with the mentally ill in the Casa de los Inocentes, founded around 1436 in the parish of San Marcos. The hospital, "where all those lacking judgment, be they furious or having manias, are sheltered and they cure them of this illness," was one of the earliest establishments in Europe dedi-

---

1. AMS, sec. 10, 1580 [2] (30 September).

cated to assisting the insane. As in the case of the prison, the city would have to act in case contagious disease broke out among the inmates of the mental hospital.[2]

During the same meeting another important issue was broached. The Count of Villar reported that many water pipes (*caños*) were spilling into the streets, and as a result "the city is very dirty and has a terrible odor, which causes great harm to health." Problems resulting from either broken or overflowing pipes and public fountains often vexed both residents and city officials. The spilled water created puddles, some of them quite large, and the standing water, combined with the usual filth found in the streets, attracted insects and produced a nasty stench. The council did not need a long debate to approve the count's recommendation to repair the caños and to punish any infractor tapping into the pipes with a penalty of ten thousand maravedís (twenty-seven ducats) and ten days in jail.[3]

In normal times the more affluent dead in Seville were interred inside parish churches or within the churches of the numerous convents, monasteries, and charitable hospitals. The poorer people were buried in the plazas adjacent to the temples. Not everyone agreed with this practice. When Licentiate Francisco de Morgaez, a priest in the Church of Santa Ana, lay dying in 1567, he was adamant about not being interred inside the temple. He insisted that "churches were founded for prayer," and only the higher ecclesiastical authorities, such as bishops or abbots, should be buried inside, along with anyone whose life was miraculous, because their bodies "give good odor rather than bad." Licentiate Morgaez cited early church canons and councils in stressing that "cemeteries were blessed to bury in them the bodies of the faithful dead" and that inside the churches, "where the Blessed Sacrament is kept and the saints and their relics and images are venerated, one should not put nearby anything foul-smelling, such as dead bodies." Unfortunately, even in the churchyards, whenever mortality rose and hurried gravediggers dug insufficiently deep, the fetid smell of decaying flesh soon followed. Only during serious epidemics, when the number

---

2. AMS, sec. 10, 1580 [2]. Quote cited in Carmona García, *El sistema de la hospitalidad,* 55. Carmen López Alonso, *Locura y sociedad en Sevilla: Historia del Hospital de los Inocentes (1436?–1840)* (Seville: Diputación Provincial, 1988), traces the foundation and functioning of this institution.

3. AMS, sec. 10, 1580 [2]; Carmona García, *Crónica del malvivir,* 81–83.

of dead would be so enormous that the usual burial grounds simply could not accommodate them, were mass graves dug outside the city.[4]

During the 5 October meeting, the councilors undertook the issue of burials and the health hazard posed by improperly interred decomposing bodies. The cabildo decided to send Bartolomé López de Mesa to ask the cathedral dean to order that "the graves where up to now the dead have been buried be bricked over." Furthermore, all new graves should be dug deeper, so that "neither from the ones nor from the others can bad odors escape." Two days later one of the chief justices, Martín Gutiérrez Cerón, who was also a health commissioner, reported that he had visited several burial grounds, and the large number of decomposing bodies was creating an unbearable stench. Gutiérrez Cerón singled out as one of the worst the cemetery of San Andrés, and he urged the council "to order a dozen cartloads of lime to be dumped there." He recommended that this be done in all the cemeteries where the dead were being buried. He went on to say that the procurador mayor, Bartolomé de Hoces, should see for himself "this cemetery of San Andrés, and that of San Lorenzo and La Magdalena and all the others he deems necessary," and decide how much lime should be spread in each "to remedy the said bad odor." Martín Gutiérrez Cerón insisted that action needed to be taken immediately regardless of cost. The councilors agreed, and all voted affirmatively.

The city council returned to the issue of the pressing meat shortage during the 7 October meeting. The governor reminded everyone of "the great need for meat, especially that which is most suitable at present for the many sick, which is that of the ram." The count stressed that although the measures that were taken "were very beneficial during the past week," they did not solve the problem in the long term, and the shortage was expected to grow. He lamented that in spite of permission to sell meat at "such elevated prices," there was still insufficient quantity coming from outside. The governor believed that because the disease was so widespread "the rams are being detained" in order to supply local markets in surrounding towns, leaving the stalls of Seville's butchers empty. Therefore, the count proposed to send procurers to "buy the rams where they are and order them to be brought to this city." As another option, the gov-

4. Carmona García, *Crónica del malvivir*, 121–23. For a 1610 copy of the cleric's will, see AHPS, Protocolos notariales, leg. 16185, fols. 515r–33v.

ernor suggested that the council could "order public proclamations in various places of some designated reward to any persons who would bring rams to market in this city." The count further told the cabildo that regarding cows, he had been informed that "the breeders of this city and its district have very good ones"; given the great shortage of rams, cows could not be exempt, and a certain percentage should be brought to the city for slaughter to alleviate the meat shortage.

The ensuing discussion was short, and the city's provision straightforward and quick. The councilors decided to send orders to the territories under Seville's jurisdiction and messengers on foot "to Extremadura, and the bishopric of Cordova and Jaén, and Jerez de la Frontera and to the Condado" to proclaim that anyone who brought merino or ordinary rams to be slaughtered in Seville would be "rewarded with four maravedís per pound above the price at which they were weighed." The officials ordered the city's steward to cover the costs of the itinerant criers as well as the rewards out of the city's propios. Furthermore, cattle breeders in the entire district were required to contribute one of every ten cows "to be brought to the butcher shops of this city."

After discussing the meat shortage the Count of Villar left. The council continued the session, and its attention once again turned to burials. The physician Licentiate Olivares presented a petition regarding "the inconveniences that exist when those who die in the Amor de Dios Hospital are buried in the cemetery of San Andrés." Licentiate Olivares reiterated the complaint about the "bad smell" that emanated from the cemetery and warned about "the infection caused by the garbage dumps within the city and outside of it, near the walls." The petition also included a plea from the hospital for "alms to buy a house."

Martín Gutiérrez Cerón advised that several members should take the petition to the Count of Villar and discuss it with him. Regarding the hospital's request to purchase a new building, the chief justice thought the issue should be brought back to the council before a final decision was reached. Diego Caballero agreed with Gutiérrez Cerón and added that the council should ask His Majesty to authorize the purchase and at the same time send the king a report by physicians and others, telling him "how important it would be for the health of this city to buy this site."

Most councilors at the session spoke in favor of the proposal, and they chose Gaspar Ruiz de Montoya and Martín Gutiérrez Cerón as deputies to move on the matter. In addition to bringing up these issues with the governor, the councilors also charged the men with exploring with the administrator of the Amor de Dios Hospital and others whether "it were good to consolidate and move this hospital to the countryside." Don Francisco del Alcázar suggested that the city should provide the site and add some money to what the hospital already had for the purpose. He also pressed the deputies to find out "the value of the house that is today the hospital."[5] As the discussion continued, Diego Mexía proposed that the city should become patron of the hospital, "considering that it always had the custom to inspect it and that every year it gives it alms for its maintenance." Others agreed, and several members recommended Don Diego de Portugal as a third deputy for the commission. As the long session closed, the cabildo voted to adopt the proposal.[6]

5. Francisco del Alcázar was the grandson and namesake of another distinguished veinticuatro. His grandfather and Melchor del Alcázar's father were brothers. See Gil, *Los conversos y la Inquisición*, 3:198–99; and Pike, "The Converso Family," 355–57.

6. AMS, sec. 10, 1580 [2].

7

TUSSLE WITH THE INQUISITION

In virtue of holy obedience and under penalty of excommunication.
—THE HOLY OFFICE OF THE INQUISITION

INCE THE MIDDLE OF AUGUST, the city had been battling the influenza epidemic, taking various measures to accommodate the sick poor, ensuring an adequate food supply as well as addressing numerous sanitation problems. But on Monday 10 October a letter from Seville's chief standard-bearer, Don Francisco Tello de Guzmán, from Badajoz, "that deals with the plague" brought the disease back to the cabildo's attention. At the same time, Sevillians were questioning some of the protections against the plague. Later in the week, on Friday, the customs duties agent (*solicitador del almojarifazgo*) Juan Ramírez requested reexamination of the orders prohibiting the import of cloth from Portugal. As the person responsible for the collection of duties on imports, he had to act to protect the various groups that survived on such income, particularly as these revenues were sold a year in advance.

Diego Ortiz Melgarejo, as usual, expressed his strong opinions. He stated that the petition should be turned over to the deputies assigned to this matter, who should decide which parts were "suspicious and from where no cloth should enter." When the officials determined which specific places the city should guard against, they ought to proclaim it publicly, given the great importance of the issue. These proclamations should only include places where there was bona fide suspicion of the plague. At the same time, the outspoken veinticuatro broached another subject. Once again a cargo of slaves had arrived in Seville, and he asked the governor to order an investigation of where the ship had sailed from. Ortiz Melgarejo proposed that unless it had arrived from Portugal, the slaves should be allowed to disembark.

Diego Caballero de Cabrera agreed, and regarding the customs duties agent's petition he argued that given what the councilors had just learned from Don Francisco Tello de Guzmán's letter describing conditions in Badajoz, "they should order what is most expedient, taking into account not the demands of tax farmers, but rather the public welfare of this city and its health." Following a general consensus, the Count of Villar indicated his support for the proposals and recommended that they should add one of the city's *letrados* (legal advisers) to the commission so he could examine what orders the city could issue regarding the tax farmers.[1]

For the next two months the municipal council turned most of its attention to topics other than disease. One event that attracted immediate notice was news of the death of Queen Anna of Austria on 26 October 1580. She was pregnant when she contracted the influenza that raged throughout Spain, and unlike Philip II, the queen succumbed to the disease. Her doctors tried in vain to save her, and her death deeply affected the king, who was still convalescing from the sickness himself. One chronicler reported that "they say that she offered herself to God, praying fervently for the king's life, so important to public welfare; He accepted her, taking her to eternal rest." King Philip, whose ten-year marriage to Anna was by all accounts a happy one, never quite recovered from the loss.[2]

Seville, like other cities in Spain, was in mourning, and the cabildo along with church authorities planned a solemn devotional service (*honras fúnebres*) for the deceased queen. The ceremony, a symbolic funeral ritual, was celebrated in many major cities in Spain as well as the viceregal capitals in the Indies whenever a royal personage died, and it served the purpose of honoring the deceased and laying them to rest at the local level.[3] During the funerary honors all the civic and religious authorities would have assigned places around the catafalque.

On the evening of 20 December, in his lodgings, the Count of Villar received an order from the inquisitors, displeased with the place they had been

1. AMS, sec. 10, 1580 [2].

2. Diego Ortiz de Zúñiga, *Anales eclesiásticos y seculares de la muy noble y muy leal ciudad de Sevilla* [1796] (Seville: Guadalquivir, 1988), 4:113; Kamen, *Philip,* 136–37, 176–77.

3. Carlos M. N. Eire, *From Madrid to Purgatory: The Art and Craft of Dying in Sixteenth-Century Spain* (Cambridge: Cambridge University Press, 1995), 287–91.

allocated for the services. Threatening him with a penalty of one thousand ducats and excommunication, they demanded that he call a special meeting of the cabildo for the following morning at eight o'clock. The count protested, declaring that the inquisitors had no right to request extraordinary meetings except with a royal provision or in case of sudden "death of a royal person or for an auto-da-fé." The governor insisted that it would be "very inopportune to call the cabildo to meet tomorrow" because it was a festive day, but he agreed to convene the council because he believed it would be of service to His Majesty.

The following morning the councilors assembled for the special meeting. The devotional services for the queen had been scheduled for that afternoon, and the governor had informed all the involved parties of the seating arrangements, which called for the Royal Audiencia to sit on the right side of the catafalque and the cabildo of the city on the left. The members of the Inquisition were to sit in the main chapel "as the most prominent place," which was the traditional order.

The veinticuatro who had been sent that morning across the bridge to the Inquisition castle in Triana, to inform the officials that the seats were being prepared, quickly returned to tell the count that the inquisitors "were discontented with the seat and place of the said main chapel." They wanted the Audiencia to sit in the main chapel on the left-hand side, while they should sit on the side of the evangelio (gospel nave), that is the right-hand side of the main altar, the most prominent spot in the cathedral. The inquisitors claimed that this was the customary seating order.

When the Audiencia learned what the Inquisition was demanding, the judges responded that the seating precedent the inquisitors were citing was a one-time special arrangement. The exasperated Count of Villar asked the cabildo to support his position regarding the seating order, pointing out that he did not want to have to suspend the honras and report to the king, because "it would not be just to remind His Majesty of the Queen Our Lady's passing or give him grief," but he felt it was unavoidable if the inquisitors persisted.

While the count and the councilors were deliberating, a secretary of the Inquisition, Antonio Ortuño de Espinosa Briceño, arrived with a message from the inquisitors. They insisted that the seating arrangement was "a novelty" because traditionally they sat on the side of the Evangelio and the Audiencia sat on the left-hand side, both inside the chapel, while the city council sat outside the main chapel. The inquisitors commanded everyone to follow the old custom, "in virtue of holy obedience and under penalty of excommunication" and two hundred ducats in fine to be paid by anyone who disobeyed. They demanded that everyone's vote be recorded, and all those who opposed the Inquisition's bidding be noted down, and they mandated that the register was to be taken "within 3 hours of the notification" to the Holy Office in the Triana castle.

The Count of Villar, who had been forced to call the morning meeting, was not amused to be threatened with excommunication a second time. He asked for legal counsel, and after the letrados and the cabildo discussed how to proceed, the governor sent the chief justice Don Gerónimo de Montalvo, the chief standard-bearer Don Francisco Tello, and the jurado Juan de Avendaño to Triana to inform the inquisitors that the seating arrangement remained in place. They were to wait for a response and then return to the city hall. The cabildo representatives left, but "within a short while the said gentlemen came back," stating that the inquisitors remained unmoved in their position.

In the end, neither the count nor the Inquisition nor the Audiencia would budge, and the devotional services for Queen Anna were suspended pending a decision by His Majesty. The king's reply, addressed to the Count of Villar, arrived on 16 January 1581. Philip II fully supported the governor, agreeing that the Inquisition was to sit in the main chapel, while the city council and the Audiencia were to sit on their respective sides of the catafalque. Furthermore, the king instructed the inquisitors to do "what the Count of Villar, our governor tells you." A similar missive went to the Royal Audiencia. The petty demands of Seville's inquisitors found no royal support, and the count's challenge of the Holy Office was validated at the highest level.[4]

A much more pressing issue had occupied the governor and the cabildo on and off since the Count of Villar assumed office: shortage of wheat and consequently bread, the main staple of the city's residents. Floods, droughts, and locusts regularly caused grain shortages, in spite of a well-provisioned depository. Seville's public granary, the *alhóndiga*, whose primary function was to supply the city with grain at reasonable prices, consisted of several buildings "with its patios and granaries, and very large upper and lower rooms, ample for all the

4. AMS, sec. 10, 1580 [3].

wheat, flour, barley and any other grain" that was stored there "for the provisioning of this great city." The alhóndiga had its own chapel, jail, and gallows to punish "the transgressors of its divine ordinances."[5]

Already in June, Diego Mexía, as chief warden of the alhóndiga, warned that there were barely 4,000 fanegas of wheat left in the storehouse, "and of those 526 are dispensed every day, given the many people in this city." A few days later, Veinticuatro Mexía informed his colleagues that the price of bread was high (two reales a loaf), and there were only 2,500 fanegas of wheat left in the public granary. He urged the city to ask the king for help. By the end of June it was becoming clear that "the wheat and barley harvest is half or less than that of previous years." It would become necessary to buy wheat from Murcia, Lorca, and Cartagena, "where there is notice of a good harvest." The officials estimated that the city would need to spend a hundred thousand ducats to buy enough grain for the year. On 8 July Diego Mexía reported that because of the poor harvest around Seville and Cordova, he was unable to find any wheat for less than two ducats (twenty-two reales) a fanega, and the lowest barley price was twelve reales a fanega. The cabildo decided to import cereals at the prices that were fixed by a royal ordinance: wheat at one ducat and barley at five and a half reales per fanega, plus transportation costs.[6]

As the shortage of grain was becoming more acute in the winter of 1581, Diego Mexía reminded the cabildo that in the 1470s the Catholic Monarchs, Ferdinand and Isabel, had confirmed the ordinances of Seville's public granary. Among them was a stipulation that no one could remove merchandise from the city without putting a *carga* of wheat or barley into the alhóndiga.[7] The goods subject to this duty included iron and ironworks and fish, though olive oil was exempt. Mexía pointed out that "at that time the Indies had not yet been discovered, and raw hides were not removed from the city." But after the Americas were settled by the Spanish, there was a huge quantity of "the said raw hides and other merchandise such as cochineal, indigo and sugar and others." He argued that up to the present time the public granary had not col-

5. Morgado, *Historia de Sevilla*, 153–54. Carmona García, *Crónica del malvivir*, 226–32, discusses some of the ordinances issued by the Catholic Monarchs to regulate Seville's public granary. He points out that in times of crisis and scarcity the rules were worthless, and the operation of the *alhóndiga* was overwhelmed by the demands placed on it.

6. AMS, sec. 10, 1580 [1].

7. A carga was equivalent to approximately four fanegas.

lected taxes on these commodities, and therefore the city was losing substantial revenues.[8]

The war with Portugal also contributed to the shortage of grain. In September 1580 the cabildo learned that Philip II had requisitioned 70,000 fanegas each of wheat and barley to provision his fleet in Málaga, grain that Seville had been authorized to purchase. The councilors petitioned the king to issue an order that no cereals that had been bought by Seville be embargoed. They reiterated that the city needed 150,000 fanegas each of wheat and barley "according to what is known of the year's sterility in this archbishopric and its district." The city's petition succeeded, and the wheat that Seville had purchased was not requisitioned in Málaga. But other places continued to embargo wheat that Seville had bought. The grain shortage was a constant theme during the Count of Villar's tenure as governor of Seville. The cabildo devoted much time to ensuring that the city and the public granary were adequately supplied with good quality wheat and other cereals and that bread was available to all who depended on it.

8. AMS, sec. 10, 1581 [1] (21 February). Regarding the rules about supplying the alhóndiga, see Carmona García, *Crónica del malvivir*, 226–27.

8

SIGNS OF CONTAGIOUS DISEASE

There is suspicion that there are contagious diseases.
—DIEGO DEL POSTIGO

T HE YEAR 1580 BECAME KNOWN as the "year of the *moquillo* [mucus]," a graphic reminder of the highly contagious disease that swept through Spain, affecting and killing rich and poor alike. The influenza epidemic lasted only three months, but if we are to believe contemporaries, the mortality was high. According to one report, twelve thousand people died in Seville by year's end.[1] Throughout that same year, the city council had faced additional challenges, ranging from food shortages, crop failures, locusts, and Morisco unrest to a tussle with the Inquisition; in addition, Seville loyally supported King Philip's claims to the Portuguese throne with men and supplies as well as by quartering and provisioning soldiers. The threat of plague, though not acute, was present throughout the year, and the governor, along with the cabildo, never lifted the measures that had been adopted to guard the city from the contagion.

During the month of January 1581, the question of payment for the plague guards surfaced on several occasions. Finally, at the end of the month, the cabildo agreed with the plague commission's decision that, with the Count of Villar's authorization, countersigned by two plague deputies, the city steward should disburse the funds necessary to cover the costs "of things related to the said plague."[2] At the same time, the cabildo debated whether to continue to safeguard entrance to the city in all the places where watchmen had been posted. The councilors decided that guards could be withdrawn from some spots because it seemed the city was now well enough protected. They also

1. AMS, sec. 11, vol. 20; Pérez Moreda, *Las crisis de mortalidad,* 252–53.
2. AMS, sec. 10, 1580 [3].

ordered that any gates that had been removed should be placed in a storage house.

The threat of contagious disease brought with it another concern for the cabildo: the condition of the boticas and the supply of medicine in the city. There were approximately forty boticas in Seville at this time, scattered throughout the various parishes; some were independent, others were associated with a hospital.[3] There was also a dispensary in the Royal Jail, and it was the city that paid for the medicines administered there. *Boticarios* (pharmacists) were trained as apprentices by another apothecary during a period of several years, receiving shelter and food in addition to the practical knowledge of how to produce numerous medicinal concoctions using plants and animal parts or products, as well as minerals and metals. In theory, the pharmacists were supposed to know Latin, but many did not. They were licensed following an examination by the Protomedicato and after paying the requisite fee for the test. It was determined that anyone wishing to become a boticario would need a large enough capital (in 1591 it was fixed at five hundred ducats) to be able to equip and maintain an apothecary's shop. Pharmacies were regularly inspected in Seville. The governor ordered these inspections, which were normally carried out by two council members, a physician, and an apothecary, who was to be an outsider. The inspectors reviewed the credentials of the boticario and the quality and freshness of his medicines and raw products. Any infractions resulted in fines.[4]

On 9 February 1581 the Count of Villar informed the cabildo that it was time to inspect the pharmacies, because "it is imperative that the medicines that they have are those that are especially useful at this time which is somewhat suspect of being unhealthy." To bring in an outside boticario for the inspection, the council would need to authorize his payment from the city's propios.

Chief Justice Martín Gutiérrez Cerón supported the count, saying that the

3. According to documents in Seville's Municipal Archive, there were forty-two boticas in 1594 (AMS, sec. 13, siglo XVI, vol. 1, doc. 114) and forty-nine in 1631 (AMS, sec. 13, siglo XVII, vol. 2, doc. 6). The exact number of pharmacies in Seville in the early 1580s is not known, but there must have been more or less forty.

4. Mercedes Fernández-Carrión and José Luis Valverde, *Farmacia y sociedad en Sevilla en el siglo XVI* (Seville: Biblioteca de Temas Sevillanos, 1985), 15–30; María Soledad Campos Díez, *El Real Tribunal del Protomedicato castellano (siglos XIV–XIX)* (Cuenca, Spain: Universidad de Castilla-La Mancha, 1999), 65–71.

council should follow tradition and pay what was given during the last inspection, in the mid-1570s, when the Count of Barajas was governor. Because it was well known that local apothecaries resented being inspected by an outsider, Diego Ortiz Melgarejo cautioned the count to send for a good outside boticario "as secretly as possible." Don Andrés de Monsalve agreed and urged the count to order that "all the gentlemen who are now in the cabildo take a pledge of secrecy."[5] A few weeks later, on 23 February, the council named Diego Caballero and Andrés Núñez Carcuela to inspect the city's pharmacies. Eventually (on 4 March) the cabildo decided that henceforth the boticas should have regular deputies assigned to inspect them at the beginning of each year.[6]

The Count of Villar, who normally presided over the cabildo sessions, was absent from 23 February to 14 March except for a brief visit on 4 March. Licentiate Diego de la Peña had been duly sworn in on 28 February to be the acting lieutenant for the count "because one of his deputies is absent and the other one is sick, and the said Count governor is also sick." But Licentiate Juan de Aguilera, one of the deputy governors, returned and would preside over many of the meetings during these weeks.

The issue of infectious disease came up at the same meeting of 28 February. It was near the height of Seville's rainy season, a dangerous time because of the possibility of flooding. Diego del Postigo, one of the plague commissioners, reported to the cabildo that "in the Islas Mayor and Menor a large number of livestock, cows as well as mares and rams, have drowned, and they give out a bad odor." He warned that "it could result in infected air and be very harmful to the city's health," particularly given the "suspicion that there are contagious diseases" in the city. He reminded the councilors that in 1561, although there was no sickness, "the city had ordered the burial of all the livestock that had died at that time." Although Jurado Postigo argued forcefully that the officials should deal with the problem immediately, the councilors decided that the question should be resolved by the plague commission.[7]

During the first three months of 1581, the cabildo vacillated between lowering its guard in taking protective measures and remaining vigilant because there were "suspicions" of disease. The devastating influenza epidemic of the past year had ended, but "signs" of contagious disease continued to surface

5. AMS, sec. 10, 1580 [3].
6. AMS, sec. 10, 1581 [1].
7. Ibid.

throughout the winter. In the sixteenth century many infectious diseases, such as smallpox, measles, and typhus periodically flared up in Seville. The physicians as well as barbers attended patients with various types of "fevers," including malaria, as well as gastrointestinal afflictions caused by poor hygiene or spoiled food. Most of these sicknesses were present and did not generate any special preventive actions. Only when the plague threatened did the city and medical authorities pay attention to foul air, filth in the streets, and other conditions believed to cause pestilence. At the beginning of March 1581 it became clear that prevention had not sufficed. Seville's cabildo received the news the council members had been dreading: there was plague in various cities in Andalusia, and there had been suspicious deaths in Seville.[8]

8. Ann G. Carmichael, "Diseases of the Renaissance and Early Modern Europe," in Kiple, *History of Human Disease*, 279–86; Noble David Cook and José Hernández Palomo, "Epidemias en Triana (Sevilla, 1660–1865)," *Annali della Facoltà di Economia e Commercio della Università di Bari*, n.s., 31 (1992): 71. Regarding the debate on the effectiveness of plague prevention, see Paul Slack, "The Response to Plague in Early Modern England: Public Policies and Their Consequences," in *Famine, Disease, and the Social Order in Early Modern Society*, ed. John Walter and Roger Schofield (Cambridge: Cambridge University Press, 1991), 167–87.

9

CARING FOR THE POOR AND NEEDY

This sickness . . . has hardly touched any person who is not poor and needy.
—COUNT OF VILLAR

N THE MEETING OF 2 MARCH, Don Diego de Portugal, one of the plague deputies, denounced the council's failure in "preserving this city from the sickness of the plague." He complained that the plague was spreading and that many people had died "without any attempts to take them outside the city to be cured, or burn the linens, or lock up the lodgings." Don Diego blamed the lax guarding of the gates, pointing out that it was common knowledge that "many people are dying of the plague in the Puerto de Santa María and Puerto Real and all their residents come to this city and freely enter." The irate commissioner urged the cabildo to establish a strict guard and to request documents from the Royal Audiencia regarding past practice in similar emergencies. He recalled that the last major plague epidemic had occurred in 1568, and a number of measures were taken then to "preserve this city." Veinticuatro Portugal advised the cabildo to cooperate with the court and order removal of the sick, the burning of infected linens, and the locking up of the residences of those found stricken with the plague. He also stressed the need for religious processions. Before finishing, he reiterated the importance of reviewing the records to see exactly what had been done in 1568–69.

Francisco de Bustillos supported Diego de Portugal's proposal and added that the council should employ "the best physician and physicians of this city to cure the sick." It was also necessary to secure cooperation from the patrons of the hospitals. Another plague deputy, García de León, reported to the cabildo that he and Melchior de Baena had been charged by the commission to go to the priors of the Monasteries of San Jerónimo and Las Cuevas to get their approval for placing "the sick with the plague in the Cinco Llagas Hospital." He would also speak to the priors of the Monastery of San Isidoro that afternoon, "since

His Lordship the Count is ill and cannot go and deal with the priors." García de León warned that they needed to move quickly to secure ample hospital space, before it became necessary "to take it by force."[1]

It is likely that the councilors reviewed the records of how the city had proceeded in 1568 when Don Francisco Hurtado de Mendoza, the Count of Monteagudo, was governor of Seville. That year the plague first appeared in the parish of San Gil, when nine people suddenly became sick on Palm Sunday, three of whom died. The afflicted exhibited the classic symptoms of bubonic plague: buboes in the groin, the armpits, and some behind the ears. The Count of Monteagudo had immediately ordered a search for a suitable building outside city walls to convert into a pesthouse, and the councilors found a *corral* (a rooming house with a central patio) across from the San Bernardo Church.

To locate those unfortunates infected with the plague, each jurado inspected his neighborhood daily to identify those who appeared stricken. Then, constables on horseback accompanied two men who carried the sick to the pesthouse in a wooden or straw litter. The city provided nurses, doctors, surgeons, barbers, and apothecaries, and it also fed the patients. The dead were removed in a straw litter, three to four corpses at a time, and buried in the two mass cemeteries behind the shrine of San Sebastián. They were accompanied by a priest and a sacristan carrying a cross. As the plague raged, more hospitals were needed, and the Cinco Llagas Hospital was used to treat the stricken. To make the transport of the sick easier, two special wooden chairs were built, and four men, dressed in distinctive clothing, were assigned to carry them. When the plague ended, the chairs were burned. Each parish had its own physician to monitor the progress of the contagion, who reported to the governor once a week. To appease God, the images of two popular Sevillian saints, Santa Justa and Santa Rufina, were taken out in a procession, which included the city's religious and secular authorities headed by the governor, the Count of Monteagudo. The documents noted that not long after the procession the plague had ended.[2]

Many of the measures that had been implemented in 1568 were again used

1. AMS, sec. 10, 1581 [1].

2. AMS, sec. 11, vol. 1, doc. 39. Perry, *Gender and Disorder*, 137, states that "a syphilis epidemic hit Seville in 1568," but there is no evidence supporting this contention. Indeed, Perry's source, Velázquez y Sánchez, *Anales epidémicos*, 65–67, notes that there was a syphilis outbreak in 1504 and a plague epidemic in 1568.

in 1581. The cabildo met on Saturday, 11 March, and the deputy governor, Juan de Aguilera, exhorted the councilors "for the good of this republic" to ensure that the order was carried out regarding the need for each official to identify the sick in his parish. He advised that those stricken should "be seen by approved doctors," and the respective jurados should officially notify "the hospital regarding the sick so that if it is the current disease they can be taken there." To ensure that the jurados complied with these orders, Licentiate Aguilera threatened a fine of ten thousand maravedís and ten days in jail.

Another item on the cabildo's agenda that day involved a troublesome crime wave in Seville. Diego Caballero de Cabrera brought up the issue of theft, complaining that "there are in this city many thieves and cloak snatchers, and they scale houses with much shamelessness and dissoluteness, something that has never been seen before." Cloak snatchers assaulted their victims in dark empty streets, stealing not only their garments but, more important, their money. The alderman argued that in order to stop these impudent criminals the city needed to improve the night patrols.

Deputy Governor Aguilera defended the current administration, insisting that the Count of Villar and the officials had paid close attention to the night patrols. He pointed out that there had been many "punishments and examples and that forty-five men have been hanged, over 440 have been sent to the galleys, which is more than what was done ten years ago." Licentiate Aguilera blamed the current crime wave on soldiers on board the galleys anchored in the river. He stressed that some had been punished and noted that the count had notified the king of the excesses. Therefore it was clear that His Majesty's officials were carrying out their duties. Caballero de Cabrera replied that he was not attacking His Lordship the count and his ministers because in his opinion they had done a fine job. He was merely concerned because the situation was worse at the moment, and they needed to improve the night patrol.[3]

Delinquents ranging from petty thieves to murderers posed a chronic nuisance for the city throughout the early modern period. The social outcasts, some organized in gangs, others acting individually, relentlessly tested the patience and abilities of the authorities. The Royal Jail was filled with criminals; many were sentenced to serve in the galleys, and executions provided a common spectacle for Seville's inhabitants. What were seen as lesser crimes such as fights and rapes were often settled with the aggressor agreeing to pay damages to the

3. AMS, sec. 10, 1581 [1].

victim and obtaining a statement of pardon. The influx of wealthy travelers to or from the Americas attracted gangs of thieves who often assaulted their victims on the roads. Robberies within the city were a daily occurrence, and the safety of the inhabitants as well as of travelers were concerns the cabildo periodically discussed.[4]

By 14 March the ailing Count of Villar had regained his health sufficiently to return to the city hall to preside over the day's meeting. The elderly governor was preoccupied with the "great necessity that afflicts the poor of this city and its district." The governor emphasized that "this sickness that has begun and exists in this city, has hardly touched any person who is not poor and needy." He reasoned that it could "be inferred that the principal cause of it is that the poor lack food." The count's observation reflected a common belief. The relationship between poverty, malnutrition, and sickness had been repeatedly noted by contemporaries and has been debated by modern historians.[5] The governor urged, for the sake of God and king, that these poor unfortunates must be helped, because it was clear how much "they missed the prelate's alms," a reference to the deceased Archbishop Cristóbal de Rojas y Sandoval, who was known among the poor as "a great alms giver."[6]

The archbishop of Seville had died the previous year, and his replacement

4. Regarding crime in Seville, see Perry, *Crime and Society;* Pike, *Aristocrats and Traders,* 192–203; and Pedro Herrera Puga, *Sociedad y delincuencia en el Siglo de Oro* (Madrid: Biblioteca de Autores Cristianos, 1974), 232–46. Miguel de Cervantes paints a vivid portrait of the criminal element of Seville in several of his short stories. See especially "Novela de Rinconete y Cortadillo," in *Novelas ejemplares,* ed. Harry Sieber (Madrid: Cátedra, 1990), 1:189–240.

5. AMS, sec. 10, 1581 [1]. Regarding the issue of poverty and disease, Mollat, *The Poor in the Middle Ages,* 194–97, suggests that deficient diet, among other factors, played a role in the susceptibility of the poor to epidemic disease. On the other hand, Massimo Livi-Bacci, *Population and Nutrition: An Essay on European Demographic History* (Cambridge: Cambridge University Press, 1991), 35–39, 104–105, argues that nutrition had minimal impact on the course of major epidemics, such as the plague, which was "devastating and there was little that individual or social defenses—the quantity and quality of food—could do in the face of it."

6. AMS, sec. 10, 1581 [1]; Ortiz de Zúñiga, *Anales eclesiásticos,* 4:112. When Archbishop Cristóbal de Rojas y Sandoval died, he and his household owed pharmacist Juan del Valle 71,000 maravedís (about 189 ducats) for medicines. The bill was dated 10 September 1580, and the question of payment was raised on 13 April 1581 as the Count of Villar conducted an audit of the archbishop's estate and finances. See AHPS, Protocolos notariales, leg. 2367, fols. 1169r–70r. There were also some outstanding debts to Dr. Nicolás Monardes. For example, the doctor was paid 10,779 maravedís (about 29 ducats) as late as 13 October 1581 as part of a salary that "the said archbishop was giving me as his personal physician." See AHPS, Protocolos notariales, leg. 2368, fol. 1108v.

had not yet been named. The count believed that the vacancy was detrimental to the welfare of the poor and told the councilors that he had urged the king to send a new prelate to fill the seat. He stressed that he had written to the king not because the Cathedral Chapter and the dean were performing badly but because the new archbishop would be able to "help the poor with part of his income." The archdiocese of Seville was one of Spain's wealthiest, and the archbishop's substantial income, mostly derived from tithes, allowed him to contribute with numerous alms to poor relief in the city.

The count's letter was followed by a plea from Seville's agent at Court, the veinticuatro Don Gonzalo de Saavedra. Don Gonzalo told the king that there was "infectious disease" in the city and indicated the great expense incurred in trying to help the poor sick, "having public houses to cure the infected with the said disease, and to give them food when they are convalescing." Furthermore, because "this sickness is so dangerous, it is necessary to give large salaries to the physicians and surgeons and other servants of the said houses." Don Gonzalo pointed out that "the sustenance and medicines . . . are very expensive" and the city's income insufficient to cover these costs. The veinticuatro lamented that as a result, "many die unable to be cured," but what was even worse, "they die without having been administered the Holy Sacraments." There were so many sick that though the local priests "do what they can, it is not enough," and it would be beneficial to send in clergymen from other places to help them.

In conclusion, the city's "lobbyist" bemoaned the current vacancy in the archbishopric and urged the king to intervene with the pope, who now "enjoys the property that belongs to the archbishop, . . . to help carry the burden of the cure of this disease and provide more priests and clergymen." Don Gonzalo expressed his belief that "His Holiness . . . as a father and a pious man and supremely Christian would provide all not only with the property of the said vacant seat . . . but from his own treasury and patrimony." He ended his plea with an exhortation to "Your Highness as king and natural lord, to whom it corresponds to give the order so that it takes effect and your subjects and vassals do not perish lacking those who aid them and administer the Holy Sacraments."[7] Certainly many of Seville's clergy were called upon to take confession from and anoint their moribund parishioners, and as the number of sick and dying increased the priests found themselves busier than usual. Lorenzo Fernández, the

7. AMS, sec. 13, siglo XVI, vol. 4, doc. 25.

parish priest of the Church of Santa Ana, provided several witnesses in May of 1581 attesting to his serving diligently, "administering the sacraments to all, even if they are sick with the plague."[8]

While awaiting the Crown's response, Seville's cabildo continued to battle the disease. During the 14 March meeting, the need for prayers was again broached, and the council decided to send four representatives to the "convents of monks and nuns so that they say prayers and make supplications so that God lifts this sickness that is presently with us." The governor and the cabildo tried to stop the disease at every front, but they also believed that the ultimate relief would come from God alone. The count even made a personal plea, a vow to erect a shrine dedicated to San Sebastián, the saint believed to provide protection against the plague, in his ancestral town of Villardompardo.[9]

Before the meeting ended, the council addressed its concern for maintaining the city adequately supplied as well as continuing unrestricted movement of people and goods from Seville. The cabildo decided to petition the royal council to order all places in the kingdom to permit the entrance of people and merchandise from Seville and not hinder the free flow of supplies for the city. To keep commerce and communications open with the outside world was vital for the city's well-being, and the councilors did not seem troubled that their request contradicted their own policy of keeping out people and goods from places suspected of having the plague. Hypocritically, Seville could impose quarantine on other communities, but others should not guard against the city, even if people were dying there from the plague.

Throughout the month the councilors continued to grapple with the question of the poor sick. They agreed to approach the cathedral dean, the highest church official in the archbishop's absence, to "beg him that it would be beneficial for the health of the city, for the infected poor not to wander around the city while there is suspicion of this disease." In order to prevent the sick from roaming the streets, they should be "distributed in the hospitals, those that provide hospitality as well as those that do not." The city's emissaries should also ask the dean "to order the parish priests not to bury anyone except in the day-

8. AHPS, Protocolos notariales, leg. 2367, fols. 1221r–31v.

9. Ibid., leg. 17720, fol. 435r. From the inserted Count of Villar's sixty-five-folio will of 12 October 1592, where among other things he mentioned this vow, which he had fulfilled. On his deathbed he begged his heirs to maintain in good repair the shrine of San Sebastián as well as other religious edifices he and his ancestors had erected in the town of Villardompardo.

time," and if in some parishes "they dump a corpse at church doors at night, the priests need to find out from which house it came and inform His Lordship the Count."[10]

Along with processions, prayers, and personal promises, the Count of Villar took other steps to appease God's wrath. Convinced that "public sin" was the cause of divine ire and hence the growing sickness, the governor decided to act and punish the sinners. On Saturday 18 March 1581, "on the eve of Palm Sunday," the beginning of Holy Week, the governor ordered the arrest of about seventy women who were taken to the Royal Jail on charges of prostitution. The women were outraged and complained to the Royal Audiencia, charging both the Count of Villar and the chief justice Gerónimo de Montalvo and their officials with having imprisoned them "without having committed any crime." The women claimed that "some were married and the others were maidens and honorable women" and complained that they were unable to appeal their arrest because the court was not in session during Holy Week and Easter.[11]

Prostitution in Seville was regulated by municipal authorities and was to be confined to a section near the Arenal, known as La Mancebía or La Pajería. The "official prostitutes," supervised by so-called "fathers," were regularly examined for venereal disease. But in addition to the sanctioned public brothels, clandestine prostitution was widespread and involved women of all ages and conditions, including married women. It was these "illegal" prostitutes whom the Count of Villar had targeted in his spring sweep. Some of the women proved their innocence by presenting testimony vouching for their honor, and the governor ordered their release. The rest remained incarcerated for several days.

Eventually the judges of the Royal Audiencia reviewed their cases and because of fear of disease they too were ultimately released, though most were placed under house arrest, only allowed to "leave to their parish to hear the Divine offices and to confess and receive the sacraments directly."[12] Three months later, on 11 June, Dr. Juan Fernández Cogollos, the president of the Royal Audiencia, wrote to King Philip justifying the magistrates' decision to release the women and a notorious gambler who had also been arrested by the Count of Villar to "punish public sin in order to appease the wrath of Our Lord."

10. AMS, sec. 10, 1581 [1] (16 March).

11. BL, Add. Mss. 28342, fols. 330r–31r.

12. Ibid. See also Perry, *Gender and Disorder*, 137–41; and Vázquez García and Moreno Mengíbar, *Poder y prostitución*, 65–93.

Dr. Cogollos argued that the magistrates were correct in freeing the women because the governor had acted "without preceding testimony regarding their guilt." The gambler, whose "sentence was to be in money and not corporal," had been released on bond at the beginning of May when "the plague began to spread in the jail." Dr. Cogollos insisted that he saw no reason to reprimand the magistrates for countering the governor's actions.[13] This was a perfect example of a jurisdictional conflict between the royal governor and the Audiencia in administering justice.

By the end of March 1581 the plague seemed widespread in Seville, and the cabildo tried to cope with the consequences of the epidemic. One of the major worries confronting city officials was tracking down those who had become sick as well as those who had succumbed to the disease. They assigned the jurados of each parish this responsibility as well as ensuring that the residences of plague victims were locked up and the sick taken to a hospital. However, the situation of the city's wealthy elite was far different; if they became sick, they remained in their homes and were cared for by private physicians.

13. BL, Add. Mss. 28342, fols. 328–29.

10

FLEE FAST, FAR, AND FOR A LONG TIME

Some left their dead wives and locked their houses and went away.
—THE COUNT OF VILLAR

DURING THE MONTH OF APRIL 1581 the crisis heightened, as the city battled sickness and death, food shortage, and financial difficulties. The president and judges of the Royal Audiencia, fearing for their lives, petitioned the king to allow them to leave Seville. They reported that people were dying of the plague "in all the parishes, and entire neighborhoods are devastated and the most prominent people have abandoned it." The panicked magistrates claimed that on 11 April in one of the plague hospitals alone, there were "more than 500 stricken with this disease." The royal council replied on 24 April 1581, telling the judges to do whatever they deemed appropriate, because the king and council had full confidence that they would act "with the required prudence."[1]

The members of the municipal council were not so lucky. When the cabildo met on Monday, 3 April, the Count of Villar ordered that no councilor was to leave the city "until Our Lord is served to restore health to it," though he did make an exception for a trip "related to the very health." The governor threatened anyone who disobeyed with a hefty fine of one thousand ducats and ordered those who were currently outside the city to return "very quickly." The count, well aware of the popular belief concerning how best to ward off the plague—"flee fast, far, and for a long time"—wanted to ensure that most municipal officials were available for duty in the city.[2]

In a letter to the royal council, the Count of Villar explained why he felt it

1. BL, Add. Mss. 28342, fols. 328–29, 252r–v.

2. AMS, sec. 10, 1581 [1]. It was known as the three *l*s: "*huir luego, lejos y largo tiempo.*" This advice was also given in the fourteenth century by exasperated physicians who felt helpless during the onslaught of the Black Death. For example, the Italian Gentile da Foligno, having recommended

was important that the veinticuatros and jurados remain in the city during the health crisis. The governor did not mind if others fled the city, because "the fewer people that are in it, the better, and thus those who leave are doing us a favor." But he believed that the presence of the councilors was "very necessary and useful because, since they are almost a hundred and have their houses scattered throughout the whole city, this disease can strike in very few places where there is not one of them, and so they immediately know it, and because it affects them they come to redress it." Furthermore, the governor noted that at the beginning of the outbreak the constables, along with his lieutenants and sometimes the count himself, were able to supervise the efforts to help the afflicted, but now that the sickness "has grown so much," he needed all the assistance he could get, though he complained that "until now [the councilors] have done it slowly and unwillingly and not without coercion."[3]

The disease outbreak was serious, and as the number of dead climbed, the city council issued strict new orders regarding burials. The officials instructed each jurado to designate a constable in his parish and to take down the name of the parish priest and where he lived. All cadavers were to be removed by four persons charged with transporting the dead. The men were to burn the infected bedding and keep a careful record of their activities, which would earn them three reales a day. The city also employed four gravediggers, who were paid two reales daily. Anyone refusing to carry out his duties would be jailed. The city's steward, Diego del Postigo, would pay the workers weekly and keep records in the "plague book." In addition, the jurados were to collect an inventory of the possessions of the deceased. On the following Wednesday, 5 April, the cabildo also set the stipend for four men assigned to take the sick to the hospital; each man was to receive four reales a day.[4] At about the same time, the city council set the price of a loaf of bread at twenty-eight maravedís to keep prices at a reasonable level. The average price of meat or fish fluctuated between

---

various remedies against the plague, in the end stated, "Finally I conclude that to flee, as I have said, is best in this particular pestilence; for this sickness is the most poisonous of poisons." At the beginning of the seventeenth century, the Spanish doctor, Juan Sorapán de Rieros, concurred: "To flee with the three LLL from pestilence is good science"; cited in Campbell, *Men of Learning*, 92, and in Luis S. Granjel, "Vida y obra de Sorapán de Rieros," *Asclepio* 24 (1972): 74, respectively.

3. BL, Add. Mss. 28342, fols. 257r–59v. The letter is dated 12 April 1581.

4. AMS, sec. 10, 1581 [1].

ten and fourteen maravedís a pound, though sardines were much cheaper. A gravedigger earning two reales, or sixty-eight maravedís, a day would be able to barely feed his family.[5]

As the sickness intensified, the need for more-frequent strategy sessions at the parish level became apparent. Conditions were constantly changing, and the municipal council wanted to remain informed regarding the individual sectors of the city. During the 5 April meeting, the officials agreed that the councilors would meet in their respective districts with the parish priest three times a week, on Monday, Wednesday, and Friday, at five o'clock in the afternoon to discuss the latest developments in the neighborhood.

As during the previous year's influenza epidemic, the city faced the problem of assuring adequate meat supplies. The jurado Alonso Núñez of the plague commission recommended the purchase and sale of calves "for the sick people." He also informed the cabildo that "there is no poultry." Gaspar Ruiz de Montoya confirmed that there were neither "hens nor chickens even at very elevated prices." He agreed that veal would be beneficial in the coming months for both the healthy and the sick. But Gaspar Ruiz warned that the meat of bulls should not be sold, because it was "so prejudicial to health." In the end, the councilors decided to butcher all the mature cattle designated for slaughter that were grazing on the pasture of the Tablada, with the exception of the bulls. They agreed that one-half of the calves should also be slaughtered. The cabildo had a financial interest in the cattle industry because the municipality allowed free grazing on its pastureland and in return received the viscera of the butchered animals, whose worth could reach thousands of ducats in revenue.[6]

Seville's cathedral canons Isidro de la Cueva and Alonso Marín paid a visit to the city hall on Friday, 7 April. They came in response to the cabildo's supplication to help place the sick poor in hospitals. On behalf of the Cathedral Chapter, "for the remedy of the present sickness," the two canons presented a proposition to establish a "special house in Triana where the sick can be sheltered." City council members supported the proposal and passed it on to the plague commission, with the proviso that veinticuatro Juan de León and Triana

5. Ibid. (31 March 1581). Less than a year earlier, in June of 1580, the price of a loaf of bread had reached a high of two reales (see Chapter 7 of this volume). For prices of meat and fish, see Morales Padrón, *La ciudad del quinientos,* 143–44.

6. See Morales Padrón, *La ciudad del quinientos,* 143.

jurado Juan Yáñez de Perea should be present at the commission meeting.[7] Yáñez de Perea, a man in his early fifties, was considered a hidalgo among his peers. He lived with his wife, Doña Catalina de Cabrera, in a well-furnished house on Sola Street in Triana, not far from the parish church of Santa Ana. The couple, like many well-to-do Sevillians, owned farmland and vineyards outside the city as well as rental property throughout Triana. In 1583 the jurado would purchase a young slave, Francisco, from an elderly widow for fifty-five ducats, though he would not enjoy such luxury for long; he died two years later. The couple's daughter Doña Catalina de Perea had married a seaman, Captain Cristóbal Romero, who would often leave his wife in charge of their estate while he was "absent in the Indies."

Juan Yáñez de Perea, as Triana's jurado, frequently crossed the bridge, riding his horse over to city hall on the Plaza of San Francisco. He knew his neighborhood well and was acquainted with many of Triana's residents. He was the ideal choice to help establish a pesthouse in Triana, which the plague deputies approved on 8 April, naming the jurado its administrator. They recommended that it should be modeled on the plague ward of the Cinco Llagas Hospital and similarly staffed and equipped. The Count of Villar informed the cabildo of the commission's decision to set up "in Triana another hospital and infirmary for the sick of this disease of the plague, with doctors, surgeons and a barber and a dispensary" as well as other necessities, including beds.[8]

The church followed up on the issue of hospitals on Monday, 10 April. Canon Antonio García arrived at the council meeting, along with the cathedral prebendary Pedro Venegas, and stated that to alleviate the suffering caused by "the present sickness" the city should "assign more hospitals and houses where the sick . . . can be sheltered and cured, as well as convalescent houses." Regarding the infected clothing and "the harm that results from returning it to the sick who have recovered," as well as "cleaning up the whole city from all types of filth," the church officials recommended a meeting with "deputies in the parishes." Heeding their admonitions, the councilors discussed further the issue of cleaning the streets. Veinticuatro Ortiz Melgarejo supported the suggestion

7. AMS, sec. 10, 1581 [1].

8. AMS, Escribanía de Cabildo, sec. 3, vol. 7, doc. 14. For Juan Yáñez de Perea, see AHPS, Protocolos notariales, leg. 2375, fols. 873r–v; leg. 2380, fols. 213r–v, 250r–51r; AMS, sec. 13, siglo XVI, vol. 7, doc. 60.

that if necessary the city should requisition "carts or draft animals" for the removal of the garbage.

Ortiz Melgarejo then raised the subject of hospital overcrowding. He informed the cabildo that there were more than double the four hundred patients that there should be in the Cinco Llagas Hospital, and the staff had increased to three surgeons and one doctor. Furthermore, four houses were set up next to the hospital "for the said convalescents." The talkative veinticuatro reiterated that the council had authorized another hospital, in Triana, organized along the same lines as the Cinco Llagas Hospital, and he urged the city to establish "a convalescent hospital nearby" as well. The pragmatic alderman proposed that the cabildo charge Jurado Yáñez de Perea with locating a suitable building for the convalescents and setting it up, as he had done with the hospital itself. He indicated that the church officials should "find administrators for these hospitals and three priests to hear confession and give the sacraments to the sick." Two of the priests should be designated for the Cinco Llagas Hospital and one for the pesthouse in Triana. Ortiz Melgarejo, mindful of the costs, suggested that the city ask both the king and the incoming archbishop for a donation.

Continuing his long discourse, the veinticuatro returned to the subject of sanitation. He believed that the cleaning should be undertaken by the parishes and paid for by the residents in each. He proposed that the city release thirty ducats to "the most honorable priest" in each parish to distribute to those charged with the cleanup. This proposal generated a heated discussion as to the appropriateness of indiscriminately allocating thirty ducats for each parish. Some members argued that the amount should be based on the size of the parish, while others felt it should be determined by the number of sick.

The governor spoke next. He endorsed a proposal that from that day forth, every discharged convalescent would receive two reales and one-half of a large loaf of white bread. Furthermore, the Count of Villar promised to determine whether two hospitals—Cinco Llagas and Triana—were sufficient, and if not, then another pesthouse, perhaps in the extramural parish of San Bernardo on the opposite side of the city, should be established. Both of the current hospitals dedicated to caring for poor plague victims were also outside the city walls. The Cinco Llagas Hospital stood outside the Macarena Gate, and Triana lay across the river.[9] Indeed, in the next few days, as sickness increased, it became neces-

9. AMS, sec. 10, 1581 [1].

sary to set up two more pesthouses, one in San Bernardo and the other one in the houses and hospital of Colón, which during the current meeting was at the center of a burial controversy.

As the 10 April meeting continued, the count informed the cabildo that he had received a petition from a vecino of the parish of San Vicente regarding burials. The governor had already spoken to the cathedral dean about the matter, asking him to order "that all the people who die from the current sickness outside the Royal Gate in the Colón district" should be buried "in the house and hospital which is in the very houses of Colón" to prevent "the harm that the republic receives with corpses being carried through the streets to the church." The house, actually a two-storied palace with beautiful gardens and a commanding view of the river and the Monastery of Las Cuevas, was built in the late 1520s by Christopher Columbus's son, Hernando Colón, and housed, among other things, his famous library. At this time the large edifice was in disrepair, its gardens neglected, and its current owner, Tomás Pesaro, was renting the property to the city to use as a hospital.[10]

Veinticuatro Ortiz Melgarejo spoke again. He had been busy visiting some of the larger rooming houses (corrales) in Seville. The corral provided cheap, often overcrowded housing for Seville's inhabitants, who rented the small rooms that surrounded a central patio. The kitchen and an outhouse were shared by all residents. There were many rooming houses in Seville, which were a favorite investment for wealthier individuals as well as institutions, such as the church or city government, and they varied in size and living conditions. Ortiz Melgarejo reported that he had inspected the Corral de los Alcaydes and that because of "the sickness that exists there, I ordered it closed immediately." He also informed the cabildo that he had instructed that the Corral de los Tromperos in Triana be "swept and the windows opened, and it should be sprayed with water and perfumed." The diligent alderman had the principal doors leading to the street shut, with signs posted on them threatening that no one was to enter, "under pain of 100 lashes," without the express permission of the Count of Villar.[11]

10. Ibid.; Juan Ignacio Carmona García, *El extenso mundo de la pobreza: La otra cara de la Sevilla imperial* (Seville: Ayuntamiento de Sevilla, 1993), 175. See also Morales Padrón, *La ciudad del quinientos*, 314, 318.

11. AMS, sec. 10, 1581 [1]. For a brief history of the corral, see Francisco Morales Padrón, *Los corrales de vecinos de Sevilla* (Seville: Universidad de Sevilla, 1997).

Ortiz Melgarejo did not stop there. He had also ordered cleaning of the water and "filth that comes out of the house of the Bishop Esquilache, where it is spoiled and becomes dirty, and bad odors come into the streets of that neighborhood."[12] Alonso Fajardo de Villalobos, the bishop of Esquilache, had vexed both secular and church authorities with his unbecoming business activities. He scandalized the city by having flour ground and hardtack baked as well as bricks and lime produced and then sold on the premises of his house. Clearly, all this production also polluted his surroundings. He had been accused of selling wheat at high prices and of buying gold, silver, and precious stones and then reselling them in finished jewelry. Indeed, there were complaints that the bishop "does not live as such, but as a usurious merchant and a man without conscience, without attending church."[13]

It was not unusual for church members to engage in business activities, though most tried to be discreet about it, often using relatives as surrogates for their transactions. For example, Alonso Xaymes declared in April of 1592 that in spite of having bought in Havana a ship in his own name, "the truth is that the said ship belongs to Licentiate Luis Ramos [cleric], my brother-in-law, and I bought it for him and by his order and commission and with his money, proceeds of the merchandise that I took for him to the Indies." Many clergymen in Seville participated in the Indies trade and owned and managed property of their own or their relatives and friends. Some were quite successful in their pursuits and grew wealthy. What was so scandalous about the bishop of Esquilache was his flaunting of his numerous business enterprises at the expense of his religious duties.[14]

At the end of Monday's meeting, the chief warden of the public granary, Diego Mexía, reported that there were eleven thousand fanegas of wheat from Almendralejo in Extremadura and places as far away as the province of León, ready to be transported to Seville. Veinticuatro Mexía affirmed that the city needed the wheat "very quickly for the deposits," and he urged the count to

12. AMS, sec. 10, 1581 [1].

13. The bishop's activities did not go unpunished. In 1582 his actions were reviewed and condemned by Seville's new archbishop, Rodrigo de Castro, and eventually by the pope; BL, Add. Mss. 28358, fols. 133–34. See also Pike, *Aristocrats and Traders*, 71–72.

14. AHPS, Protocolos notariales, leg. 8440, fol. 847r–v. There are numerous examples in Seville's notarial records of churchmen managing property and engaging in trade. See also, Pike *Aristocrats and Traders*, 70–71.

permit the draft animal drivers to pass freely to Seville through Alanís, Cazalla de la Sierra, and Constantina, small towns to the northeast at the edge of the foothills of Sierra Morena that fell within the city's jurisdiction. He also requested that more wheat be purchased in the Maestrazgo of Calatrava (a territorial domain of the Order of Calatrava) and elsewhere in La Mancha and quickly shipped to Seville. Local crops were in danger because again locusts and drought had severely affected the winter wheat.

When the councilors next met, on Wednesday, 12 April, the first item of business was the new plague hospital across the river, in Triana. Deputy Governor Aguilera informed his colleagues that a complaint had been lodged about the location of the pesthouse, which "is the last house in Triana" on the street that led to the Carthusian Monastery of Las Cuevas. The monks were unhappy about the close proximity of the plague hospital and stressed that their monastery "is a most principal house where they offer much hospitality, and such a multitude of people frequents it." At the moment the monastery hosted an illustrious guest, the papal legate, "who also desires that the hospital is moved and put in another house in Triana, where there will not be the said inconvenience."

As often happened, Diego Ortiz Melgarejo was first to speak. He concurred that a pesthouse would be better situated in a more isolated spot and proposed that Jurado Yáñez de Perea, who had found the original site, should "look for another place." He advised that it "should be in a part where it will not be so unsuitable." Ortiz Melgarejo urged the jurado to proceed immediately, because now "there are few sick, and it could be done easily before there are more." The talkative veinticuatro added that once Yáñez de Perea found the appropriate building, he should arrange for the sick to be "moved there and all the provisions and supplies." There was little discussion, and the cabildo voted in support of the proposal.

Two days later a frustrated Yáñez de Perea appeared before the council and defended his original site for the pesthouse, flatly stating that "there is no other [house] in all of Triana where it can be done, except in this one." He argued that the building "is as comfortable as it is because of the lodgings as well as having water nearby and being far away from the inhabitants," and he insisted that it was located some distance from the monastery. Yáñez de Perea affirmed that the hospital "has at present fifty-four sick in it, and the house is set up." He informed the cabildo that he had searched for another place with the help of the priests from the parish church of Santa Ana, and they have "not only been unable to find a comfortable house, but even any that is not." The councilors re-assured the exasperated jurado that he had done his job well; nevertheless, they instructed him to continue searching.[15]

Two months later, in June, the city had to defend its decision to appropriate private property for the pesthouse. The council received a royal provision de-manding to know the reason why the city had "taken a house in Triana of Don Juan Pardo Tavera," who had complained to His Majesty. Diego Ortiz Melgarejo recommended that the Count of Villar explain to the royal council that the house was appropriated for "the sick of this disease because it is an old build-ing with a bit of kitchen garden and because it is suitable and convenient for it." At the same time the councilors agreed to consult the city's legal adviser re-garding the requisitioning of private property during the epidemic. The dispute continued, and several months later, on 18 September, the cabildo learned that Don Juan Pardo Tavera had filed a lawsuit against the city, demanding payment of two thousand ducats "for a house taken for the plague."[16]

During the 14 April meeting the councilors also discussed another hospital. Don García Cerezo noted "the confusion that he saw in the Cinco Llagas Hos-pital in curing these sick" as well as its excessive expenses. He informed his col-leagues that "physicians and men of science and conscience" had recommended a solution for the problem. They indicated that in every parish in the city "there are many and well built hospitals, so that there is no parish which does not have one or two or more." The physicians believed that "without having to carry a sick person throughout the entire city," cures would be more effective in these local hospitals. The alderman suggested that a clergyman should be placed in charge of each of these pesthouses, which should include a physician and a barber. The cabildo returned to this proposition ten days later, when Don Pedro Tello de Guzmán affirmed that the city had established four hospitals, "which are capable of receiving all the sick poor." He added that the system was working as it had in the past. Veinticuatro García Cerezo stated that the matter should be turned over to the plague commission and urged the cabildo to sum-mon the doctors Monardes, Francisco Sánchez, and Daza y Valdés to report on the issue.

The number of plague-related deaths was substantial enough for the cloth dealer Rodrigo de Écija to petition the municipal council on Friday, 14 April,

15. AMS, sec. 10, 1581 [1].
16. AMS, sec. 10, 1581 [3].

in his name and that of the other members of the profession, to drop the tax (*encabezamiento*) levied on textiles "because many cloth dealers have died and trade has ceased." The council members denied the request, possibly fearing the repercussions for the city's coffers if other merchants insisted on similar waivers.

As the epidemic continued, the number of sick and dying edged upward. With insufficient late-winter and early-spring rainfall for crops, city officials became desperate. It was time to turn to higher powers for help. When the cabildo met on 12 April, Deputy Governor Aguilera had suggested that the municipality turn to the Convent of San Agustín, outside the city walls near the Carmona Gate, and ask the friars to bring out their famous image of the crucified Christ for a procession. The powers to end drought and plague embodied in the Christ of San Agustín were renowned throughout the early modern period. Diego Ortiz Melgarejo, always ready to add his opinion, believed that the image should be carried either to the cathedral or past the Church of San Bernardo and continue all the way to the Cruz del Campo Monument, at the eastern edge of the city.[17]

During the 14 April meeting, the cabildo's emissary, Juan de León, returned from his discussions with church authorities regarding the procession. They had agreed that during past episodes of similar crisis God had aided the city, giving health and water, "which is especially needed." Church officials recommended that following a confession "all the gentlemen of this cabildo" should receive communion at the cathedral's main altar, "to give this good example." Indeed, they expected that "all the residents of this city should do the same, and with the necessary contrition to supplicate Our Lord to assist with remedying such great affliction as there is in this place." The cabildo decided to take communion the following Wednesday and to pay for the necessary candles out of the "plague account." To ensure that no one failed to attend, the council agreed

17. According to Ortiz de Zúñiga, *Anales eclesiásticos*, 2:53–54, the image of the crucified Christ was found in 1314 in a "cellar or cave near the very convent," with its left arm loose from the cross and "hanging over the wound on the side and then many witnessed it to miraculously extend," and that is how it remained. Ortiz de Zúñiga dismissed Alonso de Morgado's claim that it was brought to Seville from the Indies. The image was destroyed during the Spanish civil war, but a modern copy can be found in the Church of San Roque. See also D. J. M. Montero de Espinosa, *Antigüedades del convento casa grande de San Agustín de Sevilla, y noticias del Santo Crucifixo que en él se venera* [1817] (Seville: Imprenta Municipal, 1995).

to levy a ten-ducat fine for any cabildo member who was absent. But the Count of Villar again became indisposed, and the procession with the miraculous image had to be postponed until Friday.[18]

Earlier in the week, on Wednesday 12 April, the Count of Villar composed an extensive letter to the president of the Council of Castile, outlining the situation in Seville and the measures being taken. As well as explaining why he had prohibited cabildo members from leaving town, he blamed the spread of the disease on initial inattention. "I somewhat believe that this fire flared up in the city so that it became inevitable, because there was such disorder in [disposing of the] clothing of those who were dying and of those who were hiding the disease." He pointed out "the fear of the living" of the plague and noted that "strange things had happened." The count described how "some left their dead wives and locked their houses and went away," and it was only discovered three days later. Furthermore, there were not enough gravediggers to bury the corpses or burn the infected clothing. "All this is remedied," he assured the council, "with the authority of the people from the cabildo," but he acknowledged that although there were many councilors, there was much ground to cover. He thanked the president of the royal council for all the advice on how to proceed during this crisis, indicating that "some of it had been put into effect" but other measures, after discussion with physicians, were decided to be "not very necessary, such as killing cats and dogs."

The Count of Villar was not a young man anymore and often missed cabildo meetings owing to recurring indisposition. He made no secret of this, and in the letter to the council president he lamented his poor health and frailty. He pledged nevertheless to continue to serve faithfully, "postponing my health and all the rest regardless of what matters to the Countess and [our] many small children." The governor admitted his apprehension, stating that "in spite of the great danger in which I find myself because of the confluence of people in my house and having to go to where they are," he felt certain that should he per-

18. AMS, sec. 10, 1581 [1]. Even in the twenty-first century, fear of losing a harvest because of drought causes people to turn to images. The Spanish newspaper *El País* reported on 22 April 2001 that in a small village in Almería province about three hundred people went out in a procession with their patron saint, Saint Gregory, "to ask him to make it rain." Even the socialist mayor of the village stated that he expected "a miracle" from Saint Gregory, who had accomplished the feat thirty-nine years earlier.

ish in the line of duty "His Majesty will favor those left behind by me," and his family would not suffer.[19] The count's fears of contracting the plague were not without foundation, and according to his later service report he was struck twice and lost two of his children to the disease. Whether or not he and his children contracted the plague is difficult to ascertain, but their sickness was serious, and the count believed it had been the plague.[20]

The Count of Villar was absent during the cabildo gathering on Monday, 17 April, when the subject of the growing food crisis was discussed. Deputy Governor Aguilera informed the councilors that there was not enough bread for all who needed it. Diego Ortiz Melgarejo then reported that the previous morning some four hundred fanegas of bread had been distributed, three hundred to the parishes and one hundred to select plazas: sixty fanegas to the Plaza del Salvador, thirty to the Plaza de la Feria, and ten to the Plaza de Santa Catalina.[21] García de León disagreed with his colleague regarding the allocation to the plazas and suggested it should be modified, with fifty fanegas of bread going to Salvador, twenty-five to Feria, ten to Santa Catalina plazas, and fifteen to Triana. García de León believed that this division was more in keeping with the general distribution of the population.

The costs related to the plague and grain shortage were mounting, and the council needed to find sources of revenue to cover the extraordinary expenditures. As the meeting continued, Diego Ortiz Melgarejo, who was also the city's procurador mayor, shared some welcome news. He had received a letter from the president of the royal council authorizing the cabildo to borrow money "in order to spend it for things of the plague." At the same time, he also reported that, according to city steward Diego del Postigo, "until today more than 10,000 ducats have been expended, and much more is being spent." He noted that the Count of Villar was already trying to identify people who could be tapped to loan the city twenty thousand ducats. The veinticuatro then proposed, and the cabildo agreed, to request from the king a loan of fifty thousand ducats to

19. BL, Add. Mss. 28342, fols. 257r–59v.

20. BL, Add. Mss. 28344, fols. 213r–19r.

21. AMS, sec. 10, 1581 [1]. The Plaza de la Feria and Plaza de Santa Catalina are today's Plaza Calderón de la Barca and Plaza Terceros, respectively. See Rafael Vioque Cubero, Isabel M. Vera Rodríguez, and Nerea López López, *Apuntes sobre el origen y evolución morfológica de las plazas del casco histórico de Sevilla* (Seville: Ayuntamiento de Sevilla, 1987), 38, 162.

cover the costs. Before the month ended, the city did secure a short-term loan of twenty thousand ducats from private parties, to be paid off by the end of the year.

A few days earlier, on 15 April, the cabildo had written King Philip complaining about the general food shortage not just in the city but in the entire province. The councilors warned that people were "dying of hunger because provisions were not coming to them," and they argued that "this danger is much greater than the disease." The current disease outbreak, they pointed out, was not nearly as serious as the one in 1568, and yet at that time food had been supplied and the quarantine sidestepped. The city council affirmed that "the cost of the cure and preservation from this disease is very high" and stressed that the propios could not sustain the financial drain. The councilors brought up the epidemic of 1568 once more, stating that at that time they were given unlimited access to the *sisa* (excise taxes) to defray the extraordinary expenses, whereas now they had not been able to secure more than twelve thousand ducats. They asked the king to issue an order that would allow the municipal government limitless revenue from the excise tax.

In closing, the officials deplored the poverty of the many communities that had quartered soldiers during the previous year's Portuguese conflict and now were facing "great shortage owing to sterility and low harvest." They complained that these places were again housing "six hundred men who say that they are going on the galleys," who were ruining the land that was "so afflicted and miserable and already is beginning to experience this very disease." The councilors asked the king to order these soldiers to go elsewhere, such as "Jerez and Écija" or any other place in Andalusia "where there are more abundant provisions and they are not suffering the calamity and misery" that communities in Seville's district were enduring.[22] The cabildo hoped that His Majesty would come to the rescue during the current crisis because the financial drain on both city coffers and local resources was substantial.

When the municipal council met on Friday, 21 April, Licentiate Aguilera again warned that the wheat deposits were running dangerously low. He urged the cabildo to temporarily stop distribution of bread to parishes and give out only 250 fanegas a day in the plazas. He noted the continued lack of rainfall and predicted a poor harvest. It was imperative that the city permit the public

22. BL, Add. Mss. 28342, fol. 270r–v.

granary to purchase wheat from places with ample grain. Martín Gutiérrez Cerón's declaration that there were no more than fourteen thousand fanegas of wheat left in the city's deposits reinforced the argument. The officials offered various solutions to the escalating grain crisis during the ensuing discussion, including the importation of wheat from Sicily or France, something that would require royal authorization and would constitute a major expenditure for the city.

The problem was compounded by the disruption of grain transports from other parts of the peninsula. Pedro Gordo, from El Espinar in the district of Segovia, petitioned the cabildo because he had been detained in Constantina, and "they took from him certain wheat that he was bringing to Seville." He complained that Francisco Duarte, factor of the House of Trade, "took his carts to go to serve His Majesty, which will be the cause of the wheat not coming to Seville." Diego Ortiz Melgarejo, always ready with an opinion, declared that because of the pressing need for wheat in Seville, the council should order the municipality of Constantina to free the shipment and demand that Duarte release the wagons. Days later, on 26 April, facing an acute crisis, the councilors decided to request authorization to import wheat from Sicily in spite of the costs.

Turning their attention from wheat to burials, the council members heard from church canons Hojeda and Cudile, who, on behalf of the Cathedral Chapter, reported that "the persons who die of this sickness in the parish of Santa Catalina" could not be buried in the church because "the dead do not fit anymore." They proposed that these unfortunates be interred "in holy ground that the Hospital of San Cosme and San Damián has incorporated in it." The church officials approached the municipal council because the hospital, also known as Bubas, or Pox Hospital, was under the city's patronage. The situation was critical; if it were not remedied quickly, "the bad odor from the dead bodies will cause much infection" and force the priests "to abandon the church."

Diego Ortiz Melgarejo immediately suggested that if indeed burial space was unavailable in the Church of Santa Catalina, then the cabildo should consult Dr. Gerónimo de Herrera, the hospital's administrator. Another councilman, Pedro Díaz de Herrera, insisted that the parish should be inspected. Furthermore, he felt that it might be enough to just add "fresh lime" to the church burials and to "deepen the graves." He pressed the councilors that "until the need is more urgent they should not inter in the said hospital of San Cosme and San Damián." But he conceded that if there were no other way, then they should contact Dr. Herrera and allow the burials in the hospital's holy ground.

The increased need for cemeteries during epidemics affected even cabildo members. The jurado Juan de Soria complained at the beginning of 1582 that the Count of Villar had confiscated the previous year a large field "that I have outside the Macarena Gate," which was used "to bury the sick with the plague," probably those from the Cinco Llagas Hospital. The field had been fenced, and Licentiate Soria asked to be compensated for the value of the land he had lost, which "could not be used any time soon because it would be very harmful to plant there."[23]

Before the month ended, the municipal government once again invoked divine assistance. Licentiate Vargas appeared and presented a report that "it would be expedient for the health of the city" to place crosses on all the church towers, including the cathedral, as had been done the previous year. The authorities should order "prayers and supplications," as they had the year before, "for health as well as for the fruits of the earth." They should send someone to the places infested with locusts to "make the usual general conjurations." Most in the cabildo supported Don Pedro Tello de Guzmán's proposal to dispatch the veinticuatro Hernando de Porras to ask church officials to authorize "Licentiate Vargas to climb the tower and to make the conjurations and to place the crosses." The month of April had passed, but the epidemic did not abate. The council was only too happy to support anyone willing to appease God's wrath and to pay the expenses.[24]

23. AMS, sec. 13, siglo XVI, vol. 6 (23 February 1582). See also Carmona García, *Crónica del mal-vivir*, 128.

24. AMS, sec. 10, 1581 [1].

11

MUCH MONEY BEING SPENT

The disease advances, and much money is being spent.
—DIEGO ORTIZ MELGAREJO

T HE GOVERNOR'S THREAT of a heavy fine for any council member who failed to attend meetings bore little result. The honorable councilors, following the age-old advice, fled fast and far. When the Count of Villar convened an extraordinary meeting of the cabildo on Tuesday, 2 May, attendance was dismal. Pedro Gutiérrez, who summoned the municipal council, testified that he had "called all the councilors who are in the city, who are few, given that they have left it because of the current sickness of the plague." The count stated that the city ordinances required that at least twelve councilmen attend an extraordinary cabildo meeting, along with the governor and his deputies. But because the situation was now critical, especially the question of food supplies, he was conducting the meeting with those present.

The officials who came to this meeting learned that the royal council had authorized the licentiate Diego de Valdivia, the magistrate of the Royal Audiencia of Seville, to transport wheat to the city. As they discussed the issue they decided that the wheat should be collected in and around the Extremaduran town of Almendralejo and shipped southward to Seville. In addition, the councilors ordered Jurado Rodrigo Sánchez, then in La Mancha, to send some of the money that he controlled to help initiate payment of the transport. They also concurred that since the king had authorized the purchase of forty thousand fanegas of wheat locally, the city should for the time being suspend attempts to import foreign cereals. The Count of Villar estimated that the city would spend at least twenty thousand ducats in La Mancha, Jaén, and the Maestrazgo de Calatrava for the purchase and transport of wheat. The special meeting ended with all present agreeing to send a letter to His Majesty, thanking him for the much needed help and noting the good news that the Portuguese had sworn an oath of allegiance to King Philip as their sovereign.[1]

With the successful close of the war with Portugal, Philip II would rule over the entire Iberian peninsula and a substantially increased overseas empire. In the settlement the Spanish king was obliged to make certain promises, especially with regard to keeping decisions about Portuguese affairs on Portuguese soil and naming only Portuguese subjects to high secular and ecclesiastical offices within Portuguese territory. Portuguese colonial trade and government was to remain in Portuguese hands. Even with these concessions, Philip II was one of the most powerful monarchs of his time.[2]

On Wednesday, 10 May, the Count of Villar shared some encouraging news with the councilors who were in attendance. According to the city's physicians and the jurados who were in charge of the four plague hospitals, "it seems, blessed be Our Lord, that there is some improvement in the current disease, at least in being cured better, and more people who become sick are recovering." But the news was not all good. The governor informed the assembled officials that there was plague in many towns under Seville's jurisdiction and that "the people who have left this city to go there, become sick with the same disease." What was worse, they returned infected, bringing their clothing, "which cannot but be detrimental and harmful for the city." Furthermore, the cabildo also received a petition from worried residents of the parish of Santiago, who demanded that "the Corral del Conde be closed because there is the sickness of the plague in it." This rooming house was one of the most densely populated in Seville, with about one hundred rooms surrounding a large patio.

Fearing spread of the disease, the council sent Don Diego de Portugal and Antonio de Tapia to investigate and to lock up the corral should they find any signs of the plague.[3] Before the meeting ended the councilors replaced the cabildo's crier, who had succumbed to the plague. They also ratified payment of salary for the jail nurse, a *beata* (holy woman), Violante de Jesús. Beatas made

1. AMS, sec. 10, 1581 [1].

2. See Lynch, *Spain under the Habsburgs,*1:309–11.

3. AMS, sec. 10, 1581 [1]; Morales Padrón, *Los corrales,* 7–15. The Corral del Conde still exists on Santiago Street.

private religious vows, including chastity, and wore distinctive dress, but unlike nuns they did not live in a convent. Although some lived in a house with other beatas, there were others who lived alone.[4]

Francisco Duarte, the House of Trade factor, arrived at the city hall on 12 May, promising to deliver forty thousand fanegas of wheat that originally came from Santander in northern Spain to supply the royal army. Some twenty thousand fanegas of this wheat were currently stored in Cádiz, and a similar quantity was on ships in Seville's Guadalquivir River. Now that the war with Portugal had ended the king did not need the wheat to feed his army, and Francisco Duarte was offering to sell it to the city "for the price that His Majesty pays." The maximum price would be nineteen reales a fanega for both the bakers and the hospitals of the city. Duarte wanted the council to guarantee payment through the city's properties. These proceedings were recorded by a substitute notary because the usual scribe, Francisco Ramírez, lay sick in bed.

Within a week some jurados complained that Duarte's wheat was "expensive and bad," but the Count of Villar insisted that the cabildo had accepted the wheat that His Majesty had favored the city with and it was necessary to use it to help alleviate the shortage. He argued that after the city had repeatedly begged the king for help it would be wrong to refuse it now. The governor pointed out that the bread was destined for "the poor of this city and its land" and stated that the wheat had been tested by two bakers. The bread "came out very good and without bad odor or flavor." The council, swayed by the count, voted unanimously to accept Duarte's wheat.[5]

The count next complained that Diego Mexía and Diego Ferrer were slacking in their duties. They had been assigned to oversee the quality of the wheat and bread in the city and conduct regular testing, but they had failed to do so. The city council agreed to reprimand Veinticuatro Mexía and Jurado Fer-

4. Regarding *beatas* in Seville, see Perry, *Gender and Disorder,* 97–117. See also Christian, *Local Religion,* 16–17; and Bilinkoff, *Avila,* 39–41.

5. AMS, sec. 10, 1581 [1]. In the end, the city bought twenty thousand fanegas of wheat from Francisco Duarte at a much higher price: 24.5 reales a fanega. The king ordered Duarte to wait for payment of up to 30,000 ducats until October, to help the financially strapped city. On 21 June 1581 Francisco Duarte asked the cabildo for immediate payment of all the debt above the 30,000 ducats that the king had postponed until October. Duarte, as the factor of the House of Trade, needed money to outfit the expedition preparing to leave for the Straits of Magellan to protect it from English pirates. Following discussion the city agreed to pay, as a service to His Majesty.

rer. Diego Ferrer defended himself, pointing out that he was just filling in for Jurado Laredo, who had left the city, and he promised to do his job well. Indeed, Laredo had fled the city without the count's authorization, and the cabildo asked Diego Mexía to send someone to find him and bring him back, though in the meantime they accepted Diego Ferrer as a temporary replacement.

Although the bread scarcity might have eased briefly, the costs stemming from the epidemic and accompanying famine rose relentlessly. On 17 May Veinticuatro Ortiz Melgarejo told the cabildo that the plague commission had discussed the use of the excise taxes, the sisa, to help cover plague-related expenses. Ortiz Melgarejo stated flatly that "the disease advances, and much money is being spent." The twenty-four thousand ducats in the sisa account were almost depleted, and to make matters worse, the tax had not been fully collected. The shrewd alderman asked the council's authorization to add to the sisa another thirty thousand ducats by levying the excise on "all the provisions that enter and leave the city," including some of the Indies exports and imports. He also wanted permission to include fifty thousand ducats from revenues collected on municipal properties. The daily costs for medicines, the hospitals, physicians, and other staff were enormous, and the veinticuatro warned that "the city does not have the possibility to get loans any more or to take it from other things." The council members decided that, given the acute need, they would grant the requests but at the same time ask the king to match these payments.[6]

While the city debated how best to meet the costs of the plague, its creditors continued to insist on payments for their services. On 26 May Licentiate Bustos, the surgeon who had been hired almost one year earlier to work in the Royal Jail, asked to be paid his salary. That same day, several widows demanded payment of salary owed to their deceased husbands, who had worked for the city in various capacities. Pedro Farfán, an apothecary in Triana, had supplied medicines to the Triana pesthouse, which by 29 May 1581 totaled 376 ducats, and the city so far had paid him only 40 ducats. At the same time Farfán owed 130 ducats for medicines that he had received from physician Francisco Díaz, who lived near the cathedral. Rather than paying his debt directly, the pharmacist and his wife María de Morales issued a power of attorney to Licentiate Díaz to collect the 130 ducats from "the deputies of the sickness of the plague

6. AMS, sec. 10, 1581 [1].

and the most illustrious cabildo and government of this city of Seville and its steward."[7]

The medicines that Pedro Farfán and other boticarios supplied to Seville's pesthouses to cure the plague included purgatives, sweat-inducing potions, traditional poison antidotes such as theriac and mithridatium, as well as various topical concoctions, including mercury, to be rubbed directly on the buboes or swellings. According to the prevailing belief, the plague was caused by "poison," and those treating plague victims focused on eliminating the bad humors from the body. There were also preparations to ease fever, headaches, and other discomforts. Patients would be given specially prepared "water," usually extracted from plants, which might or might not have been distilled. Aside from administering medicine to plague patients, the treatment also included bloodletting and cauterization of the buboes.

Nicolás Monardes, who counted among his patients some of Seville's most prominent citizens, was a firm believer in the bezoar stone, a rare concretion found in the stomach of certain mountain goats, as a cure not just for the plague but also for other diseases caused by "poison." He wrote in his treatise on the bezoar stone that for pestilential fevers it "is a marvelous thing, the good work it does, because it removes the harmfulness that [the fevers] have, and extinguishes and kills the bad quality of the poison, which is the principal and first thing a physician must do."[8] It was usually pulverized and could be mixed with herbal water or added to compound medicines.

Because of its rarity the bezoar stone would not have been administered to the poor in a pesthouse. There were other more common remedies. Theriac was an ancient compound medication that included a wide number and variety of ingredients, ranging from snake venom to various medicinal plants as well as minerals and metals. Mithridatium was another popular compound medicine, though it contained fewer ingredients than theriac. The success rate of these cures was based more on luck and the patient's immune system and natural propensity for recovery than on any restorative properties of the remedies. But people did recover from the plague, as demonstrated by the need for convalescent hospitals alongside the pesthouses.[9]

7. Ibid.; AHPS, Protocolos notariales, leg. 2367, fols. 1357r–58r.

8. Monardes, *Historia medicinal*, 146v.

9. Betrán, *La peste en Barcelona*, 415–23, provides an excellent overview of plague remedies. See also Fernández-Carrión and Valverde, *Farmacia y sociedad*, 42–43; and Laurence Brockliss and

Although the disease might have been loosening its grip on the city, the shortage of grain, and consequently bread, continued. The cabildo agreed during its session of 31 May that "the best wheat that there is in the depository should be given to the hospitals of those sick with the plague." At the same time, the councilors took the unpopular step of allowing the wheat supplied to bakeries and monasteries to be mixed with equal parts of local and overseas wheat.

Mixing of local wheat with grain that had been transported by ship always produced protests because the imported wheat was often wet and rotting. Dr. Rodrigo de León, the administrator of the Amor de Dios Hospital, at one point during the year launched a complaint that the weekly rations of wheat the hospital had been receiving were not of the usual quality: "I have been given half of it in wheat of the sea and the other half in local wheat." Dr. León grumbled that because the overseas wheat was "of bad quality the sick in the said hospital cannot eat it." Most of the patients suffered from "fevers," and they "lose their appetite."[10]

Complaints about the poor quality of overseas wheat were also heard within the municipality when the jurados composed a petition to the governor sometime in 1581. The jurados argued that according to the physicians the best way to remain healthy and to prevent "the plague and other contagious diseases is to eat good sustenance that is not spoiled, rotten, or smelly." Because "the principal sustenance is bread," they maintained, if people eat it "spoiled and smelly," clearly disease will ensue. The jurados affirmed that "the bread from the depository that is presently given and distributed in this city for the sustenance and aid of the poor is made from overseas wheat so bad" that it could cause "the said contagious diseases." Aside from the overseas wheat being spoiled, the bakers continued to put damp wheat out to dry in the sun and then mixed the good

---

Colin Jones, *The Medical World of Early Modern France* (Oxford: Oxford University Press, 1997), 159–64. Slack, *Impact of Plague*, 30–32, 173–77, examines morbidity and mortality rates between 1570 and 1670 in various English towns and villages and concludes that mortality rates varied widely from epidemic to epidemic (not just in England but elsewhere in Europe and Asia), anywhere from 40 to 80 percent. He also notes (176) that in Salisbury in 1604, "twice as many people may have been infected by bubonic plague as died of it."

10. AMS, Escribanía de Cabildo, sec. 3, vol. 10, doc. 15.

local wheat with the spoiled grain, in spite of fines levied to prevent the practice and efforts by officials to stop it. Moreover, they did not even bake the bread thoroughly enough to destroy some of the "bad odor and flavor that it has." The jurados contended that all this was done for profit, because the product weighed more if underbaked. They proposed to the governor that the spoiled wheat should be sold to the hardtack bakers, who could sell it to the shipmasters, because the "high fire and the process that they put it through will consume the bad odor and flavor."[11]

The plague affected not only the sick and those directly involved in caring for them; other Sevillians felt its repercussions as well. The food shortage and general trade disruption caused hardships throughout the community. Quarantine was a double-edged sword. Now that Seville was clearly infected, nearby towns such as Écija, Utrera, and Carmona blocked entry to anyone coming from Seville, including those charged with collecting a shipment of wheat for the beleaguered city. The failure of workers and officials to carry out their normal duties, whether because of sickness or flight or death, also left its mark. Even house rental contracts carried an added clause. When the widow Marina de Hoces rented a house on Santo Domingo Street in Triana on 24 May 1581, she agreed to pay "full rent" to her landlord, Juan Estevan, "even if there is plague in the said houses, God forbid, and any person dies there of the said disease and even if it is closed up by the magistrates."[12]

The prolonged hunger and sickness had a negative impact on manufacturing productivity, though the guilds often found little sympathy from city officials. For example, when on 29 May in two separate petitions the stocking makers and the shoemakers asked the cabildo to "lower the price of the alcabalas because of the plague," they were rebuffed with a curt, "there is no place." Nor did a petition asking the city to lower the fee on market stalls and tables in the Feria district "because of the plague" fare any better.[13] The city's financial difficulties made the councilors wary of easing taxes; on the con-

11. Ibid. Regarding the toxins in poorly stored grain, see Mary Kilbourne Matossian, *Poisons of the Past: Molds, Epidemics, and History* (New Haven, Conn.: Yale University Press, 1989). The author argues that mycotoxins in cereals caused severe food poisoning in premodern populations dependent on bread as their main staple and influenced both fertility and mortality rates.

12. AHPS, Protocolos notariales, leg. 2367, fols. 1357r–58r.

13. AMS, sec. 10, 1581 [2].

trary, they were looking for ways to collect more money through excise taxes on certain basic items. After assiduously researching the city records, they found that such tax hikes had been permitted almost a century earlier, during the reconquest of Granada.

12

ALMOST A MIRACLE

It would be almost a miracle to collect any wheat.
—RODRIGO SÁNCHEZ

HE MONTH OF JUNE BROUGHT some relief in the severity of the epidemic, but the food shortage and economic difficulties showed no sign of improving. The cabildo continued to receive petitions begging for the easing of taxes. On 2 June a tax farmer, Gonzalo Sánchez de Morales, asked the city to have his share of the meat tax payment lowered, "given that the outside stalls have been closed because of the plague" and he therefore collected fewer taxes. The councilors discussed the issue, and although they were sympathetic they did not take any action but instead agreed to take up the matter at a later time.

During the same meeting the councilors authorized payment for street cleaning, which was to come from "the account of the plague expenses." Although earlier the cabildo had tried to shift the costs for the removal of garbage to the residents of the respective parishes, in the end they relented. They all agreed that keeping the streets clean "was one of the most needed things for the health of the city, according to what the doctors say." Unfortunately, some of the people who had been charged with trash removal were remiss in their assignment. On 7 June the council heard complaints against Juan Alonso Negrón, who had not cleaned "a certain place."

The person who denounced him wanted Negrón to be fined six hundred maravedís, but Diego Ortiz Melgarejo proposed that the fine should be only 150 Melchor del Alcázar argued that the fine should be revoked and the man forgiven. During subsequent discussion, Deputy Governor Aguilera pointed out that the Plaza of San Francisco and other places Negrón had been charged with cleaning "are very dirty," making them "especially harmful to health at the present time of the plague." The deputy governor insisted that Negrón should be fined and ordered to remove the waste as he was required. Nevertheless, when the councilors voted on the matter they sided with Melchor del Alcázar and absolved the offender of all charges and fines. By not punishing Juan Alonso Negrón, the cabildo contradicted all its resolutions about the importance of keeping the city clean in order to stop the spread of the plague. It would seem that the right connections at city hall protected negligence even at a critical time.[1]

Two days earlier the Count of Villar had addressed the councilors, stressing once again the acute need for food supplies, especially bread, for "the healthy as well as for the sick and those who had been sent to the hospital to be cured at [the city's] expense because they were poor." The governor noted that "all the places of Andalusia have been closed" to commerce with Seville and would not permit entrance of any person coming from the city. Furthermore, these communities prevented people from leaving to bring provisions to Seville. The count lamented that "they guard against the plague of this city with such prudence and rigor," as a result of which Seville suffered "many more deaths from hunger than from the said disease of the plague." He reported that he had already written to the king asking him to order all of Andalusia to resume shipments of food to Seville, and he had also sent the chief justice Don Gerónimo de Montalvo to Court to petition His Majesty.

The governor was irritated. In spite of all this effort, the only result so far had been confusion regarding which of two Royal Audiencia officials had been authorized to go with the staff of justice to the countryside and collect whatever provisions were to be found. In early June the cabildo heard from Licentiate Diego de Valdivia, one of the judges of the Royal Audiencia, who claimed that he had been given a sixty-day commission to ship grain to Seville. He complained that the king had later authorized another judge, Licentiate Benito Rodríguez Valtodano, to ship the wheat and to prevent Valdivia from fulfilling his orders. Licentiate Valdivia insisted that he would continue his original commission because he had already started shipping. The Count of Villar was frustrated and blamed the city's emissaries at Court for improperly carrying out the

1. This Juan Alonso Negrón was probably a member of the prominent Sevillian Genoese Negrón family. Descended from a Genoese merchant who had settled in Seville at the beginning of the sixteenth century, the Negróns' wealth, partly acquired in slave trade, and influence would explain the leniency shown the negligent entrepreneur. See Pike, *Enterprise and Adventure*, 4–5, 64.

king's order. The governor replaced them and refused to pay any salary for "this business."

One of the men who had infuriated the count was Don Gonzalo de Saavedra, the city's official agent at Court. He had written to the cabildo on 27 May from San Clemente in La Mancha, but his letter did not reach Seville until Wednesday 7 June, two days after the governor's outburst. Don Gonzalo informed the cabildo that he had shipped five hundred fanegas of wheat to Seville that very day, though he warned that "the land is turbulent and its people are not well intentioned." He noted that there were tertian fevers and that because of the bad harvest the price of wheat stood at eighteen reales a fanega, and with the costs of transportation it would come to twenty-nine reales. He claimed he had purchased altogether twelve thousand fanegas of wheat. At the same time the city council received a letter from the jurado Rodrigo Sánchez, who also had been sent to purchase grain. He too was in San Clemente and stressed the high prices and difficulties in buying wheat because the year was so sterile. "The land is so lacking in grain," he wrote on 30 May, "and given the way the year is going, it would be almost a miracle to collect any wheat."

Upon hearing the contents of Veinticuatro Gonzalo de Saavedra's missive, Diego Ortiz Melgarejo urged the councilors to abide by the decision they had reached two days earlier and recall Don Gonzalo and the others. The Count of Villar agreed, though he again bemoaned the confusion caused by the existence of conflicting royal orders regarding wheat procurement for the city. In the end, the officials asked Diego Mexía, the chief warden of the public granary, to write to Judge Rodríguez Valtodano and instruct him to continue on to Murcia and other places along the Mediterranean coast, where he would buy both wheat and barley and send them to Seville after he completed the shipment from La Mancha.[2] The councilors hoped that by sending the judge elsewhere they could defuse the conflict created by the contradictory royal orders and at the same time increase the city's chances for getting an adequate supply of cereals for the public granary.

Seville's convents and monasteries also felt the effects of the plague, which spread rapidly in closed communities. The nuns of the Convent of La Encarnación asked for and received permission to move to "a house that they have

2. AMS, sec. 10, 1581 [3].

on the Alameda, given that the convent is at present sick with the plague."[3] The religious houses traditionally provided food for the poor, and during a crisis such as the current grain shortage combined with a plague epidemic, the monasteries played an important role in poor relief. The contemporary historian Alonso de Morgado reported that the monks of the Carthusian Monastery of Las Cuevas were regularly distributing wheat to "110 designated poor and honorable widows, giving one-half fanega a month to each one." He further described how four hundred to five hundred poor came daily to the monastery's door, and "some days they count more than 1,000," to get "bread and some soup, water and other alms." A petition by an early-seventeenth-century prior of Las Cuevas supports Morgado's narrative. Friar Juan de Polanco stated that "this year more than 1,700 people have received alms at the door, not counting those who eat inside in the refectory and those [alms] given in bread to particular people."[4]

Administering the sacraments to the poor sick during an epidemic was not uncommon among certain monastic orders. In early May the cabildo had been "very grateful" for the offer by the provincial of the Monastery of Los Remedios in Alcalá de Henares, near Madrid, to send additional Discalced Carmelites to Seville "to confess in the hospitals the sick with the plague." The provincial, Gerónimo Gracián, had sent four friars earlier, and the city "was very content" with their services.[5] When a fire destroyed the Carmelite Monastery of Los Remedios in Triana, the monks' plea to the city for alms to help rebuild was looked upon favorably. During the 16 June 1581 meeting of the cabildo, the outspoken alderman, Diego Ortiz Melgarejo, proposed that the monks be disbursed one hundred ducats from the plague account, "given that these friars are very poor and confess many sick and go to the hospitals to visit them."

3. Ibid. (5 June 1581). This house is not to be confused with the Augustinian Convent of La Encarnación, which stood on the plaza of the same name and was founded in 1591 by Don Juan de la Barrera. The petitioners in this case came from the Carmelite Convent of La Encarnación de Belén, founded in 1513 near the Macarena Gate and permanently moved in 1585 to the Plaza de Belén in the Alameda de Hércules. The community was forced to move again in 1837, this time to the Convent of Santa Ana, where some of the art work from the old convent can still be contemplated. See María Luisa Fraga Iribarne, *Conventos femeninos desaparecidos: Sevilla—siglo XIX* (Seville: Ediciones Guadalquivir, 1993), 31, 79–86.

4. Morgado, *Historia de Sevilla*, 422–23; AMS, sec. 13, siglo XVII, vol. 5, doc. 28 (30 October 1617).

5. AMS, sec. 10, 1581 [1] (5 May).

He furthermore nominated Jurado Martín Santofímia Riquelme to go to "the houses of all the aldermen and jurados and other people of the city and beg for alms for this purpose."

Don García Cerezo agreed with Ortiz Melgarejo but suggested that the city should award five hundred ducats from the propios to help rebuild the monastery, in gratitude to the impoverished friars for ministering to victims of the plague. Don Pedro de Cespedes agreed in principle but wanted to give them only three hundred ducats. Luis de Herrera declared that the cabildo should first inspect the fire damage and determine "what obligation the city has . . . because they had offered themselves in the service of the plague poor." He proposed that Don Juan Pérez de Guzmán, accompanied by another councilor, visit Los Remedios and survey the destruction. Don Juan, who was present, agreed it was an excellent idea, but he would rather see Luis de Herrera carry out the inspection instead of himself. Otherwise, he too supported Ortiz Melgarejo's original proposal.

As was customary, the Count of Villar closed the discussion. He voiced his support of Diego Ortiz Melgarejo's motion and reminded the councilors "that some of the religious who are in the said house have come from Castile to confess the sick in the plague hospitals."[6] The governor stressed that "some of them had caught the plague there and had died," which was all the more reason for the city to send the inspectors to assess "the damage the fire had done and their need and poverty" and then inform the cabildo so that the officials could take adequate measures to assist the needy friars. The motion was approved unanimously. It is uncertain how many ducats the city contributed in the end to repair the Monastery of Los Remedios, but we do know that it was rebuilt, only to be destroyed again in 1595, this time by the raging flood waters of the Guadalquivir River.[7]

The councilors also discussed the question of administering the sacra-

6. Administering sacraments to plague victims was a brave act, and some parish priests fled rather than face infection. It was not unusual for monks to step in and help in times of crisis, earning gratitude from not just city officials but ordinary people as well. See, for example, James S. Amelang, trans. and ed., *A Journal of the Plague Year: The Diary of the Barcelona Tanner Miquel Parents, 1651* (Oxford: Oxford University Press, 1991), 48–49.

7. AMS, sec. 10, 1581 [2] (16 June); sec. 10, 1595 [1] (22 December). The monastery's location on the river bank in Triana made it vulnerable to repeated flood damage until its dissolution in the nineteenth century. Only the church building survived; it is now a museum.

ments to the sick in the extramural neighborhood of the Cestería. They decided that the Blessed Sacrament should be placed in the district's Hospital of Las Vírgenes, so that the whole area could be served from there. Cestería received its name from its major industry, basket weaving, and it lay directly across the river from Triana, with most dwellings built close to the wall. Five days later, on 21 June, the cabildo provided money from the plague account and sent the jurado Melchior de Baena to the Cestería to prepare in the hospital "at the back of the altar a comfortable and decent place where the Blessed Sacrament can be kept." The councilors also entrusted the jurado with finding "a house or lodgings where the chaplain who will administer the Holy Sacrament to the sick will live."[8]

Absenteeism during the epidemic was common, but if an important official of the public granary could not be found, his colleagues grumbled. One of the deputies of the alhóndiga complained to the cabildo on Friday, 23 June, that there were ten thousand ducats that needed to be deposited in the "coffer with three keys," but because the chief warden, Diego Mexía, was absent from the city, it could not be done.[9] Indeed, several guards had to be hired to protect the money until it could be deposited. He complained that the chief warden should reside in the alhóndiga and the municipal council should do something, since Mexía "is too busy with other things and out of the city."

Diego Ortiz Melgarejo, always ready with a solution, proposed that they should let Diego Mexía know what had occurred and remind him "that his assistance here every day and every hour would be opportune." The veinticuatro added that they should also inform him "that after all, the city is much improved and every day more so" and warn the renegade that if he did not return immediately he would be replaced as warden. Furthermore, Mexía should be advised that the city would charge him for the salary of the guards. García de

8. AMS, sec. 10, 1581 [2]; José María de Mena, *Las calles de Sevilla* (Seville: Editorial Castillejo, 1994), 179–80.

9. The coffer of three keys (*arca de tres llaves*) contained the money that the alhóndiga received either from the sale of grain or from taxes due to the granary from merchandise removed to be sold outside the city. Three people each held a key, and all needed to be present to open the coffer: the chief warden, who was a member of the city council; an inspector of the granary; and the prior of the Carthusian Monastery of Las Cuevas. See Carmona García, *Crónica del malvivir*, 229–30. As noted in the text, Las Cuevas was one of the major donors of bread to the poor of the city.

León agreed, pointing out that this was not the first time that Diego Mexía was absent from office, and called for his replacement.

The Count of Villar concurred, with the exception of telling Mexía who would pay for the guards. The governor preferred to warn him that he would be held responsible for the safety of the money. The count contended that the city was not obligated to tell the chief warden what his duties were, since he knew them well. Regarding the replacement of Mexía, the count wanted to discuss it during the next meeting of the cabildo.

The letter must have produced the desired effect, because when the council met next on Monday, 26 June, Diego Mexía was back in attendance at city hall. One of the items on the agenda that day was his job performance. The officials were concerned not only with Mexía's absenteeism but also with some irregularities in the accounts of the public granary. The cabildo decided to thoroughly investigate Diego Mexía's tenure.

Two days later, the Count of Villar addressed the question. He reminded the councilors that the city traditionally named the chief warden of the alhóndiga. The governor noted that Diego Mexía could not continue in the post because "he was [warden] longer than His Majesty mandates" and was therefore violating the royal provision; moreover, "the said Señor Diego Mexía had abandoned this post." Nevertheless, the count argued that Mexía should not be dismissed in July and August, because that was peak time for buying grain for the public granary and he had already begun the process. Therefore the governor proposed that the city postpone the naming of a new chief warden until the first cabildo meeting in September. A heated debate followed the count's words.

Martín Gutiérrez Cerón, one of the chief justices, supported the motion. Diego Ortiz Melgarejo disagreed and insisted that a meeting be called in two days, on Friday, to name a new chief warden. After all, Mexía was very busy, and the city should not violate the royal provision regarding the length of the warden's term. Juan de León supported Ortiz Melgarejo's position but believed that in the meantime Mexía should continue to buy grain. García de León agreed that a new warden needed to be named immediately, and he pointed out that Diego Mexía had asked many times in the past to be replaced because of "his age and indispositions and undertakings."

After all the councilors finished speaking, the Count of Villar tabled the issue until the next meeting. When the cabildo began its Friday meeting, a heated

Diego Ortiz Melgarejo demanded that the matter should not be decided by a secret vote. Furthermore, His Majesty had clearly ordered that the chief warden of the alhóndiga could only hold the office for one year, not for four, as Mexía had done. Unless a new warden was named, Ortiz Melgarejo threatened to formally protest, because the city must follow royal decrees. The persuasive alderman prevailed, and his motion passed. Next, the councilors moved to choose a new chief warden of the public granary. They nominated Chief Justice Martín Gutiérrez Cerón, but the Count of Villar recommended instead Juan de León and again stressed that he should assume his post on 1 September 1581. In the end, the councilors supported the governor's candidate and the veinticuatro Juan de León was formally named the new chief warden of the alhóndiga.[10]

10. AMS, sec. 10, 1581 [2].

13

ACCUSATIONS OF MISMANAGEMENT

The city had done everything that was humanly possible.
—MELCHOR DEL ALCÁZAR

T HE CABILDO AND THE COUNT OF VILLAR were dealt an unpleasant surprise at the beginning of July. The king advised the officials that he had received a complaint about their handling of the plague crisis. The accuser was anonymous, but the charges were serious. King Philip included a copy of the document, asking Seville's officials to respond to the denunciation and to send him a detailed report regarding the situation in the city. The complaint contained eleven specific points. The anonymous writer acknowledged the governor's poor health, though he hardly seemed to consider that an excuse as he unleashed a barrage of accusations against the cabildo. He charged the count's deputies with shirking their duties as well as absenteeism and general inattention to the well-being of the community. The accuser grumbled that because the chief constable and his deputies had been assigned to act outside the city, crime had risen within. Night watches were disorganized, he complained, and therefore there were more "house robberies and extraordinary deaths" as well as other improper activities. The man accused the councilors of leaving the infected city with their families and appearing at cabildo meetings only when it suited their personal interests or business, abandoning the defenseless population to filth and disease.

"There are so many who die of the plague," the writer complained, and their infected belongings were dumped by survivors "at night in the plazas and the streets in order to rid their houses of the clothing and the beds of the sick," believing that they would thereby escape the disease. These discarded items were often picked up by "poor beggars" who took them to their homes, spreading the deadly contagion to their families and neighbors. Furthermore, he denounced the authorities for mismanaging the crisis and for carelessly standing by while residents of some parishes collected the plague-infested clothing and bedding in huge piles and burned them in the plazas. The writer insisted that these bonfires polluted the neighborhoods and posed a serious fire hazard that could destroy houses and property. He also noted that greedy relatives of the plague dead put the infected possessions up for sale rather than properly disposing of them.

The accuser complained that city officials did nothing to prevent communication between the sick and their families, who then spread the disease to their friends and neighbors. He charged that the city failed to lock up plague victims' residences and that houses were carelessly reopened without purification and cleaning. The writer alleged that those convalescing from the plague were allowed to return to their homes without any special precautions. He blamed the city officials for the chaos that reigned in the plague hospitals and for the high death toll and was especially critical of the failure to provide adequate spiritual services to the dying. Finally, the accuser charged that gates were poorly guarded and that many people from infected places snuck into Seville, often already sick with the plague, hoping to find better treatment in the city than in their home villages.[1]

The councilors listened to the king's missive during their meeting on 7 July and grew increasingly indignant as they heard the details of the anonymous attack. They resolved to act without delay in their own defense. Before embarking on a lengthy discourse, Diego Ortiz Melgarejo advised that the documents be placed in the archive and that the councilors meet with the Count of Villar to respond, point by point, to the charges. He spoke for a long time. Ortiz Melgarejo argued that the report to King Philip should include every action the city had taken during the plague outbreak and stress "how well-ordered it was regarding hospitals as well as everything else." The veinticuatro was particularly incensed by the allegation of absenteeism. He demanded that the report contain the governor's mandate regarding the issue and emphasize that the cabildo was never unable to hold a meeting because of lack of officials. The alderman insisted the report be sent quickly so that His Majesty "knows the truth." At the same time, he urged his colleagues to also inform the king how much conditions had improved; already, of the four pesthouses that had been established,

1. AMS, sec. 3, vol. 7, docs. 9 and 10; Velázquez y Sánchez, *Anales epidémicos,* 99–101.

two were closed. Ortiz Melgarejo wanted the king to know how well Seville had protected itself, making sure that "no diseased or sick people entered it."

Continuing his speech, the loquacious veinticuatro urged the city council to convey to the king all the actions it had taken regarding cleaning "at its own cost and the number of times that it had done it." The cabildo should also indicate the measures it took to ensure that the sick received their sacraments. Ortiz Melgarejo wanted the report to include the efforts the municipal government made to secure funds to pay for all the plague expenses. He exhorted the councilors to tell the king that individual jurados and veinticuatros visited the sick who had refused to go to the hospitals in order to learn of their condition and that they had given them alms. Finally, the city should explain to His Majesty the details of the cabildo's cooperation with church authorities regarding processions to end the plague.

Ortiz Melgarejo's proposal was so thorough that most of the councilors simply voiced their support. Melchor del Alcázar, one of the more esteemed aldermen, advised the Count of Villar to prepare "on behalf of His Lordship and his ministers and the city a report of all that had been done from the beginning of this disease for its remedy and the care that had been taken in the execution of everything." He also recommended that Juan de León should write to the king urging him not to give credit to the complaint and stressing that the count and his ministers had done an excellent job. Melchor del Alcázar emphasized that His Majesty should know that the city had done "everything that was humanly possible" and that "by God's mercy because of these endeavors this city is on this day almost free of the plague."[2]

Philip II was in Lisbon, and the officials sent their extensive report to him through Don Gerónimo de Montalvo, one of Seville's chief justices. The city's defense satisfied the king, who from the beginning had seemed wary of the anonymous accusations. He wrote back to the governor and the cabildo on 31 July, expressing his pleasure at learning that they had acted properly with regard to combating the deadly disease, as he had every confidence they would. The king thanked the officials for their work and indicated that Don Gerónimo would convey the details of his contentment with Seville's government.[3] It is difficult to assess who the anonymous denouncer was. It could have been a

2. AMS, sec. 10, 1581 [2].

3. Velázquez y Sánchez, *Anales epidémicos*, 102.

clergyman or even a disgruntled councilor. Although there was much truth to his complaints, some seem exaggerated, and city officials had no difficulty in refuting them, aided by the fact that the disease was loosening its grip.

At the end of July the city's plague deputy, Rodrigo de Jerez, affirmed that "many doctors and barbers of Seville who are not salaried by the city, and who are those who truly speak the truth by being disinterested, say it is well known that there is no more plague and it has ended." Rodrigo de Jerez proposed that since the city was unable to meet all its plague debts, they should dismiss most of those who cared for the afflicted, "leaving only one hospital where those who are sick can be collected." It should be served by only one doctor, one barber, and those necessary to minister to the sick. The jurado further proposed that no new patients be admitted. He pointed out that this would "serve God and His Majesty and this republic and the city would not fall into even greater need than it has today."

14

SETTLING ACCOUNTS

I do not have the means to provide and pay the
large sum of maravedís that is owed.

—DIEGO DEL POSTIGO

HE PLAGUE MAY HAVE BEEN EASING, but the city's financial difficulties were growing. On 19 July the city's steward, Diego del
Postigo, duly reported that the amount "that he has disbursed
from the plague account until 15 July of this year [1581] totaled
17,416,000 maravedís [46,443 ducats]." Jurado Postigo pointed out that the
money raised through loans totaled 13,676,000 maravedís (36,469 ducats) but
warned that "3,740,000 maravedís [9,973 ducats] are still owed." The city's treasurer swore "to God and on this cross that this account is accurate and true";
he lamented that he was short of funds and did "not have the means to provide
and pay the large sum of maravedís that is owed to the pharmacists, physicians
and surgeons, and nurses."[1] He did not even have the money to cover "the ordinary expenses" of the plague hospitals. Diego del Postigo implored the cabildo
to provide the necessary resources to cover these costs because he "does not have
where to take it from anymore."

The frustrated city paymaster was backed by Jurado Yáñez de Perea, the
administrator of the Triana pesthouse, who confirmed the shortage of funds
there too. The administrator of the Colón Hospital, Cristóbal Suárez, echoed
the Triana official, complaining that he had no money and was pestered by
people demanding payment. Jurado Suárez appealed to the city council for help
"so that he would not be bothered."

1. These debts were often reflected in wills. For example, Pedro de Villalobos had been hired
by the cabildo to work as a nurse in the Cinco Llagas Hospital to care for the plague victims. He
instructed the executors of his will (dated 2 June 1581) to collect the money the city owed him for
forty days of work at nine reales a day. See AHPS, Protocolos notariales, leg. 17670, fols. 1276r–7v.

Uncharacteristically, Diego Ortiz Melgarejo provided no solution other than to recommend that the problem of finding adequate sources of revenue to pay the bills be turned over to the deputies of the excise tax. Melchor del Alcázar argued that the issue should be handled by the plague deputies, who could perhaps tap into the income from the alcabalas sales taxes or into the wheat account in the public granary, as His Majesty had authorized. These funds might be enough to cover the soaring plague expenses until October. Following a long discussion, the councilors adopted Melchor del Alcázar's proposal.[2]

During the same meeting, the question of sanitation was again broached. Baltasar de Aguilar complained that although some cleaning had been done, "many streets are impassable because of the many garbage piles." He pointed out that "Madrid and other cities and towns and places in these kingdoms are clean because they take care." Jurado Aguilar argued that Seville's streets should be as clean as they had been in the past. He insisted that the city put in place the same system that had been used in prior years or, if necessary, fund a better one.

This time, Diego Ortiz Melgarejo spoke at length, covering various aspects of the problem. He recommended the establishment of a committee, which would include the Count of Villar, to determine whether it would be worthwhile to "clean the city all at once," having each parish assigned to a different councilor who would supervise the work and "order it done promptly." The cleanup costs should be paid from the plague account. Ortiz Melgarejo urged that from this point on the city should regularly clean the streets and find the means to pay for it. Furthermore, the municipality's rental agreements should be reviewed to ensure that they included provisions for cleaning. The veinticuatro proposed that the city give "a license to twenty-five carters, . . . one or two in each parish," to haul away garbage. In closing, Ortiz Melgarejo returned to the question of expenses. He believed that the cleanup should be funded using the excise taxes because "indeed, it affects all the estates and is so expedient for the good of this republic and her health." In the meantime, street cleaning should be paid for from the plague account.

The councilors voted unanimously to accept Ortiz Melgarejo's proposal. Their action in this matter might have been influenced by the recent anonymous accusations sent to the king. Although they had dealt with sanitation on

2. AMS, sec. 10, 1581 [2].

a regular basis, this time their measures seemed more comprehensive and in the short term probably were more successful.

As the month of July was coming to a close, there were several important issues to consider, some plague related, others not. There was also some welcome financial news. On Friday, 28 July, a letter arrived from Veinticuatro Saavedra, Seville's agent in Madrid, informing the cabildo that the city had been authorized to borrow fifty thousand ducats to cover "the plague expenses" until it was able to collect the money from the excise taxes.

During the course of the meeting Rodrigo de Jerez brought up the misconduct of the city guards. He complained that "as is notorious and some of Your Lordships know it," the constables who had been assigned to guard the gates "take many bribes and cause much bother"; to make matters worse, "no one is stopped from entering even if he is bringing contagious disease." The jurado suggested that the city should turn to the citizens of each parish and order them, under penalty, to guard the gates, either without salary or, if necessary, with pay of one real a day. He argued that the residents, fearful of losing their businesses, would comply, and he promised that he would see to it that one vecino would be guarding each gate for one day, and thus "a lot of money would be saved." Although the poor performance of the city guards had been one of the points raised in the anonymous letter to the king, the council members decided to pass the whole issue to the plague commission to review and make a recommendation, rather than deal with it themselves.[3]

The councilors then turned to another matter, not directly related to the plague. Clean water was scarce in the city, and what could be found was expensive. Most of it came from two springs. The water from one, in Alcalá de Guadaíra, was brought into the city over the Carmona aqueduct, and the other, known as the Archbishop's Spring, was right outside the city, on the left bank of the Tagarete stream. Some houses had private wells. People also took their water from the river, but that was hardly clean. The spring water that was piped into the city from Alcalá de Guadaíra supplied the Royal Alcázar and the numerous palaces of the nobility and houses of the elite. Not surprisingly, enterprising citizens tried to siphon off some of that precious liquid. It had come to the cabildo's attention that certain prisoners, jailed for illegally opening aqueducts carrying water to the house of Hernán Ponce, had been released by order

3. Ibid.

of a judge of the Inquisition. Therefore, the councilors sent García de León and Juan Yáñez de Perea to the Triana castle to seek an explanation from the inquisitors and to insist that "the said prisoners are returned to jail."[4]

The two men returned the following Monday and reported to the cabildo. They did indeed complain to the inquisitors about the actions of Licentiate Alfaro, the judge presiding over cases of confiscated property, who had released the prisoners jailed by Deputy Governor Aguilera. The inquisitors replied that "they were amazed that the judge of confiscated property would have done anything which would upset the city, particularly to order release of prisoners who had been incarcerated by order of another judge." The inquisitors also pointed out that the judge could only act regarding cases within his jurisdiction and that "for other extraordinary things that might occur, he cannot do anything without first discussing it with [the inquisitors]." The inquisitors promised to summon and question the judge and, "if necessary, reprimand him," because they wished to "serve and please the city." The councilors were satisfied with leaving the investigation up to the inquisitors but agreed that if there appeared to be any delay they would send García de León to remind them. There was no follow-up in the documentation, but it is not improbable that the kind judge who released the water thieves might have been the one who hired them in the first place.

On the last day of July the cabildo heard from another man whom Deputy Governor Aguilera had imprisoned. Cristóbal Suárez, a plague commissioner, who just a few days earlier had advised the city council that he had no money to pay salaries at the hospital he administered, now complained that he had been unfairly accused of "adjusting the salaries of the servants in the Colón Hospital" and had been thrown in jail for it. The jurado defended himself, claiming that "he did this to benefit the city and with the authority to do this as such an administrator." He asked the city's procurador mayor to look into the problem, particularly now that people were demanding to be paid the difference, which he agreed to do in order to get out of prison. Jurado Suárez worried about his reputation at Court because reports of his imprisonment had been sent there. He lamented that he "had served the city in this business with so much risk to

4. Ibid. Regarding the city's water supply and quality, see Carmona García, *Crónica del malvivir*, 72–83.

his life and his whole estate, and it is unjust that the prize and reward for this is that he is disgraced at Court and elsewhere for something that was not his fault."

Thorough deliberations on the merits of his plea ensued, with many councilors favorable to his position. But Bartolomé López de Mesa felt that Cristóbal Suárez should meet with the veinticuatro Hernando de Porras and bring all "the collections and agreements that had been made with the people" and settle the accounts with them, "paying them exactly what they are owed." He recommended that the city should move to satisfy the claims "so that there is no dispute." The Count of Villar agreed, stating that the city should honor the agreements, ensuring that "no one loses their work or money that they should have received according to what will be evident from what they had concerted with Jurado Cristóbal Suárez." When the vote was taken, all concurred with López de Mesa's and the count's positions.[5]

In spite of repeated efforts by city officials, there were some who tried to circumvent the order that all clothing and bedding from anyone infected with the plague be burned. This was also one of the charges made by the anonymous writer to the king, although he had put the blame directly on mismanagement by the councilors. The reselling of clothes was a common enterprise, but at a time when the city was battling the spread of the plague, dealers of used clothes vexed the authorities. The Count of Villar would complain that "many people with little fear of God and their consciences have sold and sell many plague infected clothes."[6]

One of the reasons it was difficult to enforce the order was that these items had monetary value. Clothing and bedding represented a sizable portion of most Sevillians' property and were invariably listed in inventories that accompanied dowry agreements and wills. When the plague was not threatening, these possessions would be disposed of at public auctions following someone's death. They were also favorite posthumous gifts to relatives, friends, or servants, even during a plague epidemic. As the widow Ana Pérez lay dying in her house in Triana on 28 July 1581, she made certain bequests in her will. In addition to ten ducats cash, she left to María de Aguila some of the clothing "that I

5. AMS, sec. 10, 1581 [2].

6. AMS, sec. 13, siglo XVI, vol. 6 (10 May 1582).

might have at the time of my death, which I wish to be given to her as payment for her service during my sickness of the plague."[7] One can only wonder who got hold of these pieces first, María or the men charged with burning infected clothing.

By the end of July it seemed to many that the epidemic had run its course, and Dr. Gerónimo de Herrera, the administrator of the Bubas Hospital and the Hospital of Las Vírgenes, advised the cabildo that the virgin saints Justa and Rufina should be given an offering "for the intercession with Our Lord in the sickness of the plague." Dr. Herrera suggested that the gift should be either a "silver lamp or a frontal" to adorn their altar. The council members agreed, "for the health that this city has from the disease of the plague," to take up to fifty ducats from the plague account to buy a suitable silver lamp. The municipality also asked the Cathedral Chapter to hold a procession on the feast day of Santa Justa and Santa Rufina (19 July) to give thanks that "God our Lord has been served to make a notable improvement in the contagious disease." The two Sevillian saints were much revered, particularly in times of the plague. Because they had the reputation of ending outbreaks of the disease, it had become customary for Seville's governor to attend Mass on their feast day in the church dedicated to them in the Bubas Hospital.[8]

On Wednesday, 2 August, while the councilors deliberated, two canons sent by the Cathedral Chapter appeared. The church officials pressed for another religious procession "for the health that Our Lord has been served to give this city in the past sickness of the plague." They planned to hold it on the day of San Lorenzo (10 August), and it would proceed from the cathedral to the Monastery of San Francisco. The councilors agreed to meet that day "in the cabildo at six o'clock in the morning in order to go with His Lordship the Count" in the procession.[9]

7. AHPS, Protocolos notariales, leg. 2368, fols. 309r–11v.

8. AMS, sec. 10, 1581 [2], meeting of 12 July and 24 July; and sec. 13, siglo XVI, vol. 9, docs. 7 and 8.

9. AMS, sec. 10, 1581 [2].

15

A GIFT TO THE CITY

God has been served to make a gift to this city.
—DIEGO ORTIZ MELGAREJO

IMPROVING CONDITIONS IN SEVILLE did not necessarily mean that the plague had ended in other parts of Andalusia. During the 4 August meeting, the Count of Villar informed the council that in Sanlúcar de Barrameda "there is more sickness of the plague and many more people die than here," and he advised that it would be prudent "for this city to guard against that one more carefully." Sanlúcar, the port at the mouth of the Guadalquivir, lay about sixty kilometers downriver, and ships entering Seville had to pass by the coastal town. The governor admonished that if they did not protect Seville against contagion from Sanlúcar, "it would be difficult to conserve the health that Our Lord has given" this city. He recommended that one or two jurados or other people set up guard with a boat, as they had done in the past. The count exhorted the councilors that now that Seville was free of plague, it was essential to closely monitor the city's health conditions by collecting testimony from physicians, pharmacists, and priests regarding how many days it had been since "no person has died, nor is there the said sickness," in their neighborhood.

Veinticuatro Ortiz Melgarejo supported the count and insisted that no cloth should come from Sanlúcar de Barrameda, "by river or land." He proposed to send out a boat with two rowers to guard the river day and night. He urged that any ship unable to prove that it had not stopped in Sanlúcar should be prevented from passing. The veinticuatro insisted that the cabildo should post guard against the towns of Coria and Puebla de Coria and order Lebrija and Las Cabezas, east of the Guadalquivir, to comply with the quarantine, in case anyone tried to go by land from Sanlúcar to Seville, thus bypassing the river controls. The boat guarding the river should carry at the stern a "dyed canvas banner bearing the coat of arms of Sanlúcar."[1] Everyone agreed, and following a short discussion about where best to set up controls, the councilors concluded that they would leave it up to the governor to decide where to station the guards.[2] During the following weeks, the city council received regular reports from Don Francisco Tello de Guzmán, Seville's chief standard-bearer, regarding the plague's progress in Sanlúcar de Barrameda.

As health conditions continued to improve in Seville, the councilors were determined to clean the city and remove all vestiges of the plague. Perhaps they were again driven by the anonymous accusations sent to the king in June. On 9 August they directed Jurado Santofímia Riquelme to "find two carts with their draft animals and have the city and walls and barbicans cleaned of all the plague clothes, rags, and wool that can be found" and take them away to a designated place, there to be burned.

While the threat of the plague seemed to abate, the shortage of wheat and bread continued to vex the councilors. In early August the city learned that the House of Trade's factor, Francisco Duarte, to provision the royal armies, once again had embargoed all the grain that the city had purchased in the archbishopric of Seville. There was little the councilors could do. Diego Ortiz Melgarejo suggested that a committee should speak with Duarte, while Diego Mexía, the outgoing warden of the public granary, proposed that they should supplicate His Majesty to stop such actions by his agents, because if the factors "take anything it will be the total destruction of this city."[3]

Given the scarcity of cereals, the city council again considered importation of foreign wheat. The Count of Villar informed the cabildo that he had learned that in Berbería, in North Africa, "there is a great quantity of wheat," which was easy to ship, and there was enough to "provision the whole of Andalusia." The count noted that most vendors from whom the city traditionally bought cereals would need to import them as well, and he declared that no place in Andalusia should be forced to export its grain. He proposed that Seville should appeal to the king for permission to import grain from North Africa and indicated that he had also taken the necessary steps "to bring wheat from France, Italy and Sicily." The count stated flatly that the authorities needed to make certain that

1. The scribe wrote "San," leaving a small space before the next word. In the context of the document it is likely he meant Sanlúcar, although alternative explanations are possible.

2. AMS, sec. 10, 1581 [2].

3. Ibid. (9 August 1581).

they imported "a large quantity, because with a small amount the present need could not be met."[4]

Seville employed an agent to represent her interests at Court in Madrid to ensure a successful outcome of her frequent petitions. Because Philip II had moved the Court to Lisbon following the annexation of Portugal, some councilors argued that they also needed an agent there to act on the city's behalf. Baltasar de Aguilar agreed that they needed a permanent representative in Lisbon but wondered about the city's ability to pay such an agent, given its present financial condition. He pointed out that Veinticuatro Saavedra, Seville's emissary in Madrid, received four ducats a day from the city coffers, and now the councilors were contemplating sending a second agent to Madrid at the same stipend and another to Lisbon, where the Court currently resided. Jurado Aguilar strongly opposed using the city's propios as the source of the money and suggested that the agents' salaries should be paid by the caballeros who had voted to send more representatives to Court. Undeterred, the cabildo voted to send Veinticuatro Bartolomé López de Mesa to represent the city in Lisbon. Baltasar de Aguilar protested and threatened to appeal the decision. To infuriate the dissenting jurado even more, the members of the council decided to take two hundred ducats from the public granary account to pay López de Mesa's salary. Before the month ended, Seville's new representative in Lisbon had reached his new post and immediately set to work attempting to secure the king's permission for the purchase of wheat from North Africa.[5]

On 14 August Francisco Duarte, hardly a popular man at city hall, came to remind the cabildo that the city had agreed to purchase from him twenty thousand fanegas of wheat. He claimed that there were still thirty-three hundred fanegas left uncollected. Duarte had stored the grain in warehouses in the city and wanted the cabildo to take immediate shipment. Following his departure, Juan de León, the new chief warden of the alhóndiga, disputed Duarte's assertion, arguing that the factor did not really have the wheat in Seville earlier but had just received it from Cádiz. Veinticuatro León cautioned that the cereal should be inspected carefully before the council accepted it.[6]

At the end of the month, on Friday, 25 August, Veinticuatro Ortiz Melgarejo was able to exclaim, "God has been served to make a gift to this city and re-

4. Ibid. (11 August 1581).
5. Ibid. (28 August 1581).
6. AMS, sec. 10, 1581 [2].

public in that the plague has stopped," but at the same time he deplored the high costs of managing the health crisis. He complained in particular about the "excessive salaries" that had been given "the pharmacists and physicians and other plague officials."[7] While the plague relentlessly attacked its victims, city authorities were primarily concerned with containing the disease and curing the sick, but as soon as the threat of death lifted, the councilors began to question the expenses. People were coming forward following a 2 August public proclamation "with trumpets on the steps and at the doorway of the cabildo" announcing that the city will "pay anyone who had made a loan and those who are owed for their work and service in the hospitals and any other thing related to this." Fifty thousand ducats were earmarked for these payments, but the cabildo needed the exact account of plague expenditures from the city's steward, Diego del Postigo, before any money could be disbursed. Although some would soon be paid, many of the physicians who had visited the sick and the apothecaries who had mixed and supplied their remedies would not be fully remunerated for months, even years.

The following Monday, 28 August, Diego Ortiz Melgarejo informed the cabildo that Hernando de Porras had collected the spending records "from the administrators who were in charge of the hospitals," and each one had accumulated more than a thousand ducats in plague-related expenditures. The veinticuatro pointed out that a total of twenty-four thousand ducats had already been spent, and the money had been borrowed. Furthermore, the city would need to dip each week into the account of the excise taxes to meet continuing expenses, and officials still needed to pay for the care of those who were convalescing. He insisted that those in charge of the plague needed to provide an account of the expenditures to date, including the costs of cleanup. The Count of Villar agreed, emphasizing that "the plague accounts should be followed through without letting go of them until it is concluded and finished."[8]

That same day the municipal authorities returned to the question of grain. The councilors generally agreed that the city needed to supply the public granary no matter how high the prices, but some expressed apprehension regarding importing wheat from overseas. Nevertheless, the Count of Villar insisted that at the present time there was "great need of this wheat, and much more, and

7. AMS, sec. 10, 1581 [3].
8. Ibid.

therefore he will not cease taking it, as expensive as it is." The governor also made clear his discontent with factor Francisco Duarte, stating that the city had made a mistake when it entered into the agreement with him to purchase surplus grain. The count's statement met with unanimous approval. Two days later a copy of the count's letter of complaint sent to the king was introduced into the record. The governor informed His Majesty that the grain purchased from Duarte was of bad quality and that the factor had not complied with the original contract.

The financial crisis the city was facing did not deter the councilors from contemplating public festivities to mark the end of the plague. The cabildo decided not only that thanks should be given through religious processions but that the city should celebrate in the traditional secular fashion. They would hold a bull fight and a jousting competition on the Plaza of San Francisco, "for the people of the city to rejoice."[9]

9. AMS, sec. 10, 1581 [2] (14 August).

16

BULLS AND JOUSTING

Let us organize a festival of bulls and jousting.
—MARTÍN GUTIÉRREZ CERÓN

EWS OF SEVILLE'S GOOD FORTUNE and improving health reached the Court, and King Philip conveyed to the city his satisfaction upon learning of "the relief from the sickness of the plague for which he gives thanks." The royal missive arrived at city hall on 14 August, and it might have inspired Seville's chief justice and plague deputy, Martín Gutiérrez Cerón, to propose a "general procession of thanksgiving," since God had given the city health, and to suggest that the council "organize a festival of bulls and jousting" to entertain the people.

Gutiérrez Cerón's proposal met with enthusiasm, as most councilors must have welcomed a distraction from the never-ending crises. Don Gerónimo de Montalvo recommended that six officials meet with the Count of Villar to choose a suitable day for the festivities. Don Gerónimo suggested that they should also indicate "the leaders [cuadrilleros] and how many squadrons [cuadrillas] there should be." He specified "that the dress be made of taffeta" and proposed that the city provide the attire as well as "the bulls and furnishing of the plaza, and the music."[1] Martín Gutiérrez Cerón concurred, though he felt that "the festivities cannot stretch beyond this month." Don Pedro Tello de Guzmán wholeheartedly agreed with both of his colleagues and added that the squadron leaders should come "from among the caballeros of the city council."

Diego Ortiz Melgarejo enthusiastically endorsed the idea and, as always, presented his fellow council members with detailed input on numerous aspects of the festivity. First came the clothing. The veinticuatro recommended that

---

1. AMS, sec. 10, 1581 [2] (14 August).

"each player be given fourteen *varas* of taffeta and three-quarters of a vara of velvet for a bonnet."[2] The fabric was to be turned over to the cuadrillero of each team, in the amount "necessary for his squadron," to have the uniforms sewn. Ortiz Melgarejo further specified that no one's attire could be embroidered: "they can only wear borders and frogging of silver and pure or false gold and flowers."

When he finished attiring the cuadrillas, the alderman turned his attention to the bulls: "Let there be twelve, and to the liking of Melchior de Baena." He also set the number of participants: there should be "eight leaders and each squadron should have six players," and he concurred with Don Pedro Tello de Guzmán that "those of the cabildo should be preferred above all others."

Next, Ortiz Melgarejo asked Don Gerónimo de Montalvo "to do the city the honor to negotiate with residents of the plaza to provide windows to the players, and each player should be given one." Windows and balconies facing the plaza were a coveted commodity whenever any spectacle took place; the players' family and friends would be guaranteed an excellent view of the action. Always concerned with the protocol to be observed in public ceremonies, the indefatigable veinticuatro admonished Bartolomé de Hoces "to carefully prepare the gallery" and to ensure "that no person regardless of his position or quality entered the gallery until His Lordship the Count had entered." Ortiz Melgarejo reminded everyone that "the stage should be made in front of the cabildo in the order that is normally followed so that His Lordship and the Countess and the other ladies could be there." In conclusion, Ortiz Melgarejo indicated that he and Bartolomé de Hoces would take out the silk hangings and "distribute them and adorn the plaza along with Melchior de Baena."

Diego Caballero de Cabrera spoke next and voiced some reservations. He was preoccupied with maintaining good relations with the city's ecclesiastical authorities, who might not be too enthusiastic about secular celebrations. He proposed sending Juan Yáñez de Perea, Melchior de Baena, and two other councilmen to speak with the "prelates and convents" of the city regarding processions. They were to tell the churchmen that they had held a procession of thanksgiving and to inquire whether they could also have "processions with a Mass." He believed "that for now no other issue should be dealt with." Another

2. A *vara* is equal to approximately eighty-four centimeters.

councilor, Luis de Herrera, had misgivings about any celebrations that might be premature and cautioned "that the festivities should not take place until the hospitals were dismantled."

At last the Count of Villar spoke. He agreed that "above all other things they should approach the prelates of the convents." The governor also recommended that Chief Justice Montalvo discuss with His Majesty "whether this were the time and occasion to have any celebration in this city." The count asked the chief justice to investigate whether the proposed festival would be viewed at Court "as unsuitable" or might "not sit well with serious ministers." In spite of the expressed caution, the governor favored holding the festivities. He felt "that it could well be done," since after all the city "had passed through so many tribulations and calamities that it is just to entertain it in some way." When the vote was called, all sanctioned the festival except three aldermen who continued to have reservations about the propriety of any celebrations: Diego Caballero de Cabrera, Luis de Herrera, and Juan de Escalante de Mendoza.[3]

The city moved quickly to set a date for the event and to choose the deputies charged with organizing the festivities. The cabildo also sent Chief Justice Gutiérrez Cerón to announce the bullfight to the Inquisition. He duly reported to the city council on 23 August that he had spoken with the inquisitors and had indicated to them "that Our Lord has been served to give this city health" and that in order to animate its people the council had agreed to celebrate, "on Wednesday the 30th, a festival of bulls and jousting."[4]

There is no extant record of a bullfight and jousting games (*juego de cañas*) during the Count of Villar's tenure as governor of Seville. Nevertheless, had the festival taken place as proposed, it would have been a grand and colorful affair, and markedly different from a modern *corrida de toros* (bullfight). Seville's Plaza of San Francisco witnessed many bullfights in spite of complaints that it was too small and "unworthy of such a notable city and such grandiose fiestas."[5]

As the councilors had discussed during their meeting, the plaza had to be prepared for the animals, stands built to accommodate as many people as possible, and the square adorned with colorful hangings. The common people

3. AMS, sec. 10, 1581 [2].

4. AMS, sec. 10, 1581 [3].

5. From a 1620 account in Francisco Morales Padrón, ed., *Memorias de Sevilla (Noticias sobre el siglo XVII)* (Cordova: Monte de Piedad, 1981), 194.

would crowd in the cheapest stands, while the most prominent spectators would secure windows and balconies with a good view of the square below. The Count of Villar and his wife, Doña María Carrillo de Córdoba, would preside over the tournament from a specially erected stage in front of the city hall, accompanied by important ladies, perhaps the wives of the competing cuadrilleros as well as other notables.

Each of the eight mounted leaders with his squadron of liveried footmen would have been assigned a spot, chosen by lot, from which he and his men would enter the plaza. Although Diego Ortiz Melgarejo had specified that each squadron leader should have six footmen, usually the number of retainers varied, depending on the importance of the caballero, and could surpass twenty. Each team wore a distinct attire, sporting different colors, and although there was to be no embroidery, surely there was enough gold and silver and other ornamentation to please the eye.

The fiesta began when the governor, accompanied by his deputies and the city's constables, entered the plaza on horseback and solemnly "rode around until it was time to occupy his seat and he ascended to it and the others to their places."[6] It was then that the first bull was released into the arena "at the sound of trumpets and wind instruments."[7] The cuadrilleros, each holding a *rejón*, a short spear with a sharp metal tip, would then follow one another in galloping toward the bull and stabbing the animal's side, breaking their spears and usually leaving the metal tips implanted. The object was not to kill the bull but to collect as many broken rejónes as possible, the winner's trophies. If the bull showed aggression toward the horseman or attacked any of the bystanders, the squadron leader would unsheathe his sword and punish the bull with "some very good stabs."[8]

The seriously injured animal, or one that had reached the end of its strength, would be finished off, mercilessly slashed and cut to pieces by the footmen to popular delight, though their performance could also meet with loud disapproval if the animals were dispatched too quickly, thereby ending the fiesta

6. Ibid., 195. In "reconstructing" the festivities planned by Seville's cabildo in August 1581, we have used two accounts of a 1620 fiesta, both published in Morales Padrón, *Memorias,* as well as Marcelin Defourneaux, *Daily Life in Spain in the Golden Age,* trans. Newton Branch (Stanford, Calif.: Stanford University Press, 1979), 132–35.

7. Morales Padrón, *Memorias,* 195.

8. Ibid., 190.

early for lack of bulls. The cabildo had agreed to acquire twelve bulls, but that number could be much higher, and depending on the strength and fierceness of the animals, the spectacle could last several hours. In the end, the bulls were rarely the only casualties. These large, strong, and specially bred animals often charged and gored bystanders and the footmen, and on rare occasions even the highly skilled mounted cuadrilleros did not escape injury or death.

The game of *cañas,* or javelin jousting, which often followed the bullfight, evolved in Spain from the medieval tournament. The squadron leaders, each carrying a javelin and an oval, leather-covered shield, would ride with their retainers into the square, where they "performed a battle, making a concerted skirmish, all shielding themselves and threatening to throw until one stayed put and the other went gallantly into combat throwing the javelin."[9] The mock battle would be repeated in various guises with much gallantry and skill by the cuadrilleros and their horses, sometimes in individual combat, sometimes in general charge, to the delight of the spectators.

As the sun set, the festivity would draw to a close, though at other times it might last several days. One wonders if on this occasion the cuadrilleros also stopped at the Monastery of San Francisco at the end of the day, where the monks might have "presented them with many and very good sweets with which they refreshed the weary spirits."[10]

When the cabildo met two days later, it was business as usual, and if the councilors and the city had enjoyed some respite participating in or watching the colorful spectacle, there was no indication of it in the town council records. It is also possible that the festival had not taken place, given the opposition of some councilors and perhaps of the church as well.

9. Ibid., 198; Defourneaux, *Daily Life in Spain,* 132.

10. Morales Padrón, *Memorias,* 198. The monks' hospitality in 1620 is documented, and they might have shown similar generosity earlier.

17

DAMAGES AND LOSSES

I demand payment for damages and losses.

—TOMÁS PESARO

T HE LAST FOUR MONTHS of the year 1581 transpired without any new reports of the plague. Nevertheless, the cabildo continued to wrestle with the high costs of the past outbreak and with demands for payment from numerous creditors. The grain shortage remained a serious problem for the city, as did high prices, and companies of soldiers descended once again on Seville. In addition, there was notice of fresh locust infestation and destruction of local wheat harvests. Yet the city's solutions varied little from those implemented earlier. The councilors regularly discussed purchasing cereals from North Africa, Portugal, France, or other parts of Spain, though Seville's attempts to import the much-needed commodity were often frustrated by royal embargoes. Facing constant obstacles, the exasperated city officials even turned to nuns for prayers "that this wheat comes safely."[1] The prayers seem to have been answered. At the end of October the Count of Villar, along with officials of the public granary, was able to supply all the parishes with wheat purchased in Lisbon, although first it had to dry in the sun for a day.[2]

A new archbishop, Don Rodrigo de Castro, had finally been appointed but still had not arrived to take possession of his archdiocese. The continued absence of the high churchman generated clear dissatisfaction among city officials, who decided to prod the king to send the new archbishop to Seville "as quickly as possible because it has been almost a year that it is without a prelate." The cabildo had aided the church in the interim in many ways, "espe-

1. AMS, sec. 10, 1581 [3] (20 October).
2. Ibid. (30 October).

cially where the plague is concerned, assisting with their persons and alms." The Count of Villar repeated his concern for the needy and the role the archbishop's alms had played in "the support and relief of the poor." The governor maintained that neither the Cathedral Chapter nor the city council "can do what the prelate can because they have neither the means nor the obligation."[3]

The effectiveness of the continuing quarantine was another persistent issue facing the municipality. On Friday, 1 September 1581, the plague deputy Don Diego de Portugal informed the cabildo that the guards stationed at the gates leading into the city "vex the persons who come from the outside even when they carry a certificate of health." Don Diego explained that the guards barred everyone from entering "unless their certificate is countersigned by Diego de Toledo, the notary of the commissions." At the same time, according to the troubled plague deputy, the guards "let those who come without certificates enter more easily," and he urged the city to take appropriate action to stop any misconduct on the part of the gatekeepers. As often happened, the councilors referred the issue to the plague commission, and the Count of Villar promised to convoke a meeting of the commission at seven o'clock the following morning. Before the final vote, Diego Caballero added that the cabildo should instruct Jurado Toledo to make certain that all people wanting to enter the city carried proper documentation.[4]

The city's notorious tardiness in disbursing funds to cover the emergency pesthouses, their personnel, and the cost of medicines resulted in numerous petitions during the fall of 1581 and beyond. The boticario Pedro de Sierra repeatedly demanded payment "for medicines that he gave for the plague."[5] Even the accountants hired by the city pressed for recompense for "the work they had done in that of the plague." They petitioned the city on Monday, 9 October, and, following a brief discussion centering on whether each one should receive ten thousand or fifteen thousand maravedís (twenty-seven or forty ducats), the councilors decided on the lower figure. It was an exceptional payment, which was to be released "this time, mindful how much they have worked and written in the things regarding the plague, which is an extraordinary business."[6]

3. Ibid. (4 September).

4. AMS, sec. 10, 1581 [3].

5. Ibid.; his petitions were read both on 6 October and 3 November 1581, and there was another one on 29 January 1582.

6. AMS, sec. 10, 1581 [3].

Notaries employed by the cabildo were also busier than usual. Juan Abarca de Carrión requested payment for the work he had done "relating to the plague." The public granary's chief warden, Juan de León, supported his petition, confirming that Abarca de Carrión "resided in this city at the time of the plague . . . and served the city in drawing up commissions and other decrees that the city mandated regarding this sickness." The alderman added that the notary had spent much time and worked diligently, and he proposed that Abarca de Carrión should be paid one hundred reales (nine ducats) from the plague account. Everyone agreed to pay the man.[7]

Cristóbal Suárez, Colón Hospital's administrator, reappeared before the council on Monday, 4 September, and complained about lack of payment. He stated that it had been more than twenty days since he had turned over the documentation detailing the hospital's operating costs to the accounting office (Contaduría) and that all was in order with correct signatures, yet he had not received any payment. Jurado Suárez found a sympathetic response to his plight, with everyone agreeing that the city needed to pay these bills. Nevertheless, the officials turned the matter over to the plague commission, since, as the Count of Villar pointed out, the original agreements regarding the four pesthouses had been negotiated there. Eleven days later, Diego de Aguilar, a surgeon at the Colón Hospital, still had not collected his salary.[8]

Tomás Pesaro, the current owner of the building that housed the Colón Hospital, also petitioned the cabildo. Pesaro had rented this large edifice to the city and was demanding a payment of six hundred ducats "for damages and losses that he has received." The council decided to refer this and similar cases to the legal experts, the letrados, to assess the claims and advise the city on how to proceed.[9] Other people whose real estate had been expropriated by the city for temporary hospitals also requested reimbursements. For example, the eminent doctor Andrés Zamudio de Alfaro, "physician of His Majesty," petitioned the cabildo for payment of fifteen hundred ducats "for the damage that he has received from having taken from him a house for the plague."[10]

The requests for payments continued as the year drew to a close. Pedro

---

7. Ibid. (10 November 1581).

8. AMS, sec. 10, 1581 [3].

9. Ibid. (20 September 1581). On 11 October 1581, the city received royal authorization to name four letrados to serve the city at an annual salary of fifteen thousand maravedís (forty ducats) each.

10. AMS, sec. 10, 1581 [3] (30 October).

Rondineli, the steward of the Cinco Llagas Hospital, which had been used for the past year to treat plague victims, petitioned the city on 15 December 1581 to cover the expenses that resulted from the overcrowding and the adjustments that had been made to the existing structure. He complained that though the plague had ended, there remained a "large amount of [used] bedding," which was detrimental to public health. At the same time, the number of sick women, for whom the hospital had originally been founded, continued to grow "every day, so that the infirmaries as well as the offices are very full." While the hospital was being used for the plague sick, some work had been done to accommodate the patients.

Detailing the costs, Pedro Rondineli stated that the hospital had purchased five hundred cargas of mixed lime for "floors and other work in the plague infirmaries," and they had used "400 cargas of sand and a large amount of bricks." The steward complained that the workers who were caring for the plague sick "caused another greater harm, because they stopped cooking the food in the kitchen and the fireplace, which was very large and adequate, and made a fire in two new and very principal parts of the hospital." He lamented both the high cost of the firewood and the damage. He also noted that the hospital had bought a thousand pine logs from Segura for the continued construction, much of which was still stacked in the countryside, exposed to the sun and the elements. Pedro Rondineli begged city officials to cover the damages.[11]

Although the authorities considered the city free of plague, fear of the disease lingered, and anxious city officials dealt swiftly with any suspicious item or activity they believed might cause a new outbreak. They were particularly fearful of anything that might corrupt the air. During the meeting on Monday, 16 October, the governor informed the councilors that the two fleets that just returned from the Indies brought "a great quantity of damaged cowhides," which were being stored in the city. He declared that as soon as he had learned of the problem he had ordered an inquiry and consulted "some physicians," who urged that "it would be very expedient that those that come thus damaged are quickly burned and others mended." The doctors warned that if this were not done "the plague that Our Lord was served to send this year could, God forbid, return to the city." The governor noted that he was sharing this information so that the city could act accordingly.

11. AMS, sec. 13, siglo XVI, vol. 6. Although the date on this petition was 15 December 1581, it was bound in a part that fell around 15 May 1582.

The Count of Villar's words produced considerable consternation and calls for immediate action. One of the most outspoken, once again, was Diego Ortiz Melgarejo, who proposed that the town criers should "proclaim tomorrow morning with trumpets" throughout the city that "no person should dare to store nor put in Seville or within its walls any cowhides that have come on these fleets." The unrelenting veinticuatro added that the proclamation should include the threat that anyone caught storing these hides in the city would be punished by "loss of the said hides and [a fine] of 12,000 maravedís" (32 ducats). The proceeds from these fines would be equally divided among "the treasury, the judge, and the denouncer."

Diego Caballero agreed, though he preferred that the announcement be confined to the entrance to the city hall, the steps of the cathedral, and the Arenal; furthermore, he suggested that the proclamations be made at the most appropriate time, that is, when most people would be congregated, rather than early in the morning. More discussion ensued, and Melchor del Alcázar recommended the formation of a commission to discuss the proposal. He cautioned that the city's action should cause "the least detriment possible to those involved with this merchandise." Leather products made from cowhides were valuable, and many Sevillians engaged in their importation from the Indies. The careful maneuvering in the cabildo session suggests that some of the councilmen may have been involved in the lucrative commerce. The prudent veinticuatro furthermore argued that one of the city's letrados should advise the commission regarding "justice in the manner in which the remedy is attempted."

Diego Mexía insisted that the guards should be immediately notified not to let anyone into the city with "the cowhides that are coming on these fleets." He urged his colleagues to name people to inspect the hides, and if they found any that were rotten, they should "order their owners to remove them two leagues away from the city." The cabildo passed the recommended measures, but on Friday, 27 October, Diego de Toledo had little progress to report, in spite of four days of public proclamations. The jurado complained that the owners "have not burnt or removed" anything, regardless of the orders to destroy "rotten and damaged and smelly" hides. Diego de Toledo warned that if no action were taken it could cause "sickness and plague" similar to what they had just experienced, and he reminded the councilors that the physicians and others had indicated that "the air could be infected with the bad odor."

Diego de Toledo prodded the cabildo to send deputies and inspectors to the places where "the damaged or wet hides are, and even if they are stored, those that seem damaged and rotten should be removed from this city." They should take them as far away as necessary and either "bury them in pits that they dig there or burn them"; those that could be salvaged should be mended. Toledo insisted that regardless of whether the hides were destroyed or repaired, it should all be done "at the cost of the owners of the said hides."

Four days later, two men petitioned the city for permission to transport on the river, to a distance of about one league outside the city, "certain hides that they had bought." They stated that the hides "are damaged and they want to restore them, in accordance with the proclamation." Diego Ortiz Melgarejo curtly rejected the petition, but others, including the Count of Villar, felt that if the men complied with the city ordinance and put the required amount of wheat into the alhóndiga, then perhaps they could be allowed to take the hides.[12] The bread shortage continued, and the city did not want to miss the opportunity to enforce the law requiring anyone removing certain merchandise, including raw hides, from the city to put a carga of grain into the public granary.

The cabildo's efforts to protect the city from recurrence of the plague led officials to order an inspection of "all the environs of this city, the parts and places where it had been mandated to dump the garbage." On 13 November the councilors directed the inspectors to survey "with their own eyes" not only the designated dumps but also those that were used illegally. The officials resolved that anyone caught tossing trash over the city walls or dumping it in unauthorized places should face legal action, jail, and a fine to pay for the cleanup. To ensure proper enforcement they also alerted the gatekeepers, particularly at the five city gates where dumping had been prohibited. The authorized spots for throwing out refuse were marked with wooden posts, and the officials instructed the inspectors to either place new ones, indicating "where to dump garbage," or repair the old posts.

Nine days later the Count of Villar returned to the question of sanitation, proposing to clean the city "because it is filled with filth." Although the plague was not mentioned during the ensuing discussion, clearly the officials were driven by their fear that dirt and foul odor caused infectious disease. Don Gerónimo de Montalvo recommended that one veinticuatro and one jurado

---

12. AMS, sec. 10, 1581 [3].

should oversee the process in each parish and argued that the cost of cleaning should be borne by the respective vecinos. Don Gerónimo added that to accomplish the task they would need to hire the necessary carts and draft animals to haul away the dirt and garbage.

Diego Ortiz Melgarejo agreed but stressed that the cost for cleaning should be equally divided "among all in general, without distinction of persons, indeed, this is neither a tax nor tribute or anything that is prejudicial to individual liberty." This was an important argument, because the nobility was exempt from taxation, and the payment of taxes implied commoner status. In the end, the councilmen approved the measure, including Ortiz Melgarejo's equality of payment proposal.[13]

The following month the cabildo returned to the problem, concentrating on the logistics of the cleanup, which was to be proclaimed throughout the city by town criers. The cleaning was to be done within three days, under penalty of jail, and the outcome inspected to ensure that it was satisfactory. As Ortiz Melgarejo had advocated, all vecinos, regardless of status and without exception, were required to contribute to the cost of the cleanup. Two residents "from the same street or streets" were to collect the money and pay it directly "without any money being given to any inspector or notary." Furthermore, any leftover piles of earth from finished buildings were "to be cleaned in the same order at the cost of the owners."[14]

Along with the challenge of keeping the city clean, safe, and healthy, and with adequate food supply, the cabildo faced another and familiar aggravation. During the meeting of 15 November, Veinticuatro Ortiz Melgarejo raised the issue of unsupervised soldiers roaming the city and the countryside. In a long speech he lamented the hardships of the city and its inhabitants, who "cannot maintain their homes and children," and to add to their troubles, there were fifty companies of soldiers "who are now being quartered" in Seville's territory. The alderman complained that these companies lacked their commanding officer, and "the soldiers create some disorders." Ortiz Melgarejo pointed out that "the territory of Seville is unable to feed them and the soldiers are not being paid," but he acknowledged that "they cannot go without food." In closing he

---

13. Ibid. (22 November 1581). Regarding taxation, see Lunenfeld, *Keepers of the City,* 63–67; and Helen Nader, *Liberty in Absolutist Spain: The Habsburg Sale of Towns, 1516–1700* (Baltimore: Johns Hopkins University Press, 1990), 32–33.

14. AMS, sec. 10, 1581 [3] (13 December).

recommended that the councilors turn to His Majesty for assistance through their agent in Lisbon. If the king forced the city to supply food for the soldiers, then the cabildo should insist that they were under a proper command to prevent any disturbances. Everyone agreed that the council needed to appeal to the king.[15]

It appears that Seville's appeals went unanswered, and the situation worsened at the beginning of the following year. On Monday, 8 January 1582, Diego Ortiz Melgarejo brought more bad news, informing the cabildo that he had learned that forty-seven companies of soldiers were arriving from Cartagena. The veinticuatro asserted that "12,000 soldiers will have to be lodged in this land and territory." He pressed the council to again plead with the king not to quarter troops in the district of the city, "indeed he knows about the lack of bread and the poverty of the people." Ortiz Melgarejo suggested that if there were no alternatives and the soldiers had to come, then they should be housed at the expense of His Majesty, and they should have their own "ration of bread and meat and wine," as in Gibraltar and other places.[16] The problem of feeding the troops was aggravated by repeated royal embargoes of cereals purchased by Seville, which the king claimed in order to supply frontier posts with Portugal and the galleys.

As the year ended, Seville remained free of plague, yet any optimism on the part of city officials was soon dampened by reports from small towns in Seville's territory, and the news was ominous. People were dying in larger numbers than normal in the hillside towns north of the Guadalquivir River: Constantina, Cazalla de la Sierra, Puebla de los Infantes, and other places. Seville's city council could not ignore the danger of disease spreading throughout the district and possibly returning to the city itself.

15. AMS, sec. 10, 1581 [3].
16. Ibid.

18

A PARTICULAR COMMISSION

I have come with a special and particular commission.
—DIEGO DE TOLEDO

FACED WITH REPORTS INDICATING that the plague was rampant in the district, the councilors discussed the ramifications of the threat posed by the infected places and ways to protect the city from a recurrence of the plague. The officials made two decisions early in 1582. First, to ensure that no "people or cloth" from infected towns or villages entered Seville, they alerted the guards to stop them at the gates. Second, in order to survey conditions in the countryside, they commissioned two councilors to go to the affected areas, take charge of local affairs, and give Seville's cabildo a first-hand account of the seriousness of the problem. The city council chose two jurados, Licentiate Juan de Perea Durán and Diego de Toledo, to travel northeast of Seville to the small towns of Constantina and Puebla de los Infantes.

The commissioners arrived in Constantina "at three in the afternoon," on Thursday, 18 January 1582. Diego de Toledo remained in Constantina several days, while Juan de Perea continued the next day to Puebla de los Infantes. The two men inspected Constantina's newly established hospital and learned that when it opened its doors on 11 January, twenty-four people were admitted. Now, one week later, ten patients were being cared for, though the Sevillian officials determined that two of them did not have "the sickness" and had been discharged. Of the remaining eight, two people died shortly, two seemed to be in relatively good condition, and the rest were sick. One girl was readmitted but "fled the hospital, running after a sister, screaming, because she was hardly sick." Licentiate Perea Durán recommended that a hospital be established on the edge of town, in the parish of Santiago, more because "it is isolated, rather than for being a healthy place."

One helpful local alerted the commissioners that someone sick with the plague was being secretly cared for by a friar, a newcomer to the town. They tried to locate the sick man with the help of the physician, Dr. Centurio, and Constantina's plague constable (*alguacil de la peste*). They found him "standing up, with a light fever, because since it was so low he was up and about." Two of his children had catarrh, and Dr. Centurio "dismissed what they were saying about these sick," who hardly appeared to have the plague.

Two days later, leaving Diego de Toledo behind, Juan de Perea Durán departed for Puebla de los Infantes, a town not far southeast of Constantina. From Puebla, Perea Durán wrote to Seville's cabildo reporting on what they had found in Constantina. He related that since they arrived, eight people had become sick, including the past magistrate, "who died from this sickness within two and a half days." Perea Durán added scornfully that he had previously had the official jailed "because being a magistrate he said that this sickness was a joke, and that he had two swellings behind the ear and they should dump him in the middle of the bedding." He noted with a certain satisfaction that "God was served to take this one as an example for these rustics." Perea Durán also mentioned two priests in Constantina, noting that "one confesses and the other does not want to and is scandalizing the village by not wanting to administer [the sacraments] within the hospital." He concluded his long missive with a stab at the local Franciscans, "who take alms from this village and sustain themselves with them and now not one friar comes nor does he want to."[1]

The commissioners quickly became aware that the plague raged not only in Constantina and Puebla de los Infantes but in nearby Cazalla de la Sierra as well. As soon as they reached Constantina a number of people mentioned that there was "contagious disease" in Cazalla. The commissioners questioned Benito García Harto, the proprietor of a local inn, who had heard "that in the town of Cazalla de la Sierra a barber named Juan del Barco and his wife and children had died." The innkeeper had learned about these deaths from Andrés Hernández, who had come to see him the day before and told him that he had just returned from Cazalla, where he had heard about the barber and his family. Furthermore, García Harto had received a letter from his brother-in-law who lived in Cazalla, who also told him that the town's barber and his wife and chil-

1. AMS, sec. 13, siglo XVI, vol. 5. The letter was received by Seville's cabildo on 29 January and was immediately turned over to the plague commission. See AMS, sec. 10, 1581 [3].

dren had died of "the sickness of contagious plague." Moreover, the brother-in-law informed him that his own son, the innkeeper's nephew, was also sick and was being treated by two physicians. One of them said that he was sick from "the swelling that he has on his head behind the ear," but the innkeeper pointed out that the one who said that "was not educated, just a barber-surgeon," though the other physician "is a licentiate and an old and experienced man."

The commissioners sought out Andrés Hernández and questioned him. He admitted having been in Cazalla de la Sierra the previous day and having heard that "people were dying." Hernández had heard that in one house six people had died and that town officials placed a lock on that building, but he was uncertain of the cause of their death.

Another man in Constantina had recently traveled to Cazalla. Luis de Andrada, a constable from Seville, related to the commissioners that while he was in Cazalla de la Sierra on Sunday, 14 January, he saw some men carrying a corpse toward the main church. The inquisitive Sevillian asked, "What is this?" and the onlookers told him that a black woman who had been "well and fat" had died suddenly, within five days. Andrada passed through later and noticed "that the men who had carried her left her next to the plaza, without anyone wanting to take her." He joined the bystanders, who "all feared that she had died from the plague," and a priest who was there told him that four people had perished from the plague. Andrada also overheard a woman say that the officials had sealed a house "because some died there of the plague."[2]

The news was incontrovertible; there was a plague outbreak in Cazalla de la Sierra, though the extent of it was not yet well understood. The commissioners could not immediately travel to the affected town, but with the information they had just obtained it was imperative that Seville be alerted to the danger in order to guard against travelers and goods from Cazalla.

The situation in Cazalla de la Sierra was complicated by what Seville's cabildo perceived as the election of unworthy town officials. As in other parts of Castile, towns and villages within Seville's jurisdiction elected their own municipal government, but the elections and local decisions were subject to the review and approval of central authorities. Some members of Seville's city council insisted that Cazalla's election be "revoked and annulled." One of the recently elected town officials, the new municipal magistrate Pedro García

2. AMS, sec. 13, siglo XVI, vol. 5.

Zorro, was singled out for special opprobrium for being "so poor, base, and low" that Seville's cabildo refused to confirm him in his post. The Sevillians ordered that a new election be held in Cazalla, supervised by two letrados from Seville, who would ensure that half of those elected were hidalgos and resident in Cazalla. Furthermore, they should be "honorable and rich men, indeed there are many in the said town."[3]

Following Juan de Perea Durán's departure from Constantina, Diego de Toledo continued the investigation. To have a basis for comparison regarding the number of people dying, Diego de Toledo culled Constantina's burial records for the period from 1 November 1581 to 19 January 1582. According to the documents, ten people died in November, twelve in December, and in the less than three weeks of January, twenty-seven people perished, clear indication of a sudden rise in mortality. Yet Seville's commissioner believed that only six or seven of these had died of the plague.

Diego de Toledo decided to visit the local pharmacy to check what medicines "appropriate for the sickness of the plague" were available and "their amount." On Monday, 20 January, accompanied by Licentiate Francisco González Perellón, Constantina's chief justice, and Dr. Centurio, he went to the botica of Pedro Ramírez, a widower who had lost his wife two months earlier. After taking the obligatory oath to be truthful, the boticario displayed a vast array of remedies, including purgatives, such as theriac of emeralds, and thick, syrupy concoctions (*lamedores*) made of pomegranates, citrons, lemons, and verjuice of grapes, to be slowly licked by the patient. Pedro Ramírez also stocked thistle and borage water, rose water, endive water, and orange blossom water, oils of chamomile, dill, lilies, rue, and wormwood, as well as scorpions. The botica was well supplied with the standard poultices, plasters, and ointments, including the *ungüento egipcio* made of honey, moss, and vinegar, a favorite caustic applied to buboes that had been cupped and bled and cleansed with salt water.

Dr. Centurio examined all the remedies and pronounced them "good for the said sickness" but added that "some amount of fermentative [substances] will be necessary." Ramírez promised to have them within three days. The officials ordered the apothecary to keep the medicines in stock and to be watchful, giv-

---

3. AMS, sec. 10, 1581 [3]. For general discussion of the evolution of Castilian municipal governments, see Nader, *Absolutist Spain,* 35–39.

ing them out only according to Dr. Centurio's prescriptions. They admonished him not to fill prescriptions from other doctors and told him to keep an account of "the price and value" of the remedies that he dispensed, because the council of Constantina would pay for them. Finally, they ordered Ramírez not to leave town "during the whole time that the said sickness lasts" or he would face a substantial fine.[4]

The following day, Diego de Toledo traveled to Puebla de los Infantes to join his partner Licentiate Perea Durán. Before he left Constantina, Toledo informed local officials that he had come with "a special and particular commission" from the Count of Villar to name Francisco González Perellón, the town's chief justice, as judge of the commission of the plague of Constantina. Licentiate González Perellón, a relatively young man of twenty-nine, was initially appointed to his post as alcalde mayor of Constantina by the governor of Seville. He represented the highest judicial authority in the town as appellate judge in all local disputes.[5]

On 21 January Juan de Perea Durán and Diego de Toledo presented their commission papers regarding "the business of the plague" before the assembled cabildo of Puebla de los Infantes. They again reviewed the local records and found that from 13 January to the present day twenty-three people had sickened. When they questioned town councilmen about the nature of the sicknesses that had befallen the local residents, the response confirmed what the commissioners suspected: "they are sick with the plague and swelling and contagious sickness." There did not seem to be any doubt that "all are stricken with this contagious sickness." Some of those who had contracted the disease were now convalescing, "and they have open wounds and carbuncles." Without delay, the commissioners ordered that all clothing and bedding of both the sick and the dead be burned. Any contaminated possessions that had not yet been disposed of were to be taken to the Church of Santiago and "locked there until such time that they could be burned more easily."

4. AMS, sec. 13, siglo XVI, vol. 5. See also Betrán, *La peste en Barcelona,* 416–19; Rojo Vega, *Enfermos y sanadores,* 72–75; Fernández-Carrión and Valverde, *Farmacia y sociedad,* 80–96.

5. Philip II, always in need of money, had sold Constantina in 1565 to Don Fadrique Enríquez de Ribera y Portocarrero, First Marquis de Villanueva del Río, for ninety thousand ducats. Seville protested, and the following year the sale was annulled after Seville and Constantina paid back the same amount to the marquis. See Domínguez Ortiz, *La Sevilla del siglo XVII,* 97–98. For discussion of the function of an alcalde mayor, see Nader, *Absolutist Spain,* 151–53.

Diego de Toledo and Juan de Perea Durán were joined by a physician sent from Seville. The Count of Villar had ordered Pedro García Arroyal, a surgeon from Triana, to assist the two commissioners. The previous summer, when the surgeon "who inspects the women of the Mancebía" had asked to be relieved of his duties, the city had hired García Arroyal as interim physician to supervise the prostitutes' health, something that he had already done at least a decade earlier.[6] During that time, García Arroyal had been concerned with the spread of venereal disease. Some of the prostitutes had been sent away from the brothel because of suspicion that they might be infected, but they continued to exercise their profession throughout the city. García Arroyal, then a young man in his twenties, had urged city officials to congregate all "such women . . . in the public house so that they can be examined and the sick ones taken to the hospitals to be cured."

During his lifetime García Arroyal would serve the city not only in the public brothel but also as a surgeon in the Royal Jail. Whenever the plague appeared the surgeon was called upon by the city fathers. He owned several rental properties, and his assets were estimated at four thousand ducats, a sizable amount. He and his wife, María de Moya, lived in Triana at the bustling Plaza of the Altozano, in a good location near the bridge and also close to the castle of the Inquisition. The couple had at least one daughter, María. Although the surgeon's salary and the income generated from the rentals were adequate, María de Moya occasionally supplemented the family income by sewing shirts.[7]

Pedro García Arroyal began his work in Puebla de los Infantes in the local infirmary. He would be paid thirty maravedís a day for his efforts and was forbidden to leave his post. The two Sevillian commissioners, probably advised by the surgeon, issued a series of regulations regarding the plague. They ordered that the sick be taken to the infirmary or a hospital and that their clothing, if in good condition, be securely stored there. Before being discharged, the patients needed to be examined by a doctor or a surgeon, who would authorize the dismissal. They might be given back their clothing, if it were "very clean and washed with a lot of soap and lye and not in any other way." The cloth-

6. AMS, sec. 10, 1581 [3] (5 June).

7. AMS, sec. 3, vol. 11, doc. 62; sec. 13, siglo XVI, vol. 5 (19 March, 1582); AHPS, Protocolos notariales, leg. 2366, fol. 330v; leg. 2365, fol. 618r; leg. 2378, fols. 68r–74r; leg. 8448, fols. 957r–60v; leg. 16132 (17 June 1598).

ing and bedding from the infirmary could not be washed in the public washing places or fountains; instead, "a trustworthy person" was to take it to be washed at an assigned place away from the town, and he was to "give account of the said clothing, that he took or brought back."

The commissioners stipulated that the convalescent house was to remain locked, with a notice placed on the door stating that no one could open it or enter it without express authorization from Licentiate Perea Durán. The house was to stay locked until "there is no sickness in this said town." The officials ordered that as long as the epidemic continued, physicians could treat only plague victims. There was a specific regulation regarding women. If any "nursing or pregnant women became sick and were to give birth in the said infirmary, the infants should be taken away from them and the said council should give them out to be nursed."

The day after the Sevillian officials arrived, they went to "the pesthouse of this town" at seven o'clock in the morning to remove infected clothing of the dead. They first made a list of all the items, which were later taken to a field outside the town and set on fire. The destroyed pieces included skirts of various colors, chemises, blue breeches, some cloaks, capes, hoods, and a veil as well as "a doublet, two shirts and a hat, all old and dirty." In addition, numerous "dirty and old" pillows were thrown into the flames. Diego de Toledo and his servant, as well as Licentiate Perea Durán and a local constable and some vecinos of Puebla de los Infantes, all duly witnessed the removal, the inventory, and the disposal of the undesirable items, and they affirmed "we saw it burn and it was burned."

Containing the spread of the plague was paramount for the officials from Seville. The commissioners were determined to prevent anyone who might be infected from entering Seville and causing a recurrence of the disease. If someone with the plague was unaccounted for, the officials made every attempt to find the person. Shortly after arriving in Puebla, Diego de Toledo discovered that a local widow, Ana de Rojas, was rumored to have the plague and "was missing from this town for about four days." Town justices had gone to her house to take her to the hospital, but she was not there; moreover, "her daughter had died in her house of . . . the plague." They asked if Ana de Rojas had clandestinely left town, and several people indicated she might have gone to the city of Cordova, "where they say she has her mother." The witnesses claimed that she had begged Licentiate Perea Durán to allow her to go there and that he was looking into it. Toledo ordered Puebla's officials to send someone to Cordova to discover where Ana's mother lived and find her. The diligent jurado also wanted someone to check whether Ana de Rojas might have gone to Seville instead.[8]

8. AMS, sec. 13, siglo XVI, vol. 5 (22 January 1582).

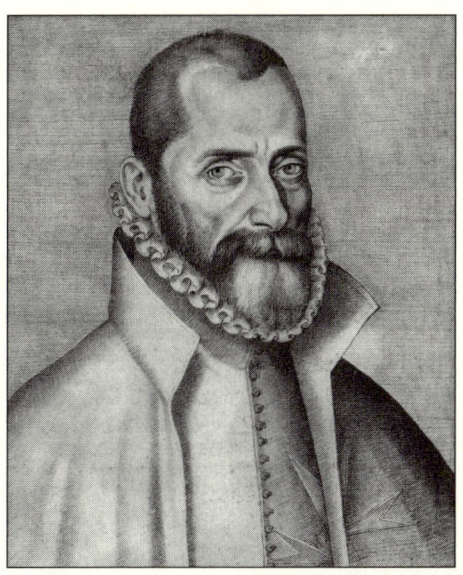

Dr. Bartolomé Hidalgo
Francisco Pacheco, *Libro de retratos de
ilustres varones, 1599*, edited by José Maria
Asencio (Seville: Litografía de Enrique
Utrera, 1886).

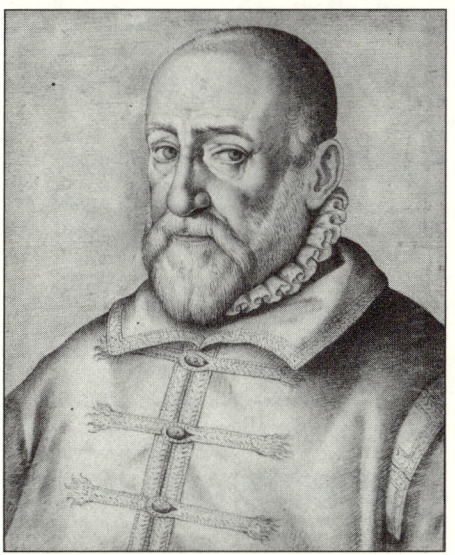

Veinticuatro Melchor del Alcázar
Francisco Pacheco, *Libro de retratos de
ilustres varones, 1599*, edited by José Maria
Asencio (Seville: Litografía de Enrique
Utrera, 1886).

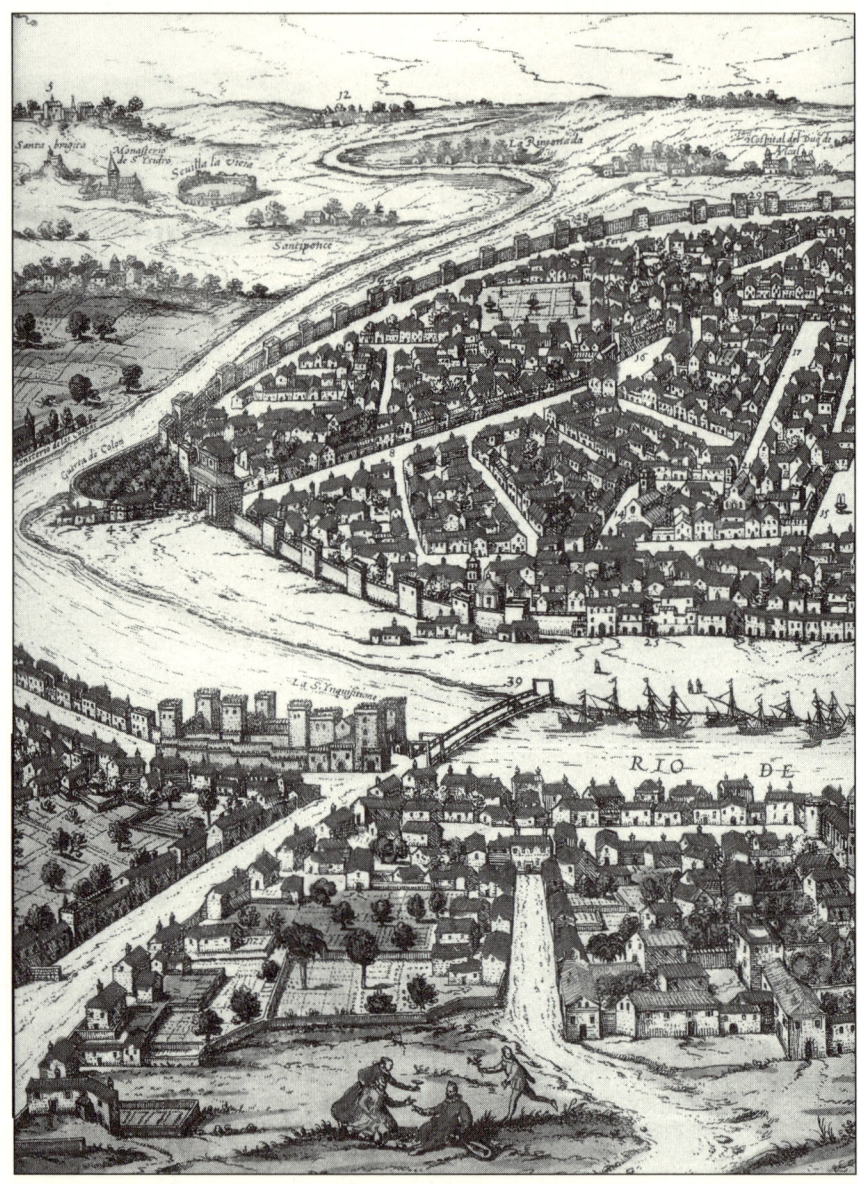

General view of north side of Seville, 1565

Georg Braun (plates by Georgius Hoefnagle), *Civitates Orbis Terrarum* (Coloniae Agrippinae, 1572–1618). Library of the Escuela de Estudios Hispanoamericanos, Consejo Superior de Investigaciones Científicas, Seville.

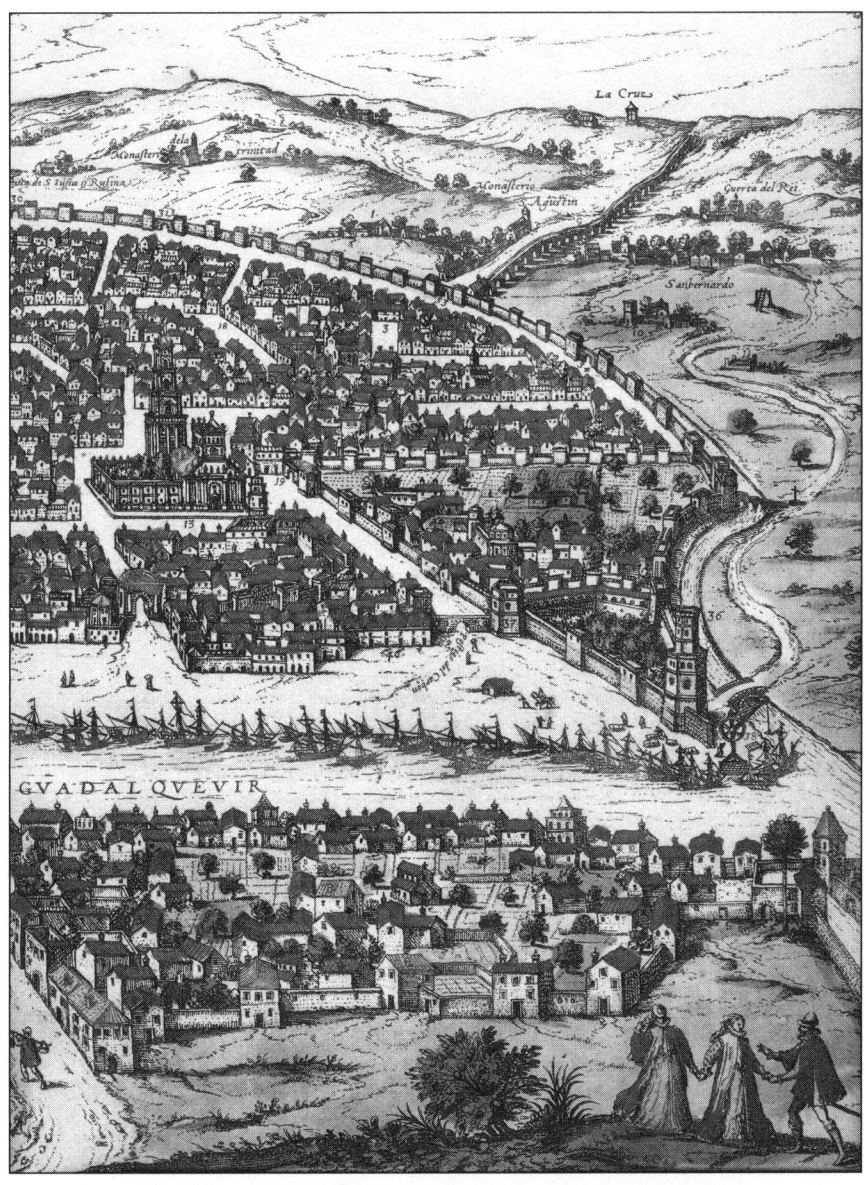

General view of south side of Seville, 1565

Georg Braun (plates by Georgius Hoefnagle), *Civitates Orbis Terrarum* (Coloniae Agrippinae, 1572–1618). Library of the Escuela de Estudios Hispanoamericanos, Consejo Superior de Investigaciones Científicas, Seville.

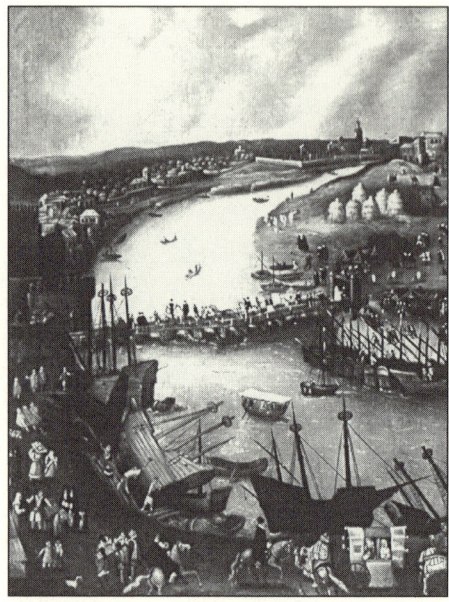

Ship caulkers near the Triana Bridge
Detail from "Vista de Sevilla," late sixteenth
century, attributed to A. Sánchez Coello.
Courtesy of Museo de América, Madrid.

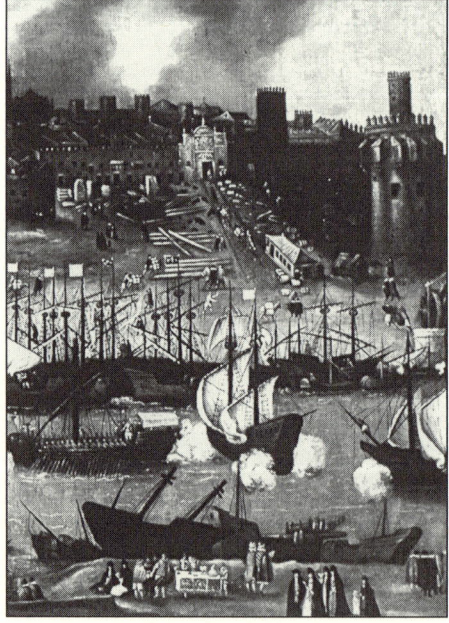

Timbers unloaded at the royal shipyards
Detail from "Vista de Sevilla," late sixteenth
century, attributed to A. Sánchez Coello.
Courtesy of Museo de América, Madrid.

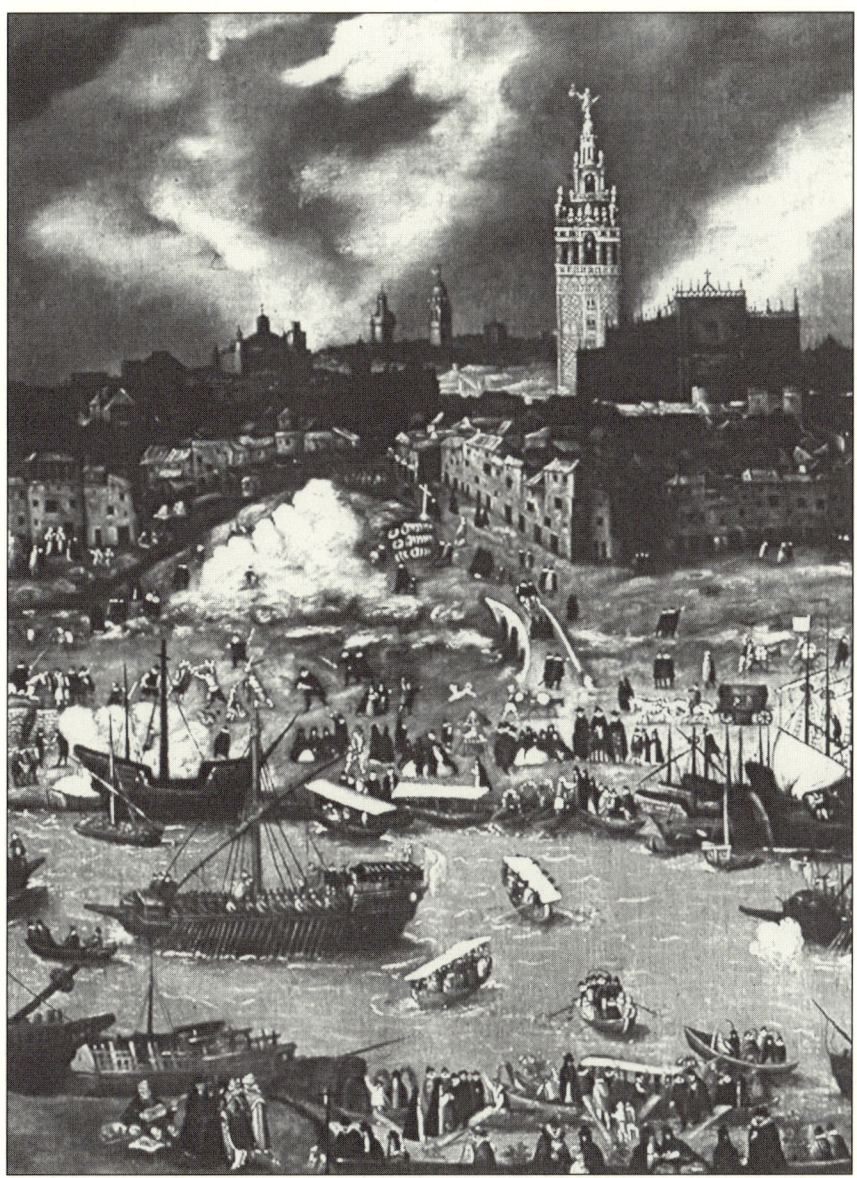

A busy day on the Arenal, with the Giralda and the Cathedral towering above
Detail from "Vista de Sevilla," late sixteenth century, attributed to A. Sánchez Coello.
Courtesy of Museo de América, Madrid.

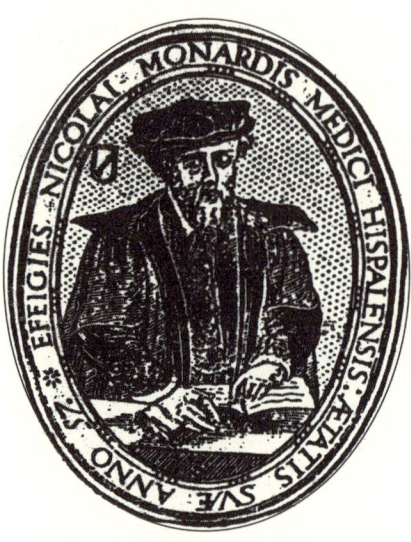

Dr. Nicolás Monardes
Primera y segunda y tercera parte de la
Historia medicinal, de las cosas . . .
(Seville: Fernando Díaz, 1580).

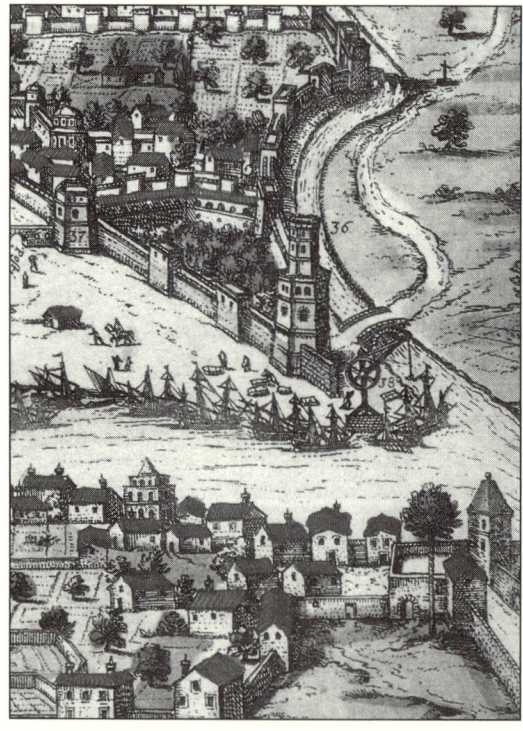

Torre del Oro and Monastery
of los Remedios (lower right).
Detail from Hoefnagle 1565.
Georg Braun (plates by Georgius
Hoefnagle), *Civitates Orbis Ter-*
rarum (Coloniae Agrippinae,
1572–1618). Library of the Escuela
de Estudios Hispanoamericanos,
Consejo Superior de Investigaciones Científicas, Seville.

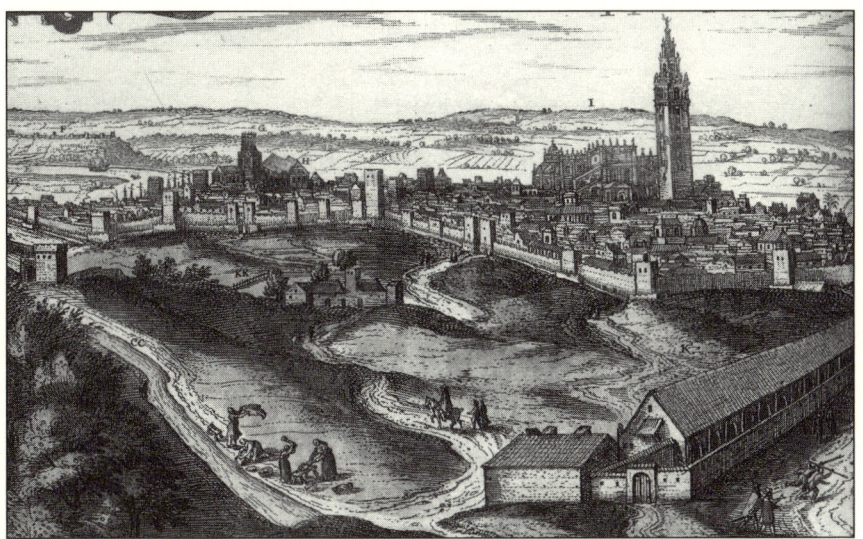

Seville from the east, the slaughterhouse

Detail from Hoefnagle 1565. Georg Braun (plates by Georgius Hoefnagle), *Civitates Orbis Terrarum* (Coloniae Agrippinae, 1572–1618). Library of the Escuela de Estudios Hispanoamericanos, Consejo Superior de Investigaciones Científicas, Seville.

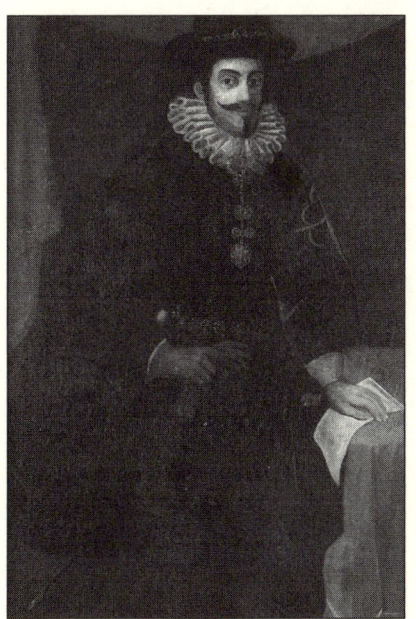

Don Fernando de Torres y Portugal, the Count of Villar

Courtesy of the Museo Nacional de Arqueología Antropología e Historia del Perú.

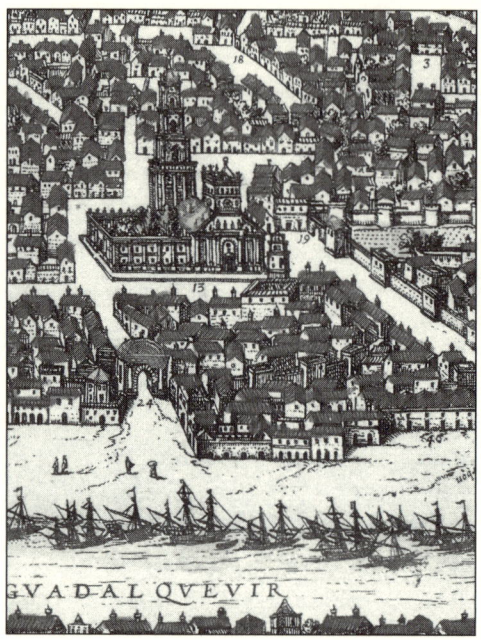

Cathedral and Arenal Gate

Detail from Hoefnagle 1565. Georg Braun (plates by Georgius Hoefnagle), *Civitates Orbis Terrarum* (Coloniae Agrippinae, 1572–1618). Library of the Escuela de Estudios Hispanoamericanos, Consejo Superior de Investigaciones Científicas, Seville.

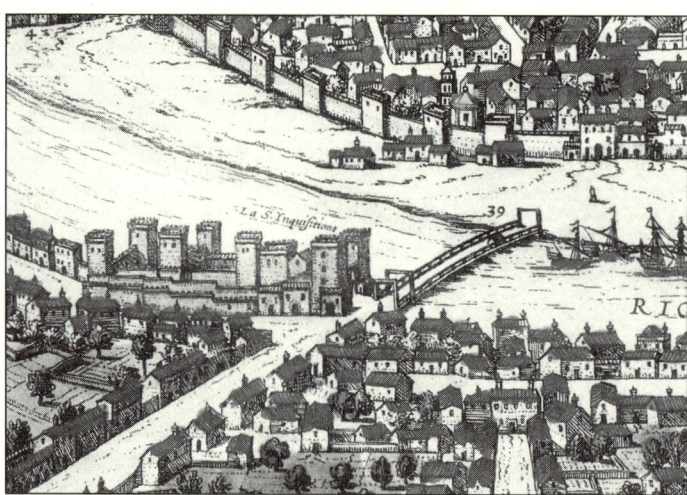

Castle of the Inquisition and Pontoon Bridge

Detail from Hoefnagle 1565. Georg Braun (plates by Georgius Hoefnagle), *Civitates Orbis Terrarum* (Coloniae Agrippinae, 1572–1618). Library of the Escuela de Estudios Hispanoamericanos, Consejo Superior de Investigaciones Científicas, Seville.

19

SOME RECOVER, THE REST DIE

Some recover, and the rest die.
—FRANCISCO GONZÁLEZ PERELLÓN

IEGO DE TOLEDO AND Juan de Perea Durán wrote regular reports to Seville's cabildo informing the governor and the municipal government of their progress. The councilors showed great interest in their envoys' missives, which often generated debates regarding what action to take. Seville's plague commission met on 23 January 1582 in the Count of Villar's residence, and the members who were present listened as letters from Diego de Toledo (still being sent from Constantina) and Licentiate Perea Durán, from Puebla de los Infantes, were read. When the deputies heard the detailed accounts of the numerous cases of the plague that the two men had encountered, they promptly ordered the guards at all the gates leading into Seville to stop any goods coming from Constantina, Puebla, and Cazalla.

On 27 January Licentiate Perea Durán penned another extensive account from Puebla de los Infantes to the Count of Villar, who received it within a couple of days, along with two letters from Constantina. Perea Durán reported that it had been cloudy for the past two days, and during that time "three or four women became sick and were put in the hospital." Consequently there were now eighteen patients, but twelve of them were recovering. Perea Durán lamented that "on this day a very good nurse died, and I have rather felt his absence," as did the patients who apparently were fond of him.

The commissioner had learned the fate of Ana de Rojas, the woman from Puebla who was suspected of having secretly gone to her mother's house in Cordova. Perea Durán informed the count that she had fled from the town "about six days ago, and today I have news that she died in Cordova." Furthermore, various people told him that "three corpses have left her house." He assured the governor that he had alerted Cordova's officials "so that they under-stand that there was a burning fire within."

The count had instructed that no one was to leave town, but Perea Durán pointed out that if the people could not go out to the fields, "they die of hun-ger, by not having anything to do, and most of them are working farmers." He pleaded with the governor to change the policy: "Your Lordship, do not allow these unfortunates to perish." At the end of the missive, he complimented the work of one of the doctors: "I am awaiting Centurio, and it seems to me that with his presence and God's help we will soon have greater health."

Dr. Centurio wrote a separate detailed account to authorities in Seville. He noted that Diego de Toledo had left Constantina on 21 January and that same afternoon two people were taken to the hospital. Shortly thereafter, local of-ficials, "those that they call of the council," confronted Dr. Centurio and "de-manded that I declare the community healthy and free of the plague." They pressed the physician to go to Seville and "give account to Your Lordship of the same." Dr. Centurio was not intimidated and refused: "what I responded to this demand will be evident from the disgust it caused."

Dr. Centurio, in keeping with Hippocratic teaching, was carefully moni-toring the weather conditions and their influence on morbidity: On 23 January "we had very stormy and therefore extremely pernicious air in this place," and that day four people sickened, including a young boy who died on the way to the hospital. The following day, however, "it cleared up once again and hence we did not have more than one [sick]." The belief that the onset of sickness or the end of an epidemic was connected to a particular season and weather condi-tions played an important role in how certain diseases were treated.[1]

Dr. Centurio did not mention the weather when he informed the Count of Villar that on 26 January four people had been brought to the hospital, and the day he was writing his report another five were discovered stricken with the disease. Nevertheless, during the five-day period only the boy had died. Meanwhile, eighteen patients were recovering, though Dr. Centurio remarked it was "not a big deal for a village like this one." In general, however, the doc-tor was less than optimistic, noting that even with all the treatment and "the four breads that are distributed to the said patients, they are dying." Dr. Cen-turio cynically observed that "it would almost be better to let the fury of the

1. See Siraisi, *Medieval Medicine*, 134.

plague flow." At the end of his missive the physician, "as the lowly servant of Your Lordship," could not hold back his contempt for the villagers, stating that he would obey the count's orders and was prepared "to just as easily take these animals as to leave them."[2]

Licentiate González Perellón, Constantina's chief justice, who had been invested with special powers by the central government to combat the plague, wrote to the Count of Villar on the same day as Dr. Centurio. He provided an identical daily tally of the sick as the physician, except on the last day, 27 January, he was aware of only two people becoming sick rather than the five reported by the doctor. González Perellón gloomily informed the governor that "the disease and contagion does not cease, it is somewhat growing," and he added that "some recover, and the rest die." Constantina's official confirmed that the town authorities had followed Dr. Centurio's instructions and burned the infected clothing and had taken the sick to the hospital. The plague costs were rising in Constantina, and González Perellón requested funds from the capital to help the local council.

Seville's cabildo members read the letters, and there was general consensus to authorize the plague commission to take the appropriate action. The councilors had little doubt that the infected towns to the north posed a serious threat to Seville's health, and they were willing to do anything necessary, and spare no expense, "so that it does not return to the city as they had it this past time."[3] They decided that no one from Jerez de los Caballeros, Cazalla de la Sierra, Constantina, or Puebla de los Infantes should be allowed to enter Seville and that those engaged in river transport should be notified. The Count of Villar alerted the gatekeepers to be especially vigilant and ordered a mounted guard to patrol Triana. The cabildo dispatched the town crier to proclaim that no "innkeeper or any other person should give neither bed nor lodging nor any abode" to anyone from the infected towns or buy or receive cloth from them. The city also sent messengers to the countryside to notify the officials and residents there of these measures.[4]

The establishment of a cordon sanitaire around the city presented immediate problems for those whose livelihood depended on commerce. Cazalla de la Sierra was a major wine producer, supplying not only the local market but

2. AMS, sec. 13, siglo XVI, vol. 5 (29 January 1582).

3. Ibid.

4. Ibid. (30 January 1582).

also the Indies fleets. Cazalla's wines were considered "among the most generous that are made in Spain, and both in Seville as well as in the Indies they occupy first place."[5] Wine entering the city was recorded for taxation. Three Sevillians, Pedro de Posadas, Juan García, and Juan Gutiérrez, had about twelve hundred *arrobas* of wine transported from Cazalla, but guards at the Macarena Gate blocked their muleteers as they tried to enter on the last day of January. The men petitioned the following day to have the wine released, arguing that it would spoil if it were not brought into the city for proper storage. The Count of Villar and the plague commission relented and allowed "these persons to bring in the wine, [since] it is being brought by persons of this city, assisted by its beasts of burden." The officials insisted that as soon as the transfer was completed, the men and their animals were to leave the city without delay.

The following day, another Sevillian wine merchant was brought to the cabildo's attention: Gonzalo Martín had just returned from Constantina, and he was sick. Without hesitating, the Count of Villar ordered the justice Licentiate Diego de la Peña to go to the wine merchant's house in the parish of San Gil and investigate. If he found that Gonzalo Martín was "sick with some contagious disease or that he came from the said town," then the justice was to remove the merchant from the city and place him, "with his clothing and bed," in a house away from the city that "was equipped for curing." The count instructed de la Peña to lock up the house if necessary.

Licentiate de la Peña, accompanied by one of the most celebrated surgeons of his time, Bartolomé Hidalgo de Agüero, went that same day to visit Gonzalo Martín. Dr. Hidalgo examined the wine dealer and found that he had "an abscess between the two buttocks and the testicles and it is open." But Martín did not have a fever or any other suspicious symptoms, leading Dr. Hidalgo to conclude that "the sickness is neither contagious nor the plague." Diego de la Peña questioned under oath both the wine merchant and his wife, María Gutiérrez, and they admitted that "on Tuesday it was eight days since he [Gonzalo Martín] came from Constantina." María told Licentiate de la Peña that shortly after he returned her husband "complained that his thigh hurt and that he had chills and fevers."

That was enough for the justice to order Gonzalo Martín to leave the city. De la Peña escorted him to a house outside the Macarena Gate, "the last one of

---

5. Caro, *Antigvedades,* 191r.

the houses on the road," and ordered him to stay there until further notification. The unfortunate wine dealer was soon joined by his wife. The authorities locked up the couple's house, and although María Gutiérrez had a key, she would be unable to enter her home because the door was barred as well. Dr. Hidalgo's diagnosis that Gonzalo Martín's sickness was not the plague did not spare the wine merchant and his wife from being banished from the city.[6] Indeed, Gonzalo Martín and his wife would not receive permission to return to their home until a month later.

Dr. Bartolomé Hidalgo de Agüero, who had studied at the University of Seville, was paid one hundred ducats a year by the city to treat the injured brought to the Cardenal Hospital, and his method of healing wounds and sores earned him both admirers and detractors. He was primarily a surgeon, but the cabildo engaged his services whenever disease threatened, along with the city's other medical practitioners. Dr. Hidalgo's *via particular* of curing open wounds included remedies for tumors and ulcers, but his writings also contained a short treatise on the plague and other contagious diseases, such as typhus and smallpox. His most famous work, *Thesoro de la verdadera cirugía,* was not published until after his death, though an earlier version entitled *Avisos de cirugía contra la común opinión* came out in 1584. Immediately, he was attacked by a fellow surgeon, Dr. Estrada, for propounding false medical doctrine to the detriment of his patients. Dr. Hidalgo had been experimenting for many years with a more soothing way to treat wounds, using ointments and powders rather than the traditional method, which involved "violent instruments and medicines."[7]

Dr. Hidalgo was about fifty-one years old when he went to examine the suspicious wine merchant. His contemporary, Francisco Pacheco, described the surgeon as a "serious person and of great authority, of lively and sharp intellect and clear understanding, of great courage and greatness of spirit, he was

6. AMS, sec. 13, siglo XVI, vol. 5.

7. Pacheco, *Libro de descripción,* 153. For the attack by the surgeon Estrada, see AMS, sec. 3, vol. 7, doc. 75. Dr. Hidalgo was also criticized by Licentiate Fragoso in 1584 for his innovative treatment. See Bartolomé Hidalgo de Agüero, *Thesoro de la verdadera cirugía y la via particular contra la común* (Seville: Francisco Pérez, 1604). See also Antonio Manuel González Díaz, *Poder urbano y asistencia social: El Hospital de San Hermenegildo de Sevilla (1453–1837)* (Seville: Diputación de Sevilla, 1997), 46–49; and Luis S. Granjel, *La medicina española renacentista* (Salamanca, Spain: Universidad de Salamanca, 1980), 37.

graceful and marvelously witty in speaking."[8] Some of the qualities that impressed the painter and humanist were condemned by Enrique Jorge Enríquez, the author of a book entitled *The Portrait of the Perfect Physician*, who complained that "there are some physicians who want more to appear as one than to be one, they always have on the tip of their tongue some witticisms, some sayings."[9] Nevertheless, Dr. Hidalgo would have pleased the author in some respects, including his appearance, as illustrated by his portrait. The ideal physician, according to Licentiate Enríquez, possessed "a good face, not ugly," and he should be well groomed, with his "hair and beard well ordered." There is no way of knowing whether Dr. Hidalgo met another personal hygiene criterion: "the doctor should also strive not to smell badly to the sick."[10]

Licentiate Enríquez believed, in addition, that the ideal doctor should be a good Christian, with good social skills and human qualities. His medical preparation was to be wide ranging and thorough, and he must not only be well read but also possess practical knowledge, because "reason and experience are the feet on which medicine walks, they are the two pillars on which it is founded."[11] Although the medical profession was generally scoffed at, and in the records and literature complaints about dishonest and ignorant barbers and physicians abound, it appears that Bartolomé Hidalgo earned admiration from his numerous patients and many of his colleagues. His reputation for successfully curing head injuries and other serious wounds led to a popular saying, "I commend myself to God and Dr. Hidalgo." His accomplishments at the Cardenal Hospital astounded his contemporaries, and it was said that out of three thousand patients admitted with head wounds during a four-year period, more than two thousand had recovered after being treated with Dr. Hidalgo's new method rather than the traditional and more perilous cure for such injuries, trepanation.[12]

8. Pacheco, *Libro de descripción*, 153. Pacheco's flattering verbal tribute and portrait of his contemporary reflect the esteem the surgeon enjoyed in Seville.

9. Enrique Jorge Enríquez, *Retrato del perfeto médico* (Salamanca, Spain: Casa de Iuan y Andres Renau, 1595) was written by the Portuguese physician in 1582 and was dedicated to his patient, the Duke of Alba. Quoted in Luis S. Granjel, *Médicos españoles* (Salamanca, Spain: Universidad de Salamanca, 1967), 131–32.

10. Quoted in Granjel, *Médicos españoles*, 127.

11. Ibid., 129. For discussion of the work of Licentiate Enríquez, see 125–32.

12. Pacheco, *Libro de descripción*, 154; Antonio Hermosilla Molina, *Cien años de la medicina Sevillana* (Seville: Diputación Provincial, 1970), 526.

On 3 February 1582, the day after Dr. Hidalgo examined the unfortunate wine merchant, the plague commission met in the governor's quarters in the Alcázar once again to discuss the measures to protect the city's health. The commissioners agreed to impose a fine of one hundred thousand maravedís on anyone who entered Seville from the four infected towns. They stipulated that the denouncer would receive one-third of the proceeds, while the other two-thirds were to be evenly divided between the king's treasury and the fund covering plague expenses. The officials ordered some city gates closed, and those that remained open had two guards posted at each. People attempting to enter Seville needed to present proof of where they were traveling from, to ensure that they did not come from the banned places. The conflictive Arenal Gate, which opened onto the riverbank, was to be closed at eleven o'clock at night. Anyone not complying with the orders was to be jailed for six days and fined six reales. The commission, faced with the recurring problem of how to pay for the expenses of protecting the city from the plague, decided to use the sisa revenues to meet the rising expenditures.

During the same meeting the plague commission ordered all physicians, surgeons, barbers, and pharmacists attending anyone with the plague to notify city officials on the first day of treatment or face a fine and exile for four years. The commission also agreed to once again close off the streets of Triana, "as had been done last year," and put gates in place, along with guards chosen from among residents of the district. The officials charged Triana's jurado, Juan Yáñez de Perea, with supervising the activities and admonished him that residents should begin patrolling Triana immediately, "night and day," while the temporary walls were rebuilt. By the end of the day, the town crier, Juan Jiménez, had made public announcements in fourteen different spots in the city, notifying residents of all the new measures and the punishments for noncompliance. The authorities informed most of Seville's physicians, surgeons, barbers, and pharmacists individually.

The plague commission, the cabildo, and the governor were all determined to prevent a recurrence of the disease, and in the following days any suspicious person who might have snuck into Seville or any report of dubious activity was investigated. The authorities paid special attention to Triana, believed to be particularly prone to illegal entry. They commissioned the constable, Cristóbal de Ayala, to patrol its streets and alleys on horseback, "watching and inquiring if any persons and cloth or any other thing that comes from the towns of

Cazalla de la Sierra and Constantina and Puebla de los Infantes and the city of Jerez [de los Caballeros] near Badajoz have entered or enter in the said Triana or pass through it to this city of Seville."[13] At the same time the officials would communicate the new regulations to the towns in question as well as to any points where commerce crossed the Guadalquivir River.

13. AMS, sec. 13, siglo XVI, vol. 5.

20

ENTER AND TRADE

Men can enter and trade in this town without danger of infection.
—SALVADOR ESTEVAN FRISADO

N EAR THE END OF THE DAY of 5 February the Count of Villar announced that he had learned that "in the corral called de la Pastrana in the parish of San Marcos, there are two women who came from the town of Constantina where there is plague." The count ordered the plague commission's notary, Cristóbal Pérez, to investigate. Pérez went to the Corral de la Pastrana the following day and took sworn testimony from Isabel de Fajardo, who lived in the rooming house with her husband. Isabel told the notary that about twelve days earlier she had noticed in the building "two women, one black and the other white," who had come from Constantina; she insisted that they appeared "well and healthy." The women had since left the corral, and Isabel had heard that they might be somewhere in Triana.

Cristóbal Pérez interviewed another resident of the Corral de la Pastrana, María de Torres. She confirmed Isabel de Fajardo's statement and added that the two women had arrived from Constantina about three weeks earlier and that before coming to the corral they had stayed in Triana. María also provided the reason for their visit. They came to "the lodging of a mulatta named Juana who is the daughter of the said black woman." The notary questioned one other person: Lorenza Gutiérrez reiterated the previous testimony but revealed that the two women "left the said corral yesterday" and seemed healthy.

The diligent notary quickly located Juana Mulata, the daughter of Juana de Llerena. She told Pérez that her mother had come to the city from Constantina along with Ana Martín about three weeks earlier. She stated that the two women first went to Triana, to the house of "Domingo de Ochoa, biscuit maker," where Juana Mulata's sister, Francisca Martín, lived. They stayed in

Triana eight days and then came to the Corral de la Pastrana to visit her. Juana assured the notary that both her mother and her companion were healthy and that they had not brought any clothing with them. They remained with her for about two weeks, "until yesterday," when her mother returned to her sister's house in Triana and Ana Martín "went to the house of Rodrigo Manan who lives near Vino Street."

When the Count of Villar learned these details, he sent a constable on horseback to find the women and "take them to the jail of the plague" outside the Macarena Gate. The constable first headed to the house of Rodrigo Manan but found neither Ana Martín nor any information that she had ever been there. When he questioned the residents of the house and their neighbors, they all denied knowing anything about any women from Constantina.

Empty handed, the constable rode toward Triana, crossed the pontoon bridge, turned left, and went directly to the house of the biscuit maker Domingo de Ochoa, who lived on the riverbank, near the Espíritu Santo Convent. Ochoa's wife, Inés de Plata, remembered that about eight days earlier Juana de Llerena had come to the door looking for her daughter Francisca, who worked as a servant in the house. But Inés could not tell the constable where Juana went after she left her house and insisted that she never returned.[1] The trail ended there, and the two women had eluded the authorities. Although all the people who had seen them declared that they appeared healthy, that must have provided little consolation to the Count of Villar and the plague commissioners.

In the meantime, authorities near the principal routes of communication leading into the capital, especially the points where commerce and people crossed the Guadalquivir River, had to be notified of the new regulations. There were few bridges to worry about, but numerous ferries operated on the river, carrying passengers and goods from one side to the other. The town crier in Alcalá del Río publicly proclaimed the council's orders on 3 February; in Lora del Río they were heard the following day, while Cantillana del Río did not learn of the orders until 12 February. The Sevillian cabildo entrusted Diego de Toledo with much of the task of ensuring that Seville's ordinances were obeyed in the rural areas. He inspected the towns of La Algaba and Alcalá del Río on 8 February, admonishing local officials and ferrymen "not to allow any outsid-

---

1. AMS, sec. 13, siglo XVI, vol. 5.

ers to cross without examining them first, even if they carry a deposition of where they came from." All travelers and any clothing they brought were to be detained.

In Alcalá del Río, Toledo learned that not all local officials had been told of the new rules, and he ordered the town council to meet the following morning, threatening to fine anyone absent. The next day the local councilors listened as the latest regulations were read. They also learned that they were required to take turns supervising the ferry. The local authorities ordered all residents to watch the roads leading into and out of the town. No people or merchandise were to pass through.

Diego de Toledo would return when necessary to ensure that town officials complied. On 13 February Toledo inspected Lora del Río and found that the guards of all four gates were performing satisfactorily. But when later in the day he checked up on the town of Tocina, he discovered that in spite of a fine having been levied against the town's magistrate for noncompliance, the local ferryman seemed ignorant as to whether "any person or cloth or another thing from these said parts had crossed on the said ferry." Toledo, infuriated, had the boatman arrested and imprisoned.

The following day Diego de Toledo went to Villanueva del Río, where during an earlier visit he had told the town magistrate Bartolomé García Zamorano to post a guard on the ferry. When he arrived he found to his dismay that García Zamorano had not established a guard either in the town or on the boat passage, nor had he "ordered anything done." Toledo demanded that the town's officials comply with the regulations and admonished them, in the name of Seville and His Majesty, "and the universal good of his kingdoms and the republic of the said city of Seville," to do it diligently. The boatman was to be particularly vigilant regarding any "poor beggar" and to make sure that none crossed on the ferry, even if he showed a certificate that he came from a healthy place, "because it has been seen by experience that they are the people who carry the said contagion and have greater disposition for it."[2]

The Count of Villar's edict that no person, cloth, wine, or foodstuff from infected towns was to enter Seville also reached the places in question. On 8 February the town crier, Gaspar Pérez, proclaimed the order in the public plaza of Cazalla de la Sierra. The punishment for disobeying the command was

2. Ibid.

high and differed according to class. A "gentleman" faced a fine of one hundred thousand maravedís, while "others of low quality" would receive two hundred lashes. All, regardless of their status, were in theory condemned to four years in the galleys, but it is likely that a "gentleman" would find a way to avoid such service.

That same day in the afternoon, the count's messenger, Juan Sánchez, approached Constantina, informing guards that he was carrying letters and other documents from the "Count Governor" in Seville. Because the town was under quarantine, he waited outside at a place called Fuente del Tejar, to be met later by local officials to whom he handed the papers. The town's magistrate, Juan Fernández, acted immediately, announcing publicly that "no person of any estate or condition" could travel to Seville, regardless of whether they were "vecinos, residents, transients or visitors" in Constantina. The count's courier had to wait until the following day, when between six and seven in the morning he was handed "sealed papers tied with a string" to be delivered to the governor in Seville. The other town that was quarantined, Puebla de los Infantes, learned of the Count of Villar's orders on 9 February.

After the messenger delivered the edicts and collected missives for the governor, he sped back to Seville. On Sunday, 11 February, the Count of Villar read the letters informing him that his orders had been proclaimed and updating him on the situation in Cazalla and Constantina. In the letter from Cazalla, Benito de Baena assured the governor that "the place is better." He reported that in the pesthouse there were only five sick, "very poor"; many people had recovered, and only a few had died. But he stressed the financial difficulties that the local city council was facing because "it is so poor." Indeed, he was unable to collect enough alms to defray mounting costs, and he begged the count "to order that some money be distributed in this place in order to be able to cure the poor."

The letter from Francisco González Perellón, Constantina's chief justice, was also dated 8 February and was more optimistic than his previous communication almost two weeks earlier. Although there had been an increase in the number of sick, he noted an improvement during the last two days. He told the count that he had taken special care to carry out all the orders and had "burned a lot of clothing [and] proclaimed that there should be no assemblies of people, school or studies, or the public house." Licentiate González Perellón assured the governor that anyone who was plague stricken was taken to the hospital "without excepting anyone." He declared that he had followed Dr. Centurio's recommendation and moved the pesthouse to a better place and locked up many houses, placing signs on their doors warning of plague inside. González Perellón mentioned that "there are many people who went to their properties in the countryside," confirming that those who had the means fled, while the poor remained at the mercy of the plague and sanitary authorities. Constantina's chief justice did express "the great fear that I have and the whole community regarding the lack of sustenance" that resulted from the interruption of commerce.

The third missive brought to the Count of Villar came from Dr. Centurio. The doctor was unsure whether his previous report had reached the governor, though he was certain that "it arrived in Seville." The physician detailed the day-to-day progress of the disease in Constantina since his last letter, indicating the number of new cases by date:

January 27	2
" 28	4
" 29	5
" 30	3
" 31	2
February 1	2
" 2	2
" 3	1
" 4	7
" 5	2
" 6	1
" 7	0
" 8	0

Dr. Centurio's list confirmed González Perellón's affirmation that the number of cases was diminishing. The physician was cautiously optimistic: "the respite of these two days invigorated and comforted the people of this land," and he added that "there is hardly anyone who does not say victory for Constantina." The doctor admitted that he would himself be tempted to "say the same, if the weather (of which I still cannot be certain) would give me guarantees to stay from here on as it has been these past two days." Dr. Centurio acknowledged that someone stricken by the plague might be secretly hidden in the community, but he assured the governor that he had been as diligent as possible in locating the sick. He lamented that "only the chief justice helps me in this cause" because the rest were not distressed "to see their community with pestilence." Rather, they were more concerned with "seeing themselves with the burden of being subjected to controls and some expenses." Dr. Centurio's contempt for the locals was barely disguised as he complained that "a large multitude of people, even the physician, went to the fields and mountains, awaiting from afar what will become of us."

The count also received letters from Puebla de los Infantes. Licentiate Perea Durán informed the governor that there were fourteen plague-stricken patients in the hospital, some in critical condition, and seven people were convalescing. Four others were being treated in their homes, and there was much hope for their recovery, because the licentiate Juan Sosa Sotomayor, "with good spirit and Christianity came in time with a remedy and medicines to cure them." Perea Durán insisted that contrary to what was being said, no one was dying at present. He assured the count that his orders were being followed and told him that he had just permitted cattle to enter the town, since fresh meat was considered beneficial. Licentiate Perea Durán complained about tax collectors from Seville vexing Puebla's residents. He was especially incensed about one Benito Falcón, who had come the previous day, disregarding the prohibitions about entering the plague-stricken community. Falcón was now in prison, and Perea Durán vouched he would jail anyone else who tried to enter Puebla.

The second missive from Puebla de los Infantes came from Licentiate Sosa de Sotomayor, who echoed Perea Durán's report. The physician observed that it seemed to him that those treated at the outset of their sickness had a better chance of survival, and he bemoaned the fact that at first the outbreak had been underestimated. The doctor praised the quality of the medicines sent from Seville and assured the governor that "the whole community understands very well the favor that Your Lordship is bestowing upon them."[3]

As the number of new cases dropped, officials in infected towns attempted to convince the Count of Villar and the central authorities in Seville to lift the quarantine that was devastating the local economy. The municipal council of Cazalla de la Sierra set up a commission to collect testimony from clerics and physicians and authorized it to send the report to the governor. The commission met on Monday, 19 February, ready to record sworn depositions.

3. Ibid.

The first witness, a sixty-year-old physician from Cazalla, Hernán Vázquez Bocanegra, who possessed the lowest university title of bachelor (*bachiller*), testified that in the past week he "had cured certain sick with pleurisy and fevers." He claimed that at present he had only three patients, all of whom were rapidly improving. The doctor swore that he "had not seen nor cured anyone sick with the said diseases (plague or other contagious disease)" and was certain that there were none in the town, because "if there were this witness would know it."

Next to testify was a thirty-year-old surgeon, Andrés Gutiérrez, who declared that although there had been plague earlier, the town "is now much better." He added that he did not have any more plague patients and knew from talking to other physicians that there were some people sick with the usual fevers but nothing more serious. The surgeon substantiated what the local authorities wanted to hear: the greatest threat to the community was "hunger as a result of the provisions not coming to this town, with which they usually sustain themselves."

The third witness was also a physician. The forty-year-old bachiller Salvador Estevan Frisado acknowledged that "since Christmas of the year 1581 there had been a disease of plague and typhus in this town," noting that only "very poor and miserable people" died from these. He concurred with the previous witnesses that the disease had "diminished" and commented that none of his patients were sick with "the said diseases." Bachiller Frisado affirmed "that men from the outside can enter and trade in this town without danger of infection" and agreed that lack of food posed the greatest threat to the community, which was dependent on outside trade for its sustenance.

The same day, the local clergy also voiced their confidence that Cazalla was a healthy and a safe place to engage in commerce. Alvaro de Valero categorically stated that "for more than eight days" there had been no contagious disease present. He testified that neither he nor the other priests had to administer the last rites to the sick. Indeed, the enthusiastic cleric proclaimed that it "has been more than fifteen years since there were fewer sick in this town and more health." Bachiller Valero too stressed that the few people who had died were "very poor and the lack of sustenance caused them to die."

The parish priest of Cazalla's principal church, fifty-year-old Pedro Gallego, also testified. Like the other witnesses, he stated what local authorities wanted to hear: there was absolutely no plague at present, and he added that he had not been called "to confess, give communion or administer extreme unction, nor has any person been buried." The priest not only attested to the seriousness of the food shortage but also pointed out that the supplies were not coming to Cazalla because "of the bad reputation that has been imposed on this said town, which is uncertain and untrue." Another cleric, Diego Sánchez Cornado, corroborated the testimony of the others, stressing that those who had died in recent days were poor and perished "from pure hunger and lack of sustenance." He too insisted that the current "reputation of contagious disease had been untrue." Seven more witnesses were questioned, all of whom provided similar evidence, buttressing the town council's position. Clearly, there was no more plague, and therefore Sevillian authorities should lift the quarantine and allow food supplies in and permit resumption of regular trade. The sworn depositions, along with a petition asking to have Cazalla declared healthy, were dispatched to Seville.

Unfortunately, even before the petition reached Seville, there was evidence that the plague not only continued in many of the infected towns but had spread to other places, "and all are close to this city." At the same time, Sevillian authorities were concerned that some city gates were not being well guarded. The governor therefore ordered that the gates should be even more carefully watched and that any citizen not taking his turn should be fined one ducat for each day that he missed serving. He recommended that each open gate should be supervised by a jurado and a veinticuatro.[4]

Other potential sites of infection came to light during Diego de Toledo's inspection. On Wednesday, 14 February, while visiting the town of Alcolea, he learned from its governor, Diego de Frías, that "the said disease is present in the towns of Guadalcanal, Alanís, and San Nicolás del Puerto." The Count of Villar immediately ordered Diego de Toledo to return to Alcolea to take testimony. He arrived there on 20 February; as he questioned the locals he learned that a certain Pedro de Voz Mediano, who was traveling through Alcolea on his way from Lora del Río to Seville, had said that the three towns were infected. Because of his statement, Alcolea's officials had posted guard, even though they had no other reports corroborating the traveler's assertion. Soon there would be other notices of the spreading plague.

4. Ibid. (17 February 1582).

21

LOOKING DEATH IN THE EYE

People have become very frightened having looked death in the eye.
—JUAN DE PEREA DURÁN

DESPITE THE OPTIMISTIC REPORTS from Constantina, Cazalla, and Puebla, disquieting news reached Seville at almost the same time. The Count of Villar announced in the cabildo on 21 February that Castilblanco de los Arroyos "has been again struck," and many people had sickened and died. The news was especially worrisome because of Castilblanco's proximity to Seville: the small town lies just a few kilometers north of the city. As in the case of the other places where the plague had been reported, the cabildo sent a commissioner to the affected area to investigate and to ensure that all the proper steps were being taken to combat the disease. The jurado Rodrigo Sánchez de Soria would be paid one thousand maravedís a day, and he would be accompanied by a constable, whose daily salary was five hundred maravedís, and a notary, who would earn four hundred maravedís. Who would be responsible for these men's payment depended on whether or not they found "the said disease." If there was plague in Castilblanco, their costs would be covered from the town's own properties and rents. If, however, the inspector did not find any contagious disease, then the payment would come from Seville's treasury.

On Thursday, 22 February, the plague commission met in the count's apartments; those present included Diego de Toledo, "jurado commissioner of the business of the plague," who had returned from his tour of inspection. There were three major items on the agenda. First, Diego Caballero de Cabrera argued that so much commerce was coming into the city that guarding the gates alone was not enough. The alderman proposed that guards should also be posted on the roads. Second, the commission planned to consider the testimony of good health sent from Cazalla de la Sierra. Finally, Diego de Toledo reported on the situation at the river crossings at Villanueva del Río, Cantillana, Alcalá del Río, La Algaba, and other places. Veinticuatro Caballero pressed the commission to send one jurado with two or three arquebusiers to establish more-effective guard at critical points, including the ferry crossings at Villanueva, Alcalá, and the Bodegón de las Cañas.

The plague commissioners discussed at length the report sent from Cazalla de la Sierra. Don Pedro de Céspedes suggested they should respond by saying how pleased they were to hear of the good health reigning in the town. But he cautioned that before lifting the commerce ban, they should send a letter to Cazalla's chief justice, requesting more information. Don Pedro also proposed that the plague commission send a secret inspector to the town to ascertain whether the threat of contagion had indeed passed. At the end of his intervention, Don Pedro de Céspedes voiced his support for Diego Caballero's motion and recommended that Don Diego write the letters to Cazalla. All the others attending the meeting assented. Diego de Toledo agreed but added that the jurado named to oversee the ferry at Alcalá del Río should also supervise "the roads that lead into this city." He also advised that in the letter to Cazalla they should inquire what had been done with all the clothing from the hospital.

In the general cabildo session the following day, the actions of the commission were ratified. The councilors added to the previous day's list a jurado to guard at El Garrobo. The high price of grain and food in general was affecting mounted guards, whose horses were fed with barley: they would now receive twelve reales a day, but they were admonished to keep track of their exact expenses. Regarding the letter to Cazalla de la Sierra, the councilors insisted that the town officials needed to send further testimony from physicians, pharmacists, clerics, and local convents to ensure that the report was trustworthy. Once again the municipal council members wrestled with fiscal matters, complicated by debts accrued during the prior plague outbreak. They decided to send an account of all the accumulated costs to the royal council and to Don Gonzalo de Saavedra, the cabildo's representative in Madrid. The city furthermore demanded that the towns and villages within Seville's jurisdiction assist in covering the current plague expenses.

Licentiate Perea Durán, who was still in Puebla de los Infantes, penned a new missive to the Count of Villar on 20 February. Unlike his previous letter of 9 February, which indicated some improvement, his present report was far from optimistic. It appears that the day after he sent his earlier dispatch, conditions had worsened. He related that from 10 to 12 February, "this disease attacked us with such force that in a very short time it killed twelve or thirteen people, and infected as many more." Since then, "every day there is one or two to be buried." Perea Durán noted the psychological effect the disease was having: "people have become very frightened having looked death in the eye." Shortages of food and other necessities contributed to a rise in crime. Perea Durán informed the count that "they have begun to rob houses and estates," observing that "it is very common in times of need." The situation was aggravated by the absence of the magistrate, who was "busy in Constantina." Perea Durán complained that because there was no one who punished the criminals, "the malefactors are exerting themselves to multiply their evil doing." He ended his missive reporting that there were ten or twelve sick in the hospital, and six patients were recovering in the convalescent house. He again praised the doctor, who, in spite of the difficulties, "cures many and there are many good outcomes." Furthermore, "the medicines are very good and have benefitted notably."[1]

While learning of the tribulations of the residents of Puebla de los Infantes, the Count of Villar and the cabildo were waiting for news from Castilblanco de los Arroyos. Jurado Sánchez de Soria had left the city along with constable Antonio de Luna and a notary, and they reached the countryside one half league outside Castilblanco on Friday, 23 February. There, before entering the town itself, the jurado cautiously conducted "a field inquiry."

The first witness was a local resident, Bartolomé Gómez. He stated that approximately fifteen days earlier the body of a man had been discovered about a quarter league outside Castilblanco and that he may have come from "Jerez de Badajoz" in Extremadura.[2] The corpse was brought into the town and buried in the Church of La Magdalena, adjacent to a hospital. Gómez added that he had heard that the man had died of the plague. Furthermore, he had seen that within two or three days after the man's burial, the *hospitalera* (hospital worker) and her daughter suddenly died, and it was rumored that the cause was the plague, "because the said woman put on a shirt of the said dead man and had gotten the plague." He commented that the hospital caretaker had infected her daughter, and they both perished. Since then, about three or four days ago, a Morisco, his wife, and his two daughters had died suddenly; they had gone to

1. AMS, sec. 13, siglo XVI, vol. 5.
2. Jerez de los Caballeros.

bed at night and were found dead the next morning, and again the rumor was that they had the plague.

The investigator from Seville certainly found an excellent source of information in Bartolomé Gómez, who told him not only how many people had perished but their names as well. He stated that "yesterday, Thursday," Alonso Esteban died, and plague was suspected. Three or four days earlier, Francisco Benítez, a vecino of Castilblanco, had been brought into town with "a carbuncle on one leg and two days later he died." Benítez's son also perished, although the opinions regarding the cause were divided: some claimed he had died of pleurisy, while others insisted it was the plague. The witness further testified that he had seen local justices lock up one or two houses where people had died, but he could not tell the jurado what had happened to the clothing of the dead.

One other witness came to the fields outside Castilblanco. Francisco de Brenes, the administrator of the hospital, provided slightly different testimony. He did not mention a dead man found outside the town, but he stated that the locals had brought into Castilblanco a woman, a stranger, and put her in the hospital. He heard the barber say that the woman had "a lump in the back of her neck." She died in the hospital, and it was her shirt that the hospitalera had put on. Francisco de Brenes confirmed that both the hospital worker and her daughter had died. He mentioned that about fifteen days earlier three Moriscos had perished—a man, his wife, and one son. Within a day and a half two more Moriscos succumbed, though "it was said that it was of hunger." The witness also knew about Francisco Benítez and confirmed that he had died of "a carbuncle that appeared on his leg"; he also revealed that Benítez's clothing was still in his house. Before finishing his testimony, Brenes told Rodrigo Sánchez de Soria that beds were kept in the hospital and were normally used for patients who suffered from "fevers."

The testimony of the two men sufficed to convince Sánchez de Soria that he needed to investigate further. Rather than flee, the brave jurado and his team promptly entered the town to collect more evidence. They went to the inn of Juan Pérez, and after they settled in, they questioned a local barber surgeon, Francisco Díaz. The barber confirmed the hospitalera's death but insisted that she suffered from "kidney disease." He was unable to explain why her daughter perished so quickly after her mother. The barber remembered that a few days before the hospital worker died a woman was brought to the hospital from outside the town who later perished, though he could not tell the investigators "what disease she died from." Francisco Díaz did corroborate that Francisco Benítez had died about ten days earlier "from a carbuncle that he had on the right leg on the knee," and his eight-year-old son had perished a few days earlier. The barber said he did not treat the boy, because he died so suddenly. The barber also revealed that another vecino of Castilblanco, Gregorio García, had died and that he had displayed "a lump in the manner of a bubo under his left armpit."

The barber also mentioned the death of the three Moriscos, but since he had not treated the family he was unable to tell the jurado any details of their ailment, other than that they were all dead within twelve days. Francisco Díaz affirmed that another Morisca died in town, but again he could not provide details. The barber corroborated that the local officials had locked up the houses of the dead, "saying that it was the plague," and that they relocated the hospital outside the town. The barber knew no more, save that he had been treating a young man "who is sick with fevers" and that "yesterday, Thursday, the 22nd . . . another man, a shepherd, died," and he had been ill a long time.

After Rodrigo Sánchez de Soria finished questioning the barber, he turned to the innkeeper, Bartolomé Pérez. The *mesonero* (innkeeper) was able to shed more light on the deaths of the Moriscos, Diego Martín and his wife Marina de Vera, because they lived on the same street as he did. Pérez recalled that some fifteen days earlier, on a Friday, Marina had brought water to his house, and she was "well and healthy, without any sickness"; suddenly, by Sunday morning, she was dead, "and they said she died of the plague." Then, three days after Marina perished, one of her children died, though "it is unknown of what," and on the following Sunday, Diego Martín was dead as well. Local officials said they had all died of the plague, and their house was locked and barred.

The jurado also questioned the innkeeper's wife, Catalina Pérez. She remembered a healthy-looking Marina bringing water to her house. Regarding the sudden demise of her neighbors, her testimony was similar to that of her husband, although she stated that two of the couple's children perished. Catalina added that the four Moriscos were buried outside Castilblanco, near San Sebastián. The innkeeper's wife had discussed all the unexpected deaths in town with Francisco Díaz, the barber, and her deposition reflected that. She provided one detail the others had missed: the stranger found dead in the fields was bringing hogs from Jerez de los Caballeros. The curious woman had asked the barber, "what did that man die of, because they say that he was killed?" The barber answered, "look señora, he only died because of the bubo he had."

Diego Martín and his wife Marina had another daughter, nineteen-year-old Juana Martín, who was married to a Morisco, Alonso García. Juana stated that her parents, her sister, and her brother Juan had all been well and then suddenly, within three days, "all were sick in bed." Juana insisted that she never went to visit her family during this time, "rather she fled from them, because it was said that they were sick with the plague." She told the jurado that as soon as they died "the justice came and locked the door." Rodrigo Sánchez de Soria asked Juana what happened to the bedding, and she stated that they only had "a blanket and a sheet." The sheet was used as a burial shroud for her brother, and the blanket was taken to the house of her aunt, called La Ballestera, along with some clothing. Juana divulged that her mother had left some "old blue skirts" and that her grandmother, Leonor de Vera, had taken them. She finished her testimony revealing that "yesterday, Thursday," a six-year-old boy died, the son of Guzmán Morisco, and he only "lasted three days," but she did not know what had caused his death.

When Jurado Sánchez de Soria heard that infected clothing had been taken by relatives, he and his team tried to find the people as quickly as possible. They hastened to where Leonor de Vera, Marina's mother, reputedly lived. There they only found the proprietress of the house, Magdalena Ferré, who informed the investigators that Leonor had left her house about six days earlier, "with all her clothing." Magdalena stated that "a neighbor who lives across the street" warned her not to let Leonor in the house because "she was carrying clothing in which Diego Martín, his wife and children had died." As a result, Leonor left and went to Alcalá del Río, "to the house of one of her daughters." Unfortunately, Magdalena did not know the daughter's name, nor exactly where in Alcalá the house was located.

The commissioners then went to the house of the Morisca Ballestera, who presumably had the blanket in which Diego Martín, her brother-in-law, had died. This time the investigators were successful. When they entered the house, they found "the said Morisca with an eight-year-old boy in her arms." The child was sick, and when they asked the woman what was wrong with him, she responded that she did not know, other than that the night before he was well, and suddenly "he got pain in one eye, a fever and vomited." The men looked at the boy and the notary certified that his "left eye was all swollen, he was not speaking and was vomiting." When the jurado had ascertained how sick the boy was, he sent for the barber surgeon Francisco Díaz to examine him and make a statement about his condition. Jurado Sánchez de Soria also ordered constable Antonio de Luna to remove from the woman "the blanket and the other clothing that was with her in order to burn them."

Antonio de Luna found the barber and ordered him to see the sick boy. To make certain that the barber obeyed, he threatened him with a fine of ten thousand maravedís. With that incentive, Francisco Díaz rushed to La Ballestera's house and examined the child. His diagnosis was not helpful. The barber stated flatly that he "did not know what caused the sickness." He found the boy "without speech, with a high fever and the left eye swollen." He described the swelling as "very black with a very large ring in it" and added that the boy's lips were black and blue. The barber concluded that he "cannot determine nor say what disease he has, other than that it seems to him to be dangerous." The barber's report, though inconclusive, sufficed to convince Jurado Sánchez de Soria to isolate the sick boy and his mother. He ordered the local constables to lock up the house and take "Ballestera Morisca and the boy, her son and the bedding" to the hospital.

The following day, Saturday, 24 February, the investigators returned to Juana Martín to take additional testimony. This time Juana provided more detail. She revealed that her sister Isabel had cared for their mother and father when they fell sick. Then, two or three days after the parents died, Isabel too became sick and went to her aunt La Ballestera's house to recuperate. But she died and left there the blanket and some of her father's clothing. The primary reason why the commissioners needed to talk to Juana again was to find out where her grandmother, Leonor de Vera, could have gone to in Alcalá del Río. Juana claimed not to know the name of Leonor's daughter, but she knew where she lived: "next to the Corral del Consejo in a small house." She was married to a Morisco, but Juana did not know the husband's name, either. This promising information would be followed up in due time.

In the meantime, Jurado Sánchez de Soria continued questioning as many people as he could in Castilblanco de los Arroyos. That same Saturday he located Leonor de Vera's son, Alonso. Alonso could not tell the investigators much about the deaths of his sister Marina and his brother-in-law because he was out of town when they died. But he confirmed that his mother was living with his sister in Alcalá del Río, and the commissioners finally learned the sister's name:

Beatriz Fernández. Alonso could not verify her address because he did not know it, other than that she lived in Alcalá. When asked whether Beatriz had visited Marina, Alonso replied that she had come to see her sister when she heard she was sick, but when she arrived Marina was already dead. According to Alonso, Beatriz returned home the next day.

There was another barber surgeon in town, Martín del Pozo, and the jurado questioned him that same day. Martín del Pozo had treated some of the dead, and his report of the symptoms was more precise. He stated that Francisco Benítez had a high fever and "on his left leg on the outer part of the knee, he had a carbuncle"; having carefully examined it, "it seemed to him to be pestilential." Benítez's twelve-year-old son had died earlier, and his body was still in the house when the surgeon visited. He noticed that the boy had "some black-and-blues on the legs, on his thigh," and he heard that he had died within two or three days of the symptoms appearing. Martín del Pozo pronounced that Gregorio García's cause of death was "a large tumor or bubo under the arm." The hospitalera and her daughter had died of "an indisposition from having worn certain clothing from a man who had been found dead."

Martín del Pozo had been called to see Marina de Vera when she became sick. The surgeon made the Morisca remove her clothes "and found her full of spots." He concluded that she suffered from typhus. At the same time, her husband, Diego Martín, was in bed with "a great headache and other great pain," and three days after the surgeon's visit he was dead. Martín del Pozo remembered the couple's daughter, who seemed well at the time and was taking care of her parents. Shortly after they died she too fell sick, and since she was alone she was taken to her aunt La Ballestera's house, where she died within two days. Furthermore, the surgeon had seen La Ballestera's young son after he and his mother had been taken outside the city. The boy had died on Friday, shortly after arriving at the hospital. The surgeon saw that he had "a ruptured abscess on the left eyelid and the eye white from the ruptured abscess." There was no doubt in Martín del Pozo's mind: it was "a pestilential abscess."

After taking the deposition from Martín del Pozo, the investigators wanted to talk to the widows of the two men who had died recently in Castilblanco. First, they searched out Isabel Ferré, the widow of Gregorio García. After her husband's death, Isabel had moved to another house, just up the street. She could not say what Gregorio died of, and as far as any garments and bedding,

Isabel claimed that there was very little. According to the widow, her husband "did not have more clothing than a coat and a mantelet and some old dark breeches and a hat." And the bed in which he died consisted of "a mattress made of wool and a sheet and an old blanket." Isabel insisted that there was nothing more. Apparently the items were still in the house, and Jurado Sánchez de Soria ordered their removal.

The commissioners then went to find Leonor Pérez, the widow of Francisco Benítez, who had lost not only her husband but her young son as well. The widow's description of her husband's affliction was more detailed than that of the barber surgeons. Francisco was sick for about five or six days, she reported, and had "a carbuncle on the left leg next to the knee, and on the same side on his genitals he had a swelling in the manner of a bubo which descended with a red line." Their son had a "headache and a fever" for about four or five days before he died. When asked about clothing and bedding, the widow replied that her husband "was very poor and did not have a bed," though he did have a blanket. As for clothing, Francisco left some old breeches and a coat, and Leonor was keeping it all "in the courtyard of her house."

As in the case of Gregorio García, the jurado ordered the meager possessions of Francisco Benítez to be removed and burned outside of town, and he charged local Moriscos with transporting the infected items to the fields. There were separate orders for the burning of all the goods, and everything was carefully inventoried to prevent townspeople from appropriating them for their own use or for sale. After everything was carried out of the houses, the doors were locked and, for added security, "nailed shut."

The following day, Sunday, 25 February, the commissioners completed their business in Castilblanco. Jurado Sánchez de Soria concluded that the town was "sick and stricken with this disease of the plague and is contagious" and mandated the usual measures when plague was suspected. He commanded that a pesthouse staffed by a barber and nurses be established outside the town and be supplied with the necessary medicines. The jurado also recommended that a convalescent hospital be set up. He admonished local officials to ensure that physicians, barbers, and pharmacists did not leave town. Sánchez de Soria stipulated that houses of the plague dead be locked up and their clothing and bedding burned. Finally, the jurado ordered all commerce to cease until further notice. Castilblanco's councilors called an emergency meeting to hear Sánchez de Soria's report and recommendations. They promised to follow the orders and decided to name the hospital Santa Lucía. The town crier soon publicly proclaimed the new regulations.

The Seville team was preparing to leave Castilblanco de los Arroyos in hopes of locating Leonor de Vera, who allegedly had gone to stay with her daughter, Beatriz Fernández, in Alcalá del Río. But before they left, the barber surgeon Martín del Pozo reappeared to report that another person had become sick that day: a Morisca named Luisa, who had dealings with La Ballestera and had "entered the house of the said Diego Martín Morisco." Jurado Sánchez de Soria ordered her removal to a pesthouse and sent Martín del Pozo to examine her and file a report on her condition. The surgeon went to see the woman in the hospital that same night. He found Luisa with high fever and vomiting and discovered that she had "a bubo on the right side of the genitals." The surgeon pronounced her "on the brink of death" and declared that she had the plague. He was sure of his diagnosis and insisted that he had experience treating the disease a few years earlier, when there was plague in Utrera, and therefore he recognized its symptoms. Martín del Pozo warned that great care must be taken because "every day they are being stricken."

The following day, Monday, 26 February, Jurado Sánchez de Soria and his team reached Alcalá del Río. They located Beatriz Fernández's house next to the church and hospital of San Gregorio, and there they finally found Leonor de Vera. She denied that she had brought any of her daughter Marina's clothes from Castilblanco, but the jurado was not convinced. Several witnesses, including Leonor's children, had told him that she had taken certain items after Marina's death, and he ordered the house searched. Nothing was found. Nevertheless, because the commissioners had information that both Leonor and Beatriz were in Marina's house while she was sick, the jurado ordered both women to leave Alcalá "with all their belongings" and return to Castilblanco, warning them that if they disobeyed they would be punished.

Rodrigo Sánchez de Soria was determined to isolate Castilblanco de los Arroyos to prevent the spread of contagion. That is why he sent both women back to the town, believing that would protect the inhabitants of Alcalá del Río and, more important, Seville. At the same time he instructed the ferryman in Alcalá not to carry across the river any goods or people coming from Castilblanco. The town was now blacklisted, along with Cazalla de la Sierra, Constantina, and

Puebla de los Infantes.[3] With the location of Leonor de Vera, the jurado and his team felt they had accomplished their mission. They had spent four days questioning witnesses and tracking people who had contact with suspected plague victims, and Rodrigo Sánchez de Soria issued the pertinent orders. It was time for him to return to Seville and inform the Count of Villar and the cabildo.

3. AMS, sec. 13, siglo XVI, vol. 5.

22

JUMPING OVER THE WALL

We have jumped over the wall to confess them.

—THE PRIESTS OF SAN VICENTE

TTEMPTS TO PROTECT THE CITY and establish quarantine had immediate repercussions in Seville, a major commercial magnet with an unceasing flow of goods and people on both land and the river. Muleteers, or carters with their oxen, were bringing in food and other necessities daily to satisfy the citizens' needs. The Indies trade generated a stream of travelers and merchants as well as ships' crews. Sevillians owned vineyards, orchards, olive groves, or just garden plots outside the city, some as far as away as Cazalla de la Sierra. Many laborers who worked on these properties or administrators who supervised the planting or the harvest also lived in the city. It was not unusual for Sevillians to leave the city walls to collect wine, vinegar, or olive oil to bring back to Seville. Families were dispersed, and relatives visited each other often. To stop this traffic was impossible, and the measures designed to keep contagion out caused hardships and delays as people tried to go about their usual business. Travelers were supposed to carry certificates proving that they were not coming from infected areas, and many did have the necessary papers. But probably just as many bribed their way into the city or falsified their documents. Furthermore, people often successfully petitioned to circumvent these orders, especially if they were able to prove that they had not come into contact with the disease.

Many individuals were affected by the quarantine. Toward the end of February the recently married Juan Bautista needed to petition the authorities in order to collect his bride's dowry. Juana de Vergara was the daughter of a farmer who lived behind the Monastery of the Santísima Trinidad, east of the city outside the Sol Gate. Unfortunately for the groom, a large part of the dowry consisted of clothing and bedding, and when Juan Bautista attempted to enter the city with these goods, the guards stopped him and refused to allow the items in. Undeterred, Juan Bautista petitioned the governor for permission to bring his wife's dowry to their house in Seville. After several witnesses corroborated the truth of the request and, more important, insisted that there was no contagious disease at the farm, Juan Bautista was granted the pertinent license.[1]

The Count of Villar received another petition at this time. The unfortunate wine merchant Gonzalo Martín, who had been banished from the city in January and whose house had been locked up in spite of a medical certificate stating that his sickness was not the plague, had fully recovered. On 24 February he begged the count to permit him to return home. He complained bitterly that he had been taken outside the Macarena Gate and forced to remain in a designated house, even though he had only "a tumor that appeared on his buttock" and not the plague as the magistrate had alleged. Moreover, although authorities had locked his house in Seville, thieves had broken in and "robbed what I had in it." Gonzalo Martín lamented his fate, decried his poverty, and claimed to be "dying of hunger" because he and his family had nothing to eat where they were being kept. He assured the governor that the tumor was gone and that he was perfectly healthy, as Dr. Bartolomé Hidalgo would surely confirm. The wine merchant pleaded with the count to allow him to go home and begged him for a "favor and alms."

Four days later Dr. Hidalgo testified that he had examined Gonzalo almost one month earlier and had seen him again six days ago and that the wine merchant was now healthy. He insisted that Gonzalo Martín never had the plague, only a harmless tumor. This time the prominent surgeon's testimony sufficed to secure Gonzalo's release and permission to return to home.

Several days later, Luis de la Serna petitioned the Count of Villar to permit his servant Christóbal Palomo and his mules to enter the city. Palomo traveled regularly between Seville, Valladolid, and Palencia in the north of Spain, transporting merchandise for his master. This time he had been on the road for more than two weeks and was bringing in wheat from Valladolid and blankets from Palencia. He had returned through Cordova and Tocina but had been stopped at Casaluenga, an outpost in the jurisdiction of La Rinconada, not far to the north of Seville. Bernaldino Ramírez, charged with guarding the place, would not let him and his mules pass through because he did not carry proof

1. AMS, sec. 13, siglo XVI, vol. 5 (20–21 February 1582).

that "Palencia was healthy," as required. The petition included testimony by Christóbal Palomo, who swore that he had traveled for some seventeen or eighteen days and that he did not go through any infected parts. Without further investigation, the count authorized the man and his merchandise to enter Seville, an indication of the arbitrariness of quarantine measures.[2]

As spring approached, the threat of plague did not fade. When the plague commission met at the Count of Villar's lodgings on 1 March they again faced a variety of issues both within the city and out in the countryside. Among the most important items on the agenda was Rodrigo Sánchez de Soria's report on the situation in Castilblanco de los Arroyos. The commissioners agreed to take several steps; no person or cloth from the town was to enter Seville, and the deputies decided to send a physician to the beleaguered community. Three days later the count named the licentiate Melchior de Rojas to go to Castilblanco to treat the sick until "God, our Lord is served that there is no longer the said disease in the said town." He was to take with him from Seville the necessary medicines, and his salary, which was to be paid by Castilblanco, was to be equal that of Dr. Centurio in Constantina.

During the 1 March meeting the deputies also heard a petition from the priests in the parish of San Vicente. They requested that the Royal Gate be opened to allow them to administer the sacraments in Los Humeros, outside the city wall. The district was actually divided by the wall, part of it located inside and the other part extending outside the gate, and its name derived from its major industry, the smoking of fish. The clerics claimed that more than two hundred residents lived outside the gate, "very poor people and frequently they are sick," and because the gates were shut, many who needed their last sacraments "die without them." The priests of San Vicente, undeterred by the closed gate, declared that "we have jumped over the wall to confess them," but alas they could not bring with them the Blessed Sacrament and holy oil to anoint them with "because it cannot be taken over the wall." The persistent priests begged the count to open the gate and post guards there, as had been done with some of the other entrances into the city. Their plea was heard and their request approved.[3]

The following day the Count of Villar received disquieting news. In spite

---

2. Ibid. (7 March 1582).

3. AMS, sec. 13, siglo XVI, vol. 5; Mena, *Calles de Sevilla*, 180.

of all his efforts to protect Seville, he learned that there might be cases of the plague within the city. The governor was told that "in the Courtyard of Doña Elvira, where plays are performed, there was a sick man on the brink of death." The Corral de Doña Elvira was one of the most popular theaters in Seville, attracting large crowds eager to see their favorite actors perform in tragedies and comedies written by the Sevillian playwright Juan de la Cueva and others. People also lived within its compound. Physicians often recommended that during plague outbreaks any large congregations of people should be prohibited, including the theater, and it is unclear whether any performances took place during this period at the Corral de Doña Elvira.[4] To find out more about the sick man, the count summoned "López, the barber, who was curing him." The barber told the governor that the man had "a very dangerous bubo" and added that he "was dying." This was hardly reassuring, and the Count of Villar sent Dr. Pedro Gómez to examine the person and report on "what the sickness was."

Dr. Gómez found a young man "at the end of his life and with symptoms of death." He took his pulse and found it "very weak and with very little temperature." Furthermore, the patient was "trembling and convulsing." The doctor then proceeded to examine the young man's body and discovered "in the upper part of his thigh a small swelling, resembling a cord." Dr. Gómez asked those present, "how did the sickness start?" and was told that the young man, who was working as a tanner, had "gone the other day to tread water from certain hides and the next day he had chills." That was when they called López the barber, who promptly bled him from the ankle because he had complained that he "felt a little pain in the thigh." After the bleeding the young man "became delirious," and so the barber bled him again, and then once more.

Dr. Gómez did not need to hear more; it was apparent to him that it was because the man had been bled, "having a cold, that the entire dangerous sickness occurred." Indeed, the physician told the Count of Villar the young man's sickness and death was "the fault of the said barber, because he should not have bled him then, but given him other remedies for the cold that he had, in conformity

4. AMS, sec. 13, siglo XVI, vol. 5; Vioque Cubero, Vera Rodríguez, and López López, *Las plazas de Sevilla*, 52; José Sánchez-Arjona, *Anales del teatro en Sevilla desde Lope de Rueda hasta finales de siglo XVII* [1898] (Seville: Ayuntamiento de Sevilla, 1994), 64–69; Luis de Mercado, *Libro en que se trata con claridad la naturaleza . . . y modo de curar la enfermedad vulgar, y peste. . . .* (Madrid: Imprenta del Licenciado Castro, 1599), fol. 61v.

with medicine." The doctor affirmed that the barber should have known better, because he was "learned and *romancista*," that is, a man who although he did not know Latin was versed in medical texts in the vernacular. Dr. Gómez knew López, and he told the count that the barber "normally treats many patients with medicine," though the physician was unimpressed with his success rate. Clearly, in the eyes of the university-trained doctor, the mere romancista did more harm than good, and he accused the barber of "prolonging sicknesses and deaths of the sick, as he had seen during the sicknesses of the past year '81."

One thing Dr. Gómez was certain about, and he declared so unequivocally: the young man "does not have buboes nor a contagious disease." Moreover, the doctor denounced the barber for spreading false rumors about his patient and telling people that he had the plague, and as a result "a large part of the city is in an uproar thinking it is so." Dr. Gómez insisted that the barber killed the young man with his excessive bleeding and "things he had done on the thigh with cupping and plasters and cuts and other things." In the doctor's opinion, this treatment caused "an inflammation which appears to be something worse than it is."[5]

The testimony of Dr. Gómez, an experienced physician who had been practicing medicine for the past thirty-six years and had seen many cases of the plague, was reassuring. But given that Seville was surrounded by places with confirmed plague, people in the city feared that the "infected air" might blow in, and any unusual sickness or death created panic. A talkative barber only added to the tensions. The Count of Villar received various denunciations of suspicious sicknesses in several parts of the city, and it was again Dr. Gómez whom he entrusted with investigating them.

The first case involved "a sick woman suspected of having the plague," who lived in the house of a dyer. Dr. Gómez found the woman in bed with "a little fever and without symptoms of pestilential sickness." She had complained that her "armpit hurt," but the doctor felt it and did not find anything unusual. He asked her a few questions, and she told him that "she had worked hard in her occupation slaughtering baby goats and killing poultry" and admitted that "she had worked more with that arm." Dr. Gómez concluded that her pain was the result of her exertion and "not because she had something else."

5. AMS, sec. 13, siglo XVI, vol. 5 (2 March 1582). At this point in the documentation there appears a note stating that "His Lordship, the Count Governor, having seen the said [report] of the said doctor ordered that it be placed in the book of the plague."

The next day, 3 March, the city officials asked Dr. Gómez to give a report about three people who had perished within the past eight days, because "there is suspicion that they died from the contagious disease of the plague." They all resided in the Magdalena parish, in the Cestería, outside the city walls. According to the information received by the Count of Villar they all lived on Galera Street, notorious for its women's prison.[6] The previous week Dr. Gómez had gone to Galera Street to examine a woman named Ana Bernal, who lived in a boarding house next to the porter of Seville's Royal Audiencia, Lázaro Núñez. According to the doctor she had "an abscess on the outside of her throat and a continuous choleric vomit and the other signs of pestilential and contagious sickness"; Dr. Gómez added that she had died "within eight days."

The doctor further stated that about two or three days earlier he had learned from "some women, her neighbors," and from the barber surgeon Diego de Sotomayor, who resided in the Cestería, that another woman who lived in the same house as Ana Bernal had died in the hospital of the same sickness. What was more, a man who was a guest at the same boarding house died just a day later. Sotomayor related to Dr. Gómez that "they had called for him from the said house to bleed this sick man." When he arrived and saw the patient, the surgeon decided that he "was already dying and did not dare to bleed him" and advised that he should be given his last sacraments. The surgeon mentioned to Dr. Gómez that the man's body was "all discolored with black-and-blues of bad color and many spots."

The women neighbors, "one of whom is called Vargas and rents out beds," who lived about three or four houses down the street told Dr. Gómez that they had seen the man "up on his feet one day before he died." All these circumstances convinced the physician that "they are all very certain signs and indications of the said disease of the plague, because it all happened in one house." The neighbors told the doctor that the man's belongings were "taken to be sold outside," but no one knew where. Dr. Gómez learned that Ana Bernal's "sister or a relative moved into the house to engage in the same occupation of renting beds with the same bedding of the said Bernal." This bit of information must have sent the Count of Villar into a frenzy, and although there is no documentation, it is likely that the city's constables were swiftly dispatched to confiscate and burn any infected items they could find.

6. Mena, *Calles de Sevilla*, 85, 179–80.

That same day, 3 March, the councilors summoned Diego de Sotomayor to testify about the three deaths. The barber surgeon stated that he had been called in to bleed Ana Bernal because she "had fallen and one of her knees hurt as a result." Furthermore, Ana had a mump-like swelling "on the right outer part of her throat and was vomiting." He bled her twice and insisted that at the time he did not think it was any "contagious disease," though he did learn about four days later that she had died. Diego de Sotomayor remembered that when he was in the house, it was just a couple of days before Ash Wednesday, "and they were cooking a little bit of shad" because one of the male boarders had asked them to prepare the fish for him. Within two days the surgeon was once again called to the house, this time to "see and cure the said man," who was quite sick. When the surgeon arrived, he found the man "delirious and he took his arm and found many spots and black welts." But one of the man's relatives who was present had assured Sotomayor that the spots were normal in him because he was "a ruddy man and he had seen them before." The surgeon did not treat the sick man, and he was later told that about half an hour after he had left, the man's "life ended while vomiting black things."

At this point the officials asked Diego de Sotomayor if he thought the man had the plague or any other contagious disease, since he was "vomiting black things," and whether that was common with people who had the plague. The surgeon answered that the man did not have "a fever nor any symptoms, rather, his life just ended," and from what he had seen during past epidemics, the people "who became sick or died from the plague never vomited black things like this man." He therefore concluded that as far as he understood, this man "did not die of the plague."[7]

The conflicting diagnoses given by Dr. Gómez and the barber surgeon Sotomayor are indicative of the obstacles facing civic authorities as they attempted to combat contagious disease. There are no indications that any special steps were taken at this time, nor were any further suspicious deaths reported in the next few weeks. Once again the count's and the plague commission's attention turned to the places surrounding Seville where the plague had been confirmed. The Count of Villar was convinced that upholding the quarantine for as long as necessary, regardless of personal hardships suffered by Seville's inhabi-

7. AMS, sec. 13, siglo XVI, vol. 5.

tants or those of surrounding towns, best protected the city from the contagion. If the governor had been considering relaxing some of the protective measures, he would have quickly banished the idea as the month of March progressed. The notices from the countryside were not encouraging.

23

EVIL MEN

Filled with evil men, enemies of each other and public fornicators.
—JUAN DE PEREA DURÁN

A T ABOUT THE TIME that the suspicious deaths were being investigated in Seville, the licentiate Juan de Perea Durán sat down
in Puebla de los Infantes and penned a report to the Count of
Villar.[1] He was frustrated not only by the course of events in
Puebla but also because his previous letters had gone unanswered. He felt isolated, without any support from the capital, and powerless to deal with the local people, whom he disdainfully characterized as "without a soul and brutes
for not going to the hospital." Perea Durán lashed out at those who refused
treatment in the pesthouse because "they rot, and even though they are extremely poor, they dissimulate and allow themselves to die." The temporary
hospitals were specifically set up to treat the poor, but their reputation as a place
of death caused many to flee or to hide, and "neither proclamations nor warn-
ings suffice." The figures he provided were not encouraging: more than fifteen
people became sick on 10 and 11 February, "most of whom are already dead." On
27 February another major onslaught of sickness occurred, and of those, ten or
twelve had perished. Nevertheless, he insisted that most of those who sought
timely treatment recovered, largely owing to the "great care of Licentiate Juan
de Sosa, in whom there is rightly much confidence."

Perea Durán again noted that most people who became sick and died were
"very poor and needy, and lacking good nourishment." He charged that Puebla's public granary had not been properly supplied and reminded the count that
he himself had ordered a review of the accounts of the town's alhóndiga "and

1. AMS, sec. 13, siglo XVI, vol. 5 (3 March 1582).

found that some people owe two years' worth of wheat and more than 300,000 maravedís." According to Perea Durán, some town councilors borrowed money from the depository's coffer and failed to repay it. They also took wheat from the alhóndiga to use for seed and never replenished it. Perea Durán complained that these men go unpunished, and now there was no more than ninety fanegas of wheat in the granary, which "are needed for the hospital." The Count of Villar had instructed Perea Durán, using the power of his commission and the authority of the city of Seville over towns within its jurisdiction, to conduct a full review of the account books and then to turn over the administration of the public granary to a local vecino. But when the Sevillian official attempted to "press some of the rich men of this village into paying what they had eaten and usurped," he was hampered by Puebla's council. To Perea Durán's chagrin, the town's councilors promptly produced a pertinent royal provision; then "they forced me not to review the accounts and they took away my scribe."

Perea Durán asked the Count of Villar for copies of this document and at the same time filed a formal denunciation of the "council's irregularities," suggesting that perhaps the present problems facing Puebla resulted from past poor governance. To support his charges, the jurado included a series of papers covering the accounting of Puebla's public granary as well as testimony of various witnesses. The books were in disarray; the wheat had been removed in a haphazard manner, people owed money, and there were questions as to whether the grain had ever been returned.[2]

It was the period of Lent, and another problem weighed on the licentiate's mind: "this community, Most Illustrious Sir, is without Christians and sermons at a Holy time such as this, which is the greatest pestilence that there can be." Perea Durán denounced the local clergy, some of whom "serve more to agitate the people than to calm them with their example." He did not hesitate to blame the plague's scourge on the general immorality of the town, "filled with evil men, enemies of each other and public fornicators." Perea Durán's plaint reflects his deep dismay. "How, given this conduct, can Our Lord grant us mercy?" the desperate official wondered. "Rather, I fear, He will have to destroy us." Perea

2. AMS, sec. 13, siglo XVI, vol. 5; Paul Hiltpold, "The Price, Production, and Transportation of Grain in Early Modern Castile," *Agricultural History* 63, no. 1 (1989): 77–78, was able to partially reconstruct annual grain production for some towns in Burgos's territory, using the accounts of periodic *residencias* (reviews) of village officials.

Durán asked the count to send "a pair of Jesuit fathers" to help rectify the situation and "many other sins," because "it is important for our total salvation." In closing he mused that when "souls are cured, remedy of the bodies is easy."

As on previous occasions, the physician licentiate Juan Sosa de Sotomayor sent a report to Seville as well, confirming the numbers of the sick and those who had died, stating that there were ten patients in the hospital and four convalescing. The doctor was also troubled by Puebla's spiritual malaise and, reinforcing Perea Durán's request, asked the Count of Villar to "send someone who would preach the Gospel to us during Lent, because there is need for many conversions, and my own, so that Our Lord lifts his wrath from this afflicted community." Licentiate Sosa de Sotomayor was concerned with the dietary needs of the inhabitants during Lent. He pointed out that "there is no fish, and whatever there is, is not good." Nevertheless, because fish was deemed to help ward off the plague, people ate the bad fish "to preserve themselves from this damned disease." Sosa de Sotomayor believed that meat would be beneficial in preventing "more people from succumbing" and argued that priests should let their parishioners know that they could eat meat, even game, in spite of it being Lent.

The officials sent from Seville to various places within its jurisdiction to assure compliance with the count's directives were generally successful. There were some parts of the district, however, that proved more troublesome. The plague commission had dispatched Francisco de Cabrera to ensure that orders were obeyed at the ferry of Villanueva del Río. On 4 March he wrote to the Count of Villar from the nearby town of Tocina, informing him that he, along with the constables, had reached the ferry at Villanueva, which operated from daybreak to sunset. Jurado Cabrera discovered in Tocina that wine and vinegar had been transported from Constantina in spite of edicts against it. He called a meeting of the local council to press the officials once more not to allow any traffic from Constantina, Cazalla de la Sierra, or Puebla de los Infantes. He also ordered that anyone with direct access from their courtyards to the common pasturelands should not go there directly but for the time being should leave and enter only through the town gates, which could be controlled.

The jurado complained bitterly about the provincial governor of Villanueva del Río, who openly challenged not only his authority but that of the Count of Villar as well. According to Francisco de Cabrera, Seville's constables had boarded the ferry at Tocina, carrying their staffs of office, "in order to fulfill the commission," but as soon as they reached the other side Villanueva's governor "ordered them to come out, leaving the staffs on the boat." He informed the constables that he would have to arrest them "because they could not carry staffs of justice on the ferry." As soon as Cabrera realized there was trouble he also crossed over to Villanueva del Río and tried to reason with the official, showing him the count's latest directives. Cabrera argued with the recalcitrant provincial governor that following the commands would be of service to the king and that the count had ordered the constables to carry the staffs, giving them the authority to enforce his mandates "to prevent that neither cloth nor people cross from the parts where it was understood there was the sickness of the plague."

The local governor replied that the constables could not carry their staffs on the ferry unless Cabrera petitioned him first, in which case he might give his permission; otherwise, the constables would have to remain on Tocina's side without setting foot on the boat. Such blatant defiance infuriated the jurado, who asked the Count of Villar to deal with the uncooperative man, declaring that "the governor of Villanueva lives with such liberty that he has become master of the river and the ferry." Cabrera denounced the official for vexing the ferrymen with "imprisonment and fines without any reason" and added, "from what I have seen they cannot earn enough to pay these fines." In closing, the jurado begged the Count of Villar to "charge me with what I must do."[3]

Disobedience of the count's orders was prevalent at all levels. People attempted to sneak into the city, to bring in unauthorized goods, and to sell or take for their own use the clothing and bedding of the dead. Those charged with guarding the gates, the bridges, and the ferries were often lax in their performance. And then there was the disobedient jurado. Rodrigo Sánchez de Soria, who had just returned from Castilblanco de los Arroyos, had been named guard of the ferry at La Algaba, slightly to the northwest of Seville. Although he had

3. AMS, sec. 13, siglo XVI, vol. 5. Villanueva del Río came under the jurisdiction of a provincial governor when Philip II in the 1560s reorganized the juridical structure of towns, such as Villanueva, still belonging to the military orders. According to Nader, *Absolutist Spain,* 148–49, the provincial governor "was, in effect, a lifetime lord" who had the power to appoint a chief justice (alcalde mayor) for the district. Villanueva had been sold by Philip II in 1565 to Don Fadrique Enríquez de Ribera y Portocarrero, the First Marquis de Villanueva del Río. Thus regardless of Francisco de Cabrera's frustration with the behavior of the district governor, there was little that the Count of Villar could do, other than to appeal to his good senses.

been duly notified at his house of his appointment, Sánchez de Soria ignored the order and stayed home, probably hoping for a few days of respite following his diligent tracking of sick Moriscos. But when the governor learned of the jurado's dallying he swiftly sent a mounted constable to take him to the Atarazanas jail, where he was to be held at his own expense because from his "tardiness there comes much inconvenience and harm to this republic."

This was an ironic turn of events, given that Sánchez de Soria had himself threatened to punish negligent ferrymen just a few days earlier. The count's wrath sufficed to convince the slacker to resume his duties, and Rodrigo Sánchez de Soria, along with two constables to help him enforce the regulations, was on his way to La Algaba within hours. The jurado redeemed himself at his post, and before the end of March he informed the Count of Villar that to secure the ferry at La Algaba during the night, "I put a chain and a padlock on it and I have the key with me."

The jurado Juan de Perea Durán had traveled from Puebla de los Infantes to oversee compliance with the count's orders in the area around the town of Carmona. He wrote the governor from the Bodegón de las Cañas on 8 March, reporting that although some places were following the orders, others were lax. Licentiate Perea Durán was particularly concerned about Carmona, a substantial town with a commanding view of the rich agricultural flatlands below, located about thirty kilometers northeast of Seville. He complained that Carmona "does not preserve itself from any of the communities that Your Lordship guards against," and people "freely enter to sell wine and other things from Puebla and the other places." The jurado remained in the area to monitor the situation, and on 21 March reported back that problems in the region continued. Perea Durán denounced the illegal traffic in wine and other commodities from Constantina and Puebla. The goods were transported "outside the route, crossing the river on a ferry that is close to Guadajoz." This ferry was also near Tocina, where a guard had been posted, but by crossing at Guadajoz the ingenious entrepreneurs were able to bypass the patrols and take their merchandise to Carmona; from there, they could continue on to Seville.

Indeed, many merchants whose livelihood depended on Seville's consumers were undeterred by the governor's prohibitions and endeavored to import goods from infected towns. A Sevillian wine merchant, Clemente Muñoz, complained to the Count of Villar on 6 February that the guards at the Macarena Gate stopped seventy-four arrobas of wine coming to him from wine presses in the area of Cazalla. Muñoz asked permission to transfer the wine from the leather wineskins in which it had been transported into casks that he would provide so the wine could be stored outside the city walls, in a house belonging to the leper hospital of San Lázaro. The count authorized the transaction, which was to be supervised by notary Cristóbal Pérez and constable Pedro Barba. The next day, two men from the city poured the wine into the new containers, and then "the skins were thrown out into the field away from the said house [of San Lázaro]."[4] The wine, awaiting permission to enter the city, would remain in the San Lázaro dependency along with wine belonging to other merchants until it could be examined by a physician. It would be a long wait.

A month later, on 8 March, both Clemente Muñoz and another wine merchant, Diego de Escobar, petitioned the count to permit the entry of their wine into Seville. For the past month and a half, 334 arrobas of wine from Cazalla belonging to Diego de Escobar had been stored in large earthen jars in San Lázaro and the nearby *venta* of Ventillas de los Solares. Escobar declared that none of "the drovers who brought it nor their beasts or containers" had entered the town of Cazalla. Escobar assured the governor that the wine had been "made and appraised in two wine presses," both located about two leagues north of Cazalla "and much closer to the town of Guadalcanal." Diego de Escobar complained about the high costs of storage and security and was anxious about the risk of damage to the wine, and he begged the count to permit him to bring it into the city. The Count of Villar once again turned to the medical profession and ordered Dr. Bartolomé Hidalgo to examine the wine and determine whether it could be injurious to public health.

Dr. Hidalgo quickly responded, stating categorically that "it is a plain thing that the liquor of wine is in itself of such quality that it cannot receive pestilential contagion, indeed it serves and aids against poison and pestilence." The surgeon's report was a short treatise on the virtues of wine and its medicinal uses against snake venom or bites of "other poisonous animals," for which wine would be given to drink or used to cleanse both "fresh and old wounds." The doctor's declaration that wine "cannot receive contagion nor give it" convinced the Count of Villar to issue the pertinent permits to both wine merchants.[5]

Livestock posed a greater dilemma for the Count of Villar. The city needed meat, but the authorities feared that the animals and their handlers coming

4. AMS, sec. 13, siglo XVI, vol. 5.
5. Ibid.

from infected places could bring in contagion. On 15 March a letter arrived from Gaspar Suárez, a plague guardian at El Garrobo, who warned that "some men who seem to live in Triana are taking this road to bring a small flock of ailing sheep to slaughter in this city." The guard pointed out that most of the animals "are sick and old," and he claimed that they came from the prohibited places where plague was suspected. Suárez took it upon himself to block their passage on to Seville and asked for further instructions.

His action may have pleased the plague commission, but those bringing the sheep swiftly protested. Livestock traders from Triana, Sebastián de Alarcón, and Francisco Ramos stated that they were transporting four hundred sheep from the towns of Fuente del Maestre and Villalba de los Barros, in Extremadura, "to sell them at the market of this city." The merchants complained that the guards in El Garrobo would not let them pass, and they asked the count for license to continue to the city. The merchants included a certificate from the town of Fuente del Maestre stating that it was plague free. Several witnesses confirmed their story. One of them, a Triana wine dealer named Juan Bernal, vouched that Ramos and Alarcón, along with two of their shepherds, had left Seville about one month earlier to buy livestock in Extremadura. The need to supply the local market with meat and the appropriate papers produced by the merchants persuaded the count to authorize the group to continue toward Seville, but he stipulated that "above all things the said shepherds should be examined by a doctor or surgeon to determine if they are healthy."[6]

The list of places with reported cases of the plague was growing. On 8 March news reached Seville's authorities that people were dying in Segura de León, a town near Fregenal de la Sierra in Extremadura, and that "the place is devastated from this sickness." The count did not wait for further confirmation and added Segura de León to the quarantine list. The presence of the plague in Segura de León was confirmed in the 15 March letter from Gaspar Suárez, the plague guardian at El Garrobo, who informed the governor that six to eight people had been found dead in a house there.

6. Ibid. (19 March 1582).

24

DENYING THE PLAGUE

There had not been nor is there now the said disease.
—DON ENRIQUE DE GUZMÁN PONCE DE LEÓN

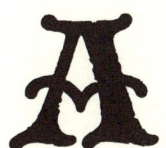T THE SAME TIME as new areas became afflicted, some of the earliest towns to have dealt with the plague were reporting recovery. Officials in Cazalla de la Sierra had been attempting for some time to convince the Sevillian authorities that their community was healthy. In mid-February they sent a thorough report to the Count of Villar. Following deliberations, the count and the plague deputies, concluding that they needed additional proof, requested more testimony. Cazalla's town council readily complied and by 2 March was able to send the required information. Cazalla's magistrate declared in a letter that accompanied the depositions that health conditions there were good. He stressed that the only ones who had died were "very poor, miserable people who had nothing to cure or refresh themselves with."

The testimony had been taken on 26 February. Bachiller Hernán Vázquez Bocanegra, a local physician who had already testified during the earlier inquiry, reiterated his observations. He declared that in all the forty years he had served as the town's physician he "had not seen so few sick here as at present." He acknowledged that at the moment he had five people under his care, two with eye injuries, one with diarrhea, and two with fevers; but no one with any contagious disease. Another physician, the licentiate Salvador Estevan Frisado, swore that Cazalla was healthy and remarked that he had not treated any patients for the past three days. The surgeon Andrés Gutiérrez, who had been practicing in Cazalla for the past nine years, concurred with his older colleagues, insisting that the town was healthy.

Cazalla's two apothecaries, Juan de Velasco and Melchior Gallardo, whose boticas were located near each other on the same street, swore that in recent days they had not dispensed any medicines for the plague. There was only one parish in Cazalla, and five of its clerics testified to the clean bill of health, as did three monks in the local Franciscan monastery. The jurado Juan de Alava, a vecino of Seville living in Cazalla de la Sierra since May of 1581 who had traveled back and forth often in the past, claimed that Cazalla was now healthier than ever. Don Enrique de Guzmán Ponce de León, who had resided there for twenty years, agreed and declared that if that had not been the case he "would have gone to live outside this said town along with many of its caballeros and wealthy people," noting that they "had not left because there had not been nor are there now the said diseases." In closing, Don Enrique affirmed that "the bad reputation that this town has acquired regarding the said disease has been neither certain nor true."

The letter and depositions reached Seville within days and were read in the cabildo on 6 March. The Count of Villar, still not entirely persuaded, decided to send someone to "secretly" survey the situation in Cazalla. He dispatched the jurado Martín de Santofímia Riquelme to the town and instructed him to remain there for eight days. Among other things, he was to determine the number of days since the last death, whether or not the infected cloth had been burned, and how many houses were locked up. Even though this was to be a secret inspection, the count ordered a constable with his staff of justice to accompany the "undercover" agent.

Taking special letters from Seville's cabildo authorizing his entrance into Cazalla, Jurado Riquelme arrived there in the afternoon of Sunday, 11 March. The following day he visited the Los Remedios Hospital, where he questioned resident physician Bachiller Hernán Vázquez, who informed him that there were presently six patients under treatment. Two had pleurisy, one had come down with fevers, one woman suffered from idiopathic illness, and two people were recovering from fevers. The physician, who had already given various depositions, insisted that he had never treated the plague. He acknowledged that at the end of January some people in Cazalla were sick, and some thought that they had buboes. He had cured several of them, and three or four of his patients had died, but Hernán Vázquez noted that because they were very poor, they probably died of hunger. He admitted that he had treated a girl with a carbuncle, applying poultice to it, "and she is already healthy."

While on his rounds, Jurado Riquelme learned that the Blessed Sacrament had been taken from the church, a sign that someone was dying. He sent constable Alonso de Torres to investigate and asked physician Hernán Vázquez to accompany him. They discovered a "*fulano* Ortega" and, after examining him, the physician diagnosed pleurisy and ordered him to be bled, a relief to all except the patient. Although bleeding was the most common treatment for a variety of ailments, it was hardly the most popular cure with those subjected to it. Indeed, Dr. Hidalgo commented in his essay on phlebotomy that he had seen some "who let themselves die rather then be bled."[1]

Jurado Riquelme also questioned the surgeon Andrés Gutiérrez as to whether there were any "plague, buboes, carbuncles and other contagious diseases" in Cazalla. The surgeon replied that everyone was now healthy, but about two months earlier there had been people with "some abscesses . . . that appeared in the groin and armpits, with their fevers." He admitted that there had been suspicion that it was the plague because "some of the sick died in a short time," but most of them, he added, were poor and "badly nourished." Gutiérrez had treated about fifteen sick people, most of whom had recovered; and the only ones who succumbed were "miserable people." Both of Cazalla's physicians had testified earlier, and their current depositions, just like their previous testimony, consistently portrayed the town as a picture of health. They insisted that whatever suspicions of plague may have existed in the past were just rumors and that those who had died perished because of their poverty, not from any contagious disease.

But the count's "secret agent" remained skeptical. When Riquelme heard that a woman had just died, he immediately set out to find her house. He took along surgeon Diego Gutiérrez, who revealed that he had been called to see the woman the day before, and he assured the concerned jurado that she had hemorrhaged to death during childbirth. The surgeon's story was confirmed by Olalla Sánchez, the woman's sister-in-law, who had assisted during the delivery.

If there were ever any "secret" as to why the jurado was in town it was dispelled the following day, Tuesday, 13 March. Riquelme met Cazalla's cabildo and ordered the town crier to proclaim that if any possessions of the dead had not been delivered to authorities, they had to be turned over within three days. Riquelme also asked the church sacristan to provide a list of all the people who had died in the previous three days.

1. Ibid; Hidalgo, *Thesoro*, fol. 70v.

The intrepid jurado next decided to inspect the town's two pharmacies. The first boticario, Melchior Gallardo, stated that he had not dispensed any medicines for the past twenty days. He assured Riquelme that he would know if there were any sickness now, "because at the time that there was the said disease they came to his pharmacy for the medicines." Cazalla's other pharmacist, Juan de Velasco, also had not served any customers for the past twenty days. By now Riquelme must have become suspicious of the town's perfect health, and he asked Velasco "if anyone had persuaded him to say that." The apothecary denied that anyone told him what to tell his questioner. But he did indicate that when the plague had been present, "about forty or fifty people might have died, who were suspected to have been sick with the disease." Riquelme also questioned the local barber, Diego Grande, who corroborated the stories of the other witnesses, though he confided that he "never wanted to go and bleed anyone with the said disease."

By the end of his busy day, Jurado Riquelme was perhaps near to admitting that Cazalla might be plague free, but he would continue his investigation. At the same time he realized that the town was suffering because of lack of foodstuffs. He noted that "wheat is very expensive and it cannot be bought." Riquelme recognized the toll the quarantine was taking on Cazalla's population: "because those from this place cannot enter the city of Seville, there is a great shortage of fish and what there is, is very expensive."

Jurado Riquelme resumed his quest the next morning. He interviewed the surgeon bachiller Salvador Estevan Frisado, who recalled that the disease that manifested itself with "buboes, spots and some carbuncles" had begun around Christmas of 1581. He related that during that time he had treated about eighteen people, most of whom were poor and undernourished, and he remarked that the disease was exacerbated by the "humid weather." Frisado confirmed that about forty to fifty people had died then, that the authorities had provided the needed medicines and hospital care, and that they made certain that the bedding and clothing of the infected had been burned. The surgeon corroborated his colleagues' depositions that for the past twenty days, "by God's mercy," there had been no new cases.

After questioning Cazalla's medical professionals, it was time to talk to the men of the cloth. The jurado went to see a local priest, Luis de Aguilar, who was also a commissioner of the Holy Office of the Inquisition. Bachiller Aguilar stated that around Christmas people started to talk about "the disease of the plague and buboes," and he recalled that "it began with a piece of clothing from the town of Constantina that was brought to this place." Luis de Aguilar checked the death register and declared that fifty people had died, all of them "poor and miserable." The priest praised the local magistrate's efforts and told the jurado that none of the clergy who had administered the last sacraments had become sick. Over the next two days Martín Riquelme questioned other priests as well as the sacristan, who all confirmed the number of deaths and the social status of those who had perished. He also spoke to the jail warden, who assured him that no one in the prison was sick.[2]

Regardless of all the favorable testimony that everyone was brimming with health in Cazalla de la Sierra, Jurado Riquelme continued to keep track of any suspicious activity for the next few days. On Friday, 16 March, he heard that the last sacraments were being administered and again sent physician Hernán Vázquez and the town constable to determine who was dying and why. After examining the patient, Vázquez concluded that although he was very sick and had been suffering from "bloody diarrhea" for the past fifteen to twenty days, his condition did not constitute a threat to public health.

Also on Friday, Riquelme learned that a widow, Francisca Ximénez, had died the day before in the house of a worker, Sebastián Muñoz. His wife, Juana Muñoz, told the jurado that Francisca had rented a room from them and that she had been sick since Monday. According to Juana, a physician came and examined Francisca and declared that she had a "lump in the armpit, which he said was a bubo." The woman had moved to the house about a month before, after her husband died, and Juana was convinced that Francisca was "fleeing from the sickness that had been around from that time."

Riquelme determined that the physician who had examined Francisca Ximénez was none other than surgeon Andrés Gutiérrez, who had sworn to him so recently that there was no sickness in Cazalla. The jurado summoned Gutiérrez and demanded to know the truth, threatening that "if any harm comes to the community it will be his responsibility and risk." The surgeon admitted that he had seen the sick woman on Monday and noted that he found her "melancholy and despairing." She told him that the evening before she had been well and had actually received a ring as promise of marriage, and she was wondering whether "it was the excitement of wanting to marry or if she felt

<hr />

2. AMS, sec. 13, siglo XVI, vol. 5.

sick from the dinner that she had eaten." Gutiérrez took her pulse and thought she had a "slight fever." The surgeon then "looked at her armpits and asked her if she had pain in any groin." Contrary to what Juana Muñoz had testified, Gutiérrez told the jurado that he did not find anything in the armpits nor did her groin hurt. The surgeon insisted that he had given her medicine to "preserve and restore her so that some sickness does not come over her." Gutiérrez affirmed that when he visited her the following day her condition was unchanged, and therefore he did not return because he "believed that it was unnecessary." He defended himself, claiming that he just discovered that the woman had died, and he did not know why.

Additional testimony was essential, and Jurado Riquelme decided to question someone who had been present at the betrothal. A tailor, Juan Martín, testified that he and other people "made an agreement to marry Francisca Ximénez with a son of a villager." The tailor told Riquelme that he took a ring to Francisca on Sunday night "and she gave him a kerchief for the groom." Apparently Juan Martín went to see the bride again on Monday morning and found her despondent. She confided that she had a nightmare in which her first husband appeared to her, exclaiming, "You whore, so now you want to marry and enjoy my property!" Furthermore, in the dream her dead little boy had begged her, "Mother, get my father off of me because he is suffocating me!" According to the tailor, the poor woman was terrified and told him that "she was going to die from fright." Juan Martín divulged to the jurado that he was concerned for her and asked Francisca if she was sick with the "sickness that there had been in this town," and she replied that she was "sick with fear." But the tailor, taking it upon himself to make sure Francisca did not have the plague, "felt her armpits and other parts of her body" but did not find anything. Just in case, he decided to call the surgeon Gutiérrez, who examined Francisca and told the curious tailor "that she did not have anything other than being very sad."

Jurado Riquelme, regardless of the surgeon's and tailor's statements, decided not to take any chances and ordered two Moriscos to collect all her personal belongings and burn them. He discovered that some other clothing had been "thrown out during the night," and he was learning that many people had kept the clothing and bedding of plague victims. The exasperated jurado asked Friar Baltasar, a Dominican from the Monastery of San Pablo in Seville, to admonish the townspeople in his sermon and warn them of the consequences of failing to destroy these items.

The jurado continued to investigate recent deaths but found no evidence of the plague. He also questioned local officials, and their stories were consistent. The town scribe told him that the pesthouse that had been established on the outskirts of Cazalla had been closed on 4 March because all were cured. The *regidor* (alderman) Don Pedro Niño Sotelo, speaking for the town's gentry, corroborated the testimony of another prominent resident, Don Enrique de Guzmán Ponce de León, whose deposition had been sent to Seville earlier. Don Pedro acknowledged that about two months before, many people had died, and the plague was suspected. But after thorough investigation conducted by doctors, among others, they concluded that "it was not the plague but acute diseases of pestilential humor." His estimate of how many had died was much lower than those of some of the others. Don Pedro claimed that twenty to thirty people had perished, and they were all "poor people and badly nourished."

Like Don Enrique earlier, Don Pedro argued that if the disease had been the plague, he and "other caballeros and wealthy people who reside and are in this town would have left and gone to their country estates." The jurado might well have accepted this as a valid argument, considering the first advice given by the medical profession whenever plague was discussed was to flee. Indeed, anyone who was able, and particularly the upper classes, traditionally abandoned stricken towns or cities where they resided and moved to the countryside, where, they believed, the pestilential air would not threaten. This and all the other testimonies, as well as his own investigation into recent deaths in Cazalla de la Sierra, convinced Riquelme that the town was plague free, and he was ready to return to Seville to report to the Count of Villar.

This was excellent news for Cazalla's authorities, and on Sunday, 18 March, a religious procession with all the local confraternities participating wound its way from the principal church to the convent of the nuns of Madre de Dios, praising God and giving thanks for "the health and happiness of this town." When the procession reached the convent a mass was celebrated. Shortly thereafter, the jurado set out on his journey back to Seville, armed with a certificate attesting that he had been in Cazalla for one week, from Sunday, 11 March, to Sunday, 18 March. When he presented his expenses to the plague commission two days later, he was authorized to receive payment for eleven days of work, which included the time that he had spent on the road.

25

CIRCUMVENTING THE CORDON SANITAIRE

If they do not carry a certificate, then they should not pass.
—DIEGO DE TOLEDO

WHILE THE JURADO MARTÍN RIQUELME was making inquiries in Cazalla de la Sierra, the town remained under orders of isolation, and travelers continued to be intercepted. On Tuesday, 13 March, another jurado, Bernaldino Ramírez, and constable Anton Alonso had stopped at Casaluenga near Seville two men and a woman coming from Cazalla. The three travelers, Cristóbal Centeno, a lawyer, his sister María Centeno, and a tax collector, Juan de la Rosa, were under orders of Jurado Riquelme and were bringing his letters to Seville. Nevertheless, the intrepid guards questioned them, inquiring about recent deaths in Cazalla. They swore that no one had died for the past twelve days, though they conceded that before then people had perished of the plague. María Centeno stated that she was from Zalamea de la Serena in Extremadura and had been in Cazalla for about one month, and during that time people had died there.[1] Now she was traveling to Seville with her brother and the tax collector, bringing letters from Martín Riquelme for the Count of Villar and the plague commission. Juan de la Rosa, a collector of His Majesty's revenues, was transporting money and wanted either to proceed to Seville or return to Cazalla. His two companions were also anxious to continue their journey to the capital or be allowed to go back to Cazalla.

Jurado Ramírez was unwilling to let them pass, in spite of his colleague's certificates. The conscientious official collected the papers the three travelers carried and sent a messenger to Seville to secure a formal decision on whether or not they could continue to the city. In the meantime, however, Ramírez or-

1. AMS, sec. 13, siglo XVI, vol. 5. Zalamea de la Serena is the setting of the 1641 play, *El alcalde de Zalamea*, by Calderón de la Barca.

dered the constable Anton Alonso to detain the three people and take them to jail in La Rinconada until the Count of Villar replied. Cristóbal Centeno protested the imprisonment and, being a lawyer, filed an appeal, arguing that his rights and those of his fellow travelers were being improperly infringed upon by Jurado Ramírez. Shortly thereafter, Francisco Sánchez, the steward of Jurado Postigo, arrived from Seville, and Bernaldino Ramírez asked him to guard the three travelers. An argument broke out because the steward refused to watch the prisoners, saying "in a very threatening way" that he worked for Diego del Postigo and "would not do anything that the said Señor Jurado [Ramírez] ordered him."

Such an attitude did not sit well with the Señor Jurado, who, "seeing the boldness and cursing of the said steward," ordered him jailed as well. Although Diego del Postigo was an important man who served as Seville's steward and thus was responsible for disbursing the city's money, the behavior of his servant offended his colleague. There were several witnesses to this exchange, and Ramírez took down their depositions as well as the testimony of the insolent steward, Francisco Sánchez. Sánchez admitted that he refused to take orders from Jurado Ramírez but denied that he was acting at the insistence of his master, Diego del Postigo.[2]

While Bernaldino Ramírez was busy with other matters, his deputy at Casaluenga, Francisco de Vergara, detained two more men at the inn. One was a shoemaker named Pedro González, from El Pedroso, not too far south of Cazalla and Constantina. The other man, Juan Esteban, had come from Azuaga, north of Cazalla, in Extremadura. Francisco de Vergara, suspecting that they were attempting to deceive the guards in order to make their way to Seville, locked them up in the house of innkeeper Gregorio Sánchez. Not long afterward, two friends of Juan Esteban arrived, and Vergara jailed them too. The deputy then proceeded to take down testimony from Pedro González, who declared that he and Juan Esteban had met each other on Sunday afternoon on the road from Cantillana to Seville. Juan Esteban confirmed they had met on the road and decided to travel to Seville together. The men claimed that in Cantillana they discovered that Seville was guarding against the plague, and therefore they resolved to go to Casaluenga to secure license to continue. Francisco de Vergara did not know where exactly Azuaga was and asked Juan Esteban, who

2. AMS, sec. 13, siglo XVI, vol. 5 (14 March 1582).

replied that it was "next to Cazalla de la Sierra." Though somewhat inaccurate, this answer was all it took for them to remain in custody.

Francisco de Vergara also questioned Juan Esteban about the two men who claimed to be acquainted with him, and Esteban admitted that he knew them and that they also came from Azuaga. He revealed that the men, Gonzalo Gallego and Santiago Rubio, were traveling to Seville "to do business and to go to the Indies." Vergara promptly questioned the men. Gonzalo Gallego stated he was a farmer from Azuaga and that on the way to Seville he had passed through Cazalla and had spent the night in El Pedroso. He acknowledged he carried no certificates, claiming to be unaware that Seville was guarding against the plague. Francisco de Vergara, not wanting to take any chances, ordered the innkeeper to keep the three men under lock and key. Jurado Ramírez returned that same day, and after listening to Vergara's report, he decided to pass the information on to the Count of Villar. While waiting for the governor's instructions, he sent the men under guard to Seville, to be kept in the jail outside the Macarena Gate, "where His Lordship orders prisoners who come from the outside be put." The constable would take them there at daybreak and turn them over to the jail warden.

The post at Casaluenga was the last important checkpoint on the left bank of the Guadalquivir River before reaching Seville, and many travelers coming from the north took that route. In addition to the others, Jurado Ramírez had stopped Manuel Rodríguez, who admitted that he had come from Cazalla de la Sierra and was bringing "a little bit of sweet wine and figs" to Seville.[3] He was originally from Portugal but had married and settled in Cazalla with his wife and children. Pressed on where and how he had secured a license to go to Seville, Rodríguez divulged that he had obtained it from a public notary in El Pedroso. Jurado Ramírez checked with the notary, Juan de Cabrera Rendón, who verified that he had issued a license to Manuel Rodríguez, whom he described as "a short man with a scar on his left cheek."

Under further questioning, Rodríguez revealed that he had been sent by Francisco Gutiérrez, a vecino of Cazalla, to take a "wineskin of sweet wine and a small hand basket with some figs" to a lady in Seville, Doña Beatriz de Alfaro,

3. The Spanish word *arrope* refers to grape must that has been cooked until it thickens into a syrup. According to the dictionary of Sebastián de Covarrubias (*Tesoro de la lengua castellana o española* [1611], ed. Felipe C. R. Maldonado and Manuel Camarero [Madrid: Editorial Castalia, 1994]), a young sweet wine was also called arrope.

along with a letter for her.[4] When Gutiérrez ordered him to undertake the journey, he also advised him where to go in El Pedroso to secure the papers. Jurado Ramírez did not allow Manuel Rodríguez to proceed; instead, he sent him to the jail at the Macarena Gate, while his donkey remained in the innkeeper's care. The unfortunate traveler joined the other inmates awaiting the Count of Villar's decision. It came quickly; on 16 March the governor ruled that all the people who had been detained were to be released from jail and return immediately to the places from which they had come.

Jurado Ramírez not only guarded his post in Casaluenga but stayed informed on the situation in nearby towns. On 17 March he learned that twelve days earlier some people from Cazalla had roomed at an inn in Cantillana. Two days later, three servants died at the inn: a woman along with a girl and a boy. The governor of Cantillana had ordered all the clothing and bedding burned, the inn locked up, and the innkeeper sent out of town. Cantillana lay not far to the northeast of Casaluenga, and people coming from there on their way to Seville would pass through Ramírez's post. His fears were confirmed when he heard from Juan Sánchez de las Ovejas, a vecino of Villaverde del Río near Cantillana, that many people in Cantillana had died of the plague. Furthermore, Sánchez and others informed the jurado that the innkeeper had taken refuge in the "shrine of San Sebastián," a fitting sanctuary given the saint's presumed power to protect against the plague. San Sebastián and San Roque were among the most popular saints invoked in times of the plague, and the poor innkeeper must have spent much of his time in fervent prayer.[5]

Cantillana was not the only town with reported plague. On Sunday, 18 March, Diego de Toledo had written a long missive from Alcalá del Río to the Count of Villar informing him that he had heard that there was plague, "much fiercer than here," in Jerez de los Caballeros in Extremadura.[6] He warned that it was essential to "put much care in the guarding of Seville." Further-

---

4. AMS, sec. 13, siglo XVI, vol. 5. According to Gil, *Los conversos y la Inquisición,* 3:222, a Beatriz de Alfaro, belonging to the important Sevillian converso family, which included prominent physicians (Nicolás Monardes and Andrés Zamudio de Alfaro) as well as booksellers and notaries, was a nun in the Convent of La Encarnación in 1582. Although we cannot know for certain who the lady in question was, it is not impossible that a letter along with gifts of figs and sweet wine would be sent to a nun.

5. AMS, sec. 13, siglo XVI, vol. 5. For discussion of "specialist saints" in sixteenth-century Spain, see Christian, *Local Religion,* 42–47; see also Betrán, *La peste en Barcelona,* 465–70.

6. The name in the document is Jerez de Badajoz, today's Jerez de los Caballeros.

more, Jurado Toledo had learned that many people continued to die in Castilblanco de los Arroyos, though many "are in the hills, who have left the place," while those who had remained in the town "suffer great need." Then the jurado shared the most disturbing information he had learned that very morning from a councilman of Alcalá del Río, who had just returned from Seville. He told Toledo that the day before he had seen in Seville people from Castilblanco who were rooming at two inns in the city. Furthermore, he believed that "many Moriscos bringing charcoal wander about in Triana saying that they are coming from the Aljarafe," the bluff overlooking the Guadalquivir River basin.

Having listened to the councilman, Diego de Toledo was convinced that the Moriscos were actually from Castilblanco, and he exhorted the Count of Villar to investigate and to order Triana's constable "not to let [Moriscos] pass unless they carry a certificate." The astute jurado cautioned that even if they did have the proper documents, they should be carefully scrutinized because he believed that "they leave Castilblanco and go to any place that they deem appropriate and taking the testimony [of health] and the charcoal from there, they enter Seville every day in this manner." Diego de Toledo also asked the governor to alert the jurado who was posted at the ferry at La Algaba, the closest one to the city, "because through there they have a direct path to Seville." He recommended that "the safest would be that if they do not carry a certificate from where they are vecinos, then they should not pass."

Without delay, the Count of Villar sent a constable to make inquiries at the inns mentioned by Diego de Toledo. The constable first went to the Mesón de la Parra and questioned the innkeeper, Juana de Arbia, who swore that it had been many days since anyone had come from Castilblanco. Next, the constable visited the Mesón del Barco, where another female innkeeper, Ana de los Reyes, also denied that anyone from that town had recently stayed at the inn. The count also instructed Triana's guard, Cristóbal de Ayala, not to allow through anyone, with or without charcoal, "who comes from Castilblanco or Segura de León, in addition to the places referred to where there is plague."

In the meantime, Diego de Toledo wrote another letter from Alcalá del Río to the Count of Villar, asking for instructions regarding four muleteers who had arrived at a local inn the night before. From the first, the jurado doubted their claim that they were traveling from the small Extremaduran town of Cabeza la Vaca and suspected that they had come from Segura de León. The two places were not far distant from each other, but plague had been reported in Segura, and as far as the officials knew, Cabeza la Vaca was healthy. The four men were transporting white wine and wool. They produced papers issued on 16 March in Cabeza la Vaca, certifying that they were vecinos of the place. Unfortunately for them, they were accompanied by a twelve-year-old boy who raised the jurado's suspicion because he was not mentioned in the documents. Diego de Toledo felt that there was something "doubtful" about the boy. He separated him from the muleteers and asked him "certain questions." The interrogation yielded the information Toledo sought as well as two letters the boy was taking to Seville. When the jurado opened the missives and read them he found out that they had both been written in Segura and that the boy also came from there. The letters provided explicit news that many people were dying of the plague in Segura, including "relatives of the said boy."

Diego de Toledo sent the boy to a house outside Alcalá del Río, and since the child did not carry any money, the jurado ordered the muleteers to pay twenty-four reales for his food. Furthermore, he demanded that the men turn over any letters they were carrying; they gave him eight missives, and when he read them his intuition was confirmed: they all came from Segura de León. The jurado interrogated them again. One of the muleteers, Diego Hernández, now admitted that he was indeed from Segura. His master, Juan Ramírez, had ordered him to pick up some wool in Cabeza la Vaca and take it to the Monastery of Santiago de la Espada in Seville. His master also advised him to get his papers in Cabeza la Vaca, and indeed, a notary there issued the document. He and his companions had brought two draft animals to transport the wine, the sack of wool, and some blankets, clothes, and the equipment needed for their journey. He had departed from Segura twenty days earlier but went first north to Zafra and then to Cabeza la Vaca. Diego Hernández confirmed there had been plague in Segura de León for some thirty to forty days. He also divulged that the boy who was traveling with them was the son of a tailor in Segura and had joined the party in Cabeza la Vaca.

The second muleteer, Rodrigo López, also confessed that he was a vecino of Segura de León and had a wife and son there. He claimed he had left thirty days before, taking a shipment of wine to Portugal. His route had taken him through Badajoz, then northwest into Portugal and Campo Maior, then south to Elvas, and then back into Castile. He traveled through Talavera la Real, west of Badajoz, and then southeast to Zafra and finally to Cabeza la Vaca. He insisted that the wine they were now transporting came from Cabeza la Vaca and was destined for the Monastery of Santiago de la Espada. He denied that they were carrying any cloth. Regarding the plague in Segura, he remembered that when he left there he had heard that a young man had died of the disease and that his parents and everyone else in the household were driven out of town. He provided testimony identical to that of his companion regarding the boy who was traveling with them.

The third muleteer, Francisco Bernáldez, affirmed that he had left Segura about a month earlier and admitted that he took some shirts with him. He insisted that he did not go back to Segura because he had heard that there was plague there and "he wants to protect himself from the said disease." His testimony regarding the wine shipment and the boy echoed those of the other muleteers. Diego de Toledo was unable to question the fourth muleteer, Juan Domínguez, because he had slipped away before the jurado could get to him.

The testimony of the boy, Tomás, confirmed Toledo's worst suspicions. Tomás stated that he was twelve years old and that his father, Juan García, was a tailor in Segura de León. He told Diego de Toledo that he had left Segura on Wednesday, 14 March, to join the four muleteers "to come with them to the city of Seville." When queried whether his father had made an agreement with the men to take him there, Tomás admitted that he had. The most devastating testimony with regard to the muleteers, who had all denied having been in Segura de León within the past several weeks, came when the boy revealed that his father had seen them preparing their transport pack in Segura on Wednesday morning, and it was then that the tailor contracted them to take his son to Seville. The men were heading for Cabeza la Vaca, and Tomás caught up with them there that very afternoon.

Diego de Toledo asked the boy whether he had heard that anyone had died in Segura of the plague and he said that he had not. But when he was directly confronted regarding his own relatives, Tomás confessed, "what happens is that there was a sick woman in the town and two of this witness's mother's sisters and her niece went to visit her and they caught the disease that the woman had." The boy added that "he heard" that his aunts and his cousin died within eight days after they became sick, and he insisted that he had not been in Segura when all this happened but just found out about it when he returned. He also heard that the woman who had infected them died as well. Then Tomás changed his story again. Actually, only one of his mother's sisters visited the stricken woman, and she became sick and was taken to the house of the other sister; while they were "removing her from the room where she was bedridden to the lodging of her sister and niece in order to administer the Last Sacrament to her," she infected them, "and so they all died."

Tomás carried two letters from his father, Juan García. One of them, dated 11 March, was addressed to Tomás's older brother, Juan Bautista, "on the steps of the shop of Señor Alonso de Cea, silk merchant in the Alcaicería," Seville's textile market. It appears that Francisco Bernáldez, one of the muleteers who was to take young Tomás to Seville, had already taken his brother there. In the missive to his older son, Juan García acknowledged that the muleteer had brought back a letter from Juan Bautista as well as "white lead and some needles." He noted the difficulty of correspondence, especially under the current circumstances. He related to his son the death of his aunt Mari Franca's entire household, consoling himself and his son with the best explanation his faith permitted: "because blessed be Our Lord for it, who does His things as He is served." Mari Franca was dead, and Ana Calañas and Anica, so "that no one remains in the whole house." Mari Franca was the last one to die, "and there was not a small or big person present at her death if it were not for your mother." The poor woman who had lost two sisters and a niece left after Mari Franca's funeral to go to "Our Lady of Los Remedios, and stayed there until now."

The tailor lamented the suffering "that we certainly have much of" yet was grateful for God's mercy "that they have not thrown us out of town," a fate that befell others who had any contact with the plague dead, because, as he noted, the women died of pestilence. Juan García also mentioned that "we have received a thistle root, which we take now in the morning while fasting," and he thanked his son for his thoughtfulness. Thistle root was believed to ward off the plague.[7] The tailor asked Juan Bautista to "tell your master that God will give him days of life and will pay him for the care he has taken of Tomás." At the same time he promised to "serve him in whatever His Honor would wish to command him." It seems Tomás was not keen to "learn a trade in Seville," and his father was concerned for him, though he hoped perhaps to teach him his own trade "because I cannot leave him any other income." At the same time, it appears that Juan Bautista was not content with his situation as an apprentice either and had complained to his father about it: "you sent word that you

7. AMS, sec. 13, siglo XVI, vol. 5. See Covarrubias's dictionary (*Tesoro*, s.v. "cardo"). Covarrubias quotes Dr. Laguna, who claimed to have saved himself and his family during a deadly plague epidemic of 1542 by drinking wine infused with ground thistle root.

were not well in the house of your master, and that they did not treat you as is customary." Juan García tried to console his older son, reminding him that his "great suffering" was allowed for by "God's great kindness and mercy as He sees necessary."

The two brothers had other relatives in Seville to turn to. Their father asked Juan Bautista to tell "your uncle Juan Franco, that I kiss his hands and relate to him all that is happening here." Juan García, who ended the letter as "Your father who wishes you well," added a postscript. First he asked his son to send him some birdseed, and then he wondered if it would be possible to send some meat as well. The other letter Tomás carried was also from his father and was addressed to Juan Calañas in Seville. The tailor informed Juan of his aunt's death and asked him to purchase an oil lamp "to put above the grave, because here there is no possibility whatever."

When Jurado Toledo finished reading all the letters he ordered the local constable to guard the three muleteers at the inn of Mari Sánchez. The boy, Tomás, was taken outside the town to the house of "Juan Martín's wife," who was told "not to let him leave nor the animal on which he comes." All four were to remain in custody until the Count of Villar sent instructions on what should be done with them.

The jurado's inclination from the start had been to send these men and Tomás back to where they came from, but to his surprise the governor ruled differently. He mandated that the muleteers with their wine and the boy could continue to Seville and that the twenty-four reales the jurado had ordered as payment for Tomás's maintenance should be returned to them. Diego de Toledo was not happy with his superior's decision, and the same day, 20 March, he wrote a full explanation and rationale for his actions. Not only that, he refused to enforce the count's ruling, insisting that all of them would remain in detention until the governor was able to reexamine all the documentation, which he felt had not been available to him when he made his decision.

The jurado pointed out the difficult conditions he was working under and contended that what he had done was justified under the circumstances. He was concerned with Tomás's fate and pondered, "consider this, Your Most Illustrious Lordship, a boy of ten or eleven years, twenty leagues away from his home, alone and without a real, entrusted to these muleteers; what would become of him being ordered to return to his home, principally coming from a part where they die with such force!" Nevertheless, the jurado was firm in his conviction that the boy and the muleteers must not proceed to Seville, and he was certain that once the count read all the material he had sent, he would agree "and would neither permit them to pass nor return the money to them." Diego de Toledo further recommended that the wine be shipped to Seville on a boat and in wineskins brought from the city.

It was a bold step to contradict the governor's mandates, but the jurado acted in the belief that the count had ruled without having all the information of the case available. There was clearly a problem of crossed communications, and the jurado's gamble proved successful. The Count of Villar changed his orders and instructed on 22 March that the wine destined for the "friars of Santiago of Seville" be brought "by people of this city and draft animals and in skins and casks taken from it."[8] There was no mention in this order of the muleteers or the boy, but given the change in how the wine was to be transported into the city, it is reasonable to assume that Diego de Toledo prevailed and that they were forced to return to Segura de León.

8. AMS, sec. 13, siglo XVI, vol. 5 (19 March 1582).

26

DEATH OF DR. CENTURIO

Dr. Centurio . . . expired with a quick convulsion.
—FRANCISCO GONZÁLEZ PERELLÓN

THE ROYAL GOVERNOR OF SEVILLE'S responsibilities were many and diverse, and in times of crisis not only was he called upon to direct the city government, administer justice, and make decisions affecting the entire province, but he or his deputies were expected to address daily emergencies, to coordinate the efforts of various officials, and to respond to letters and petitions from vecinos and visitors alike. While Diego de Toledo was pressing the count for a ruling regarding the travelers from Segura de León, the governor was asked to intervene in other matters as well. One of the people petitioning the Count of Villar on Monday, 19 March, was María de Moya, the lonely wife of the surgeon Pedro García Arroyal, whom the governor had sent in January to Constantina and Puebla de los Infantes to treat the sick. The surgeon, who had served the city for many years, had finished his tour of duty but could not return to Seville directly. Instead, he was languishing in Paradas, a small town near Marchena, which belonged to "Señor Rodrigo Ponce de León, the Duke of Arcos." María de Moya begged the count to permit her husband to join her once again in their home in Triana because his absence "causes me great harm and injury," and she included her husband's testimony certified by the notary of the cabildo of Paradas.

Pedro García Arroyal stated that he had come to Paradas on 6 February, after the Count of Villar had refused to let him enter Seville so soon after leaving the two plague-infected towns. The exasperated surgeon claimed that as of Saturday evening, 17 March, he had been in Paradas for forty-one days, living in "the house of one of his daughters and his son-in-law." García Arroyal assured the governor that "by God Our Lord's mercy" everyone in town, including his family, was well. Quarantine, as its name implies, was normally imposed for forty days, and clearly enough time had passed since the physician had left the infected towns; therefore the count issued the license for his return to Seville.

Another physician in the city's employ did not fare as well. On 20 March the count received the sad news that Dr. Centurio, who had been treating plague victims in Constantina, "died and passed away from this present life." The licentiate Francisco González Perellón, Constantina's chief justice, sent a brief notice of the loyal doctor's death with a promise that a more detailed account would follow. The main reason for the short missive was to ask the governor to send a replacement, because the plague was still raging. The count obliged and ordered Bachiller Miguel Díaz, a surgeon from Seville, to travel to Constantina.

It would be several days before Licentiate González Perellón's follow-up letter, penned on 25 March, reached the count and the plague commission. González Perellón, who on many occasions had praised Dr. Centurio's skill and his services to Constantina's sick, related the circumstances of the physician's death. He died on Saturday, 17 March, "while making his will," before he could finish instituting his father, Blasio Cirozio, as his heir. González Perellón noted that to convince the sick doctor to make his testament, "my persuasion and exposing myself to danger and enter his lodgings was not enough, until the very necessity compelled him to do it." Dr. Centurio came from the mountainous border region between Italy and Austria. González Perellón commented that although the doctor was dying, he dictated the information of his origins "with such spirit that he spelled what he was saying in order for it to be understood." Lest there be any doubt, the chief justice declared that Dr. Centurio died "of two buboes and two carbuncles" and remarked that he "expired with a quick convulsion."

There was no mention of an executor of the will, but Dr. Centurio probably chose Licentiate González Perellón to safeguard and eventually distribute the property according to the doctor's directives. In his letter to the governor the chief justice listed some of the physician's possessions, which included a hefty gold chain and about 640 reales in cash as well as a promissory note for 1,200 ducats authorized by the city of Seville to be paid to the doctor by Diego del Postigo. Some 600 reales had been used for funeral expenses, and the rest was kept safe until Dr. Centurio's debts and bequests could be paid. The physician, who had seen many dead in his career, earmarked 1,000 ducats with which to "buy land in this city where the charity's poor could be buried." In addition, he left 1,000 reales for masses to be administered by the prior of the Carmelite monastery. The chief justice reminded the count that the city still owed 3,000 reales of the doctor's salary.

González Perellón complained that the Mercedarian friars had come to him with an order issued by Deputy Governor Aguilera demanding Dr. Centurio's possessions as "abandoned property." The Mercedarian order, founded to ransom Christian captives, still pursued this vocation in the late sixteenth century when North African corsairs continued to raid Spain's coast or attacked merchant vessels to kidnap hapless victims. The ransoming, which had become a lucrative business, was carried out usually by the Mercedarians or the Trinitarians, and the money for it came from pious clauses in wills or special privileges, such as claiming property of people with no known heirs.[1]

In closing, González Perellón lamented the town's poverty and the high cost of wheat, at forty-four reales a fanega, a price the local town council could ill afford to pay. Furthermore, plague expenses were growing, and local revenues were insufficient to cover them. The chief justice tried to work with local officials, but as he pointed out to the governor, "the council of this town does not help in this at all, nor does it want to, and I have had much aggravation over it."[2]

Several days later he sent another letter, detailing his "aggravation" with Constantina's magistrate, Alonso Martín del Rincón, and town councilors Juan Hidalgo de Reina and Juan Yáñes de Ureña. González Perellón complained that his attempts to help the afflicted had been "badly received with much displeasure and arrogance as from people known for their lack of spirit and fervor to help the poor, who in this town suffer much hunger and need." Local officials were not only ignoring his admonitions, they were also acting like "predestined people," that is, people who believed that they could do nothing to change God's will. Although the chief justice did not specifically mention Protestant beliefs, there were adherents in the region about this time, whom the Inquisition managed to ruthlessly suppress. González Perellón told the count that Constantina's authorities dismissed the priest's urging to alleviate the suf-

1. AMS, sec. 13, siglo XVI, vol. 5 (19 March 1582). Ellen G. Friedman, *Spanish Captives in North Africa in the Early Modern Age* (Madison: University of Wisconsin Press, 1983), 110–23, discusses the ways in which income was procured for the redemption of captives.

2. AMS, sec. 13, siglo XVI, vol. 5.

fering of the needy using the excuse that "the council is poor." The town officials unabashedly stated that whatever money was in the community coffer was
"for their [own] deliverance and that it is inopportune to have a physician or
give out food, rather let [the poor] die of hunger." Furthermore, he accused the
men of avarice, because they "are fond of consuming the maravedís of the poor
themselves," and he pressed the count to send a judge "because he is needed."

Just before writing this letter, González Perellón tried to obtain money to
help the poor, but the officials refused. There were now thirteen people "sick
with the plague," not counting those who were treated by "the barbers among
whom there are those of the infirmary who have gone out dragging their knees
on the ground from house to house to beg a piece of bread." González Perellón
ended his letter reiterating the heartbreaking hunger in Constantina and im-
ploring the governor to order the release of funds from the town's propios.

Constantina, unlike Cazalla de la Sierra, still could not declare itself plague
free, in spite of the efforts of Dr. Centurio, himself a victim of the disease. Physicians were not immune to contagious diseases, and although bubonic plague
did not spread from person to person, there were plenty of migrating fleas to fa-
cilitate the task. Those in close contact with a sick person were advised to carry
either smelling apples or pieces of aromatic wood or plants to purify the air
and thus ward off the plague. Physicians did the same. Dr. Nicolás Monardes
claimed that carrying and smelling a sassafras stick and chewing on small
pieces of citrus rind preserved him from the plague.[3] We do not know what precautions, if any, Dr. Centurio took to protect himself as he visited his patients,
but in the end he succumbed, like many others who bravely treated a sickness
whose best-known deterrent at the time was flight.

3. Monardes, *Historia medicinal,* 62r–63r; see also Chapter 7 in this volume.

27

SWELLING IN THE RIGHT THIGH

A swelling in the right thigh slightly below the groin,
greatly inflamed, with color and pain.
—JORGE SUÁREZ

HE COUNT OF VILLAR and the plague commission continued to receive notices of suspicious sickness throughout Seville. On 22 March they learned that there was a sick girl on Sol Street, in the parish of San Román. They ordered the surgeon Bachiller Jorge Suárez to visit the child and to take along constable Alonso Rodríguez. Isabel, about eight or nine years old, had "a burning fever and irregular pulse." The surgeon concluded that her fever was "malignant and poisonous," especially since she also had "a swelling in the right thigh slightly below the groin," and he characterized the swelling as "greatly inflamed, with color and pain." Moreover, Isabel was "weak and prostrated," and given all these symptoms, Bachiller Suárez declared that it had to be "buboes and contagious disease," that is, the plague. The authorities acted quickly and the same day notified the apothecary Juan Martínez, of nearby Santa Catalina parish, asking him to provide the necessary medications. The plague commission also wanted a second opinion.

Dr. Pedro Gómez examined Isabel the next day and gave a distinctly different report on her condition. He found that she had "a *bubón*" in the right groin, but unlike Bachiller Suárez he concluded that it was a tumor without "pestilential properties or contagious disease." Dr. Gómez categorically stated that although the girl had "a little bit of fever," she did not have "a disease from which there can be danger of contagion, because it is maturing like a tumor." Dr. Gómez's diagnosis might have soothed the plague commission's concerns, but more cases were being reported.

Three days later, on 26 March, the Count of Villar learned of suspicious deaths on Galera Street, in the Cestería neighborhood near the Triana Gate. About three weeks earlier the physicians had examined some people on the same street who had subsequently died, and at that point the doctors had also given conflicting opinions as to whether they had been stricken with the plague. This time the governor was alerted to a sick woman, a shopkeeper named Juana de Ribas, whose mother had died in the same house three weeks earlier and with similar symptoms. Juana de Ribas was not the only one afflicted, for there was another sick woman nearby as well. The count ordered three physicians who had treated these woman—Dr. Pedro Gómez; Dr. Bartolomé León, "El de Granada"; and Licentiate Alonso López—to report on their condition.

Dr. Gómez acknowledged that on 23 March he had gone to a house on Galera Street. There, in a shop, he spoke to a man who told him that his mother-in-law had died three weeks earlier with "symptoms of buboes," and he and his wife were worried because the mother-in-law had "felt a pain and a lump in one side of the groin and a pimple in the other." Dr. Gómez then carefully examined Juana de Ribas, the woman he had come to see; he "felt her pulse and found her with a fever of pestilential quality and other signs of contagious disease." Dr. Gómez never mentioned the woman's name in his report, though he attended her for about three days while she continued to display dangerous symptoms. Furthermore, she had been nursing her baby boy, who also became sick "with another fever of the same pestilential quality." Gómez felt that since the woman's mother had died of what appeared to have been the plague, and she herself had developed a "carbuncle behind the ear," it was likely that she also suffered from the same disease.

The second physician's report was brief. Dr. Bartolomé de León, "El de Granada," recalled that about three weeks earlier he had visited Juana de Ribas's mother, but only once. He remembered that she suffered from "a continuous fever and languor and a small swelling in the groin," and Dr. León was fairly certain that given her symptoms she had died of the plague.

Licentiate Alonso López, a surgeon, had visited Juana de Ribas's mother about fifteen to twenty days earlier and had found her with "very high fever." The surgeon thought that the fever was "pernicious," and so he asked the woman "if she felt anything," and she told him that all she had was the fever. Licentiate López returned another day to see her but was told that she had been taken to the house of one of her nieces. As he was about to leave, another shopkeeper inquired about her neighbor, and when the surgeon replied that he did not know because his patient had been taken away, "the said shopkeeper and two or three other women that were with her told him that it was a lie, that they did not take her away, because Dr. León de Granada just visited her." Licentiate

López subsequently heard that the woman had died, "full of spots and with two buboes."

Diego de Sotomayor, the barber surgeon from the Cestería, also testified. He did not know whether "Juana de Ribas's mother had died of the plague or another contagious disease." The surgeon related that he had been called about four days earlier to bleed Juana and examine her. He found that she had "a carbuncle on the left hip" and "a swelling on the right side of the genitals." When he returned the next day, he discovered "another swelling on the left side under her throat," which appeared to have "the qualities of the plague." Diego de Sotomayor assured the officials that he had been "curing and assisting her until yesterday," and she had been improving.

The surgeon also reported that he had been called to a nearby house the day before in the afternoon "to put some cupping glass on a boy or a girl," but the child did not have the plague. Diego de Sotomayor, however, examined another person in the house, an adolescent girl about fifteen years old, who did have a "carbuncle on the left side of her back and a swelling in the throat on the same side and with pestilential qualities." The surgeon stated that when he returned to bleed her "today," he found her covered with spots.

Dr. Pedro Gómez again visited Juana de Ribas on 27 March. She had "burning fever and it seems that she had been delirious, though at present she is somewhat better." Nevertheless, she did have "two bubones in the groin," one on each side, and after questioning Juana as well as her husband, Dr. Gómez concluded that she had "the sickness of the past year of the plague" and recommended that she should be isolated "so that there is no contagion from her, because it is dangerous." The physician was also concerned because the previous day, in the house next door "a boy and an adolescent girl had died in three or four days." Declaring himself "very scrupulous," he believed that it was "the said disease," even though he did not actually examine them.

The following day the Count of Villar ordered the constable to find the house where the girl and boy had died, remove their bedding and clothing to the Arenal, and burn them. The constable must not have felt great urgency in disposing of the contaminated possessions, because he did not arrive at the house until two days later, 30 March. The constable found two women there who pointed out what he was looking for: "one mattress, one sheet, one pillow, one blanket," and some clothing. Following the count's instructions, he transported them to the Arenal and there, "near the river," burned them.

On 30 March the count and the plague commission learned of yet another potential focus of sickness. A woman who lived on the "principal street" of the San Isidoro parish had died, and another woman was reportedly sick. The governor asked surgeon Alonso Sánchez Lescano from the nearby parish of San Nicolás, who had treated the women, to report. Sánchez Lescano stated that one of the women had "six carbuncles on her legs which are large pustules, and inflammation and burning." He also noted that she had a fever and two bubones and suffered from great "nausea and fainting." When he returned to check on her condition he learned that she had died. The other woman had a fever and a carbuncle "in the middle of her chest and a swelling under the right armpit." The surgeon informed the count that another physician, Licentiate Gerónimo de Burgos, who also lived in the parish of San Nicolás, had seen them too.

The governor sought out and questioned Licentiate Burgos, who confirmed that he had examined the two women. One had been sick for twenty days with a fever and carbuncles on her legs. But unlike surgeon Sánchez Lescano, Burgos did not find any "lump or a tumor in the groin or armpits" and rejected the notion that her sickness was of "pestilential nature." He gave a different explanation for the woman's demise, saying that she had been feeling better "and went up to the roof on a very hot day and combed her hair and became lethargic, and died from it."[1] Licentiate Burgos argued that her symptoms did not prove the woman perished from any contagious disease "because to have carbuncles is a very conceivable thing in the spring when blood flows so forcefully." As in some other cases, the physicians disagreed on the diagnosis, but it appears that the plague commission accepted Licentiate Burgos's assurances that this was not a "pestilential" disease: there was no follow-up order to burn the woman's belongings.

While the physicians were reporting on suspicious disease and death in Seville, the Count of Villar received news that the plague had also made its appearance to the west and south of the city. The plague commissioners met at the governor's lodgings on 26 March and read a letter from Cristóbal de Ayala, the constable assigned to guard Triana. He wrote that he learned that "many people are dying from the plague in Cartaya," a town west of Huelva in the Condado region, and that Lepe and other places were guarding against anyone coming

1. AMS, sec. 13, siglo XVI, vol. 5. The doctor stated she died of *modorra*, that is, encephalitis. When directly quoting, we choose to translate *modorra* as "lethargy" rather than the modern medical designation, "encephalitis."

from there. He asked the count for instructions and promised that in the meantime he would not allow anyone from Cartaya to enter Seville. There was also a
brief note from Hernando de Parraga reporting plague in Tarifa, on the Atlantic
coast of Spain on the Straits of Gibraltar. After consulting with the commissioners, the governor ordered all the guards, and especially those of Triana, to
stop any people, boats, or goods from Cartaya and Tarifa.

There was other business, mostly demands for payment, that the count and
the plague commission needed to resolve that day as well. There were petitions
from pharmacists Gerónimo Ortiz, Mancio Gasco, Pedro Farfán, and Pedro de
Sierra asking to be paid for the medicines each had dispensed. Another apothecary, Pedro Colorado, requested payment of salary for his servant, who carried the medicines to the pesthouse of San Bernardo. This was not the first nor
the last time these men asked for compensation, and before any money was disbursed, the commissioners insisted that the pharmacists provide exact accounts
of how much medicine they had provided and at what price. The cabildo also
owed 488 reales to the cleric Antonio de Villaroel for administering the sacraments at the pesthouse in Triana. Villaroel claimed he was needy "because of
the sickness I got from that house." Licentiate Manuel de Hojeda, the physician
who worked at the same hospital, requested payment of 1,650 reales the city
owed him for his services there.

The Count of Villar received a petition from Leonor de Morales, a nurse
who worked in the Cinco Llagas Hospital caring for plague victims, for the re-
mainder of her pay. She had already collected half of the one hundred ducats and twenty-eight reales that the officials had authorized as wages, but now
she wanted the rest of her salary because "I am a poor woman and I come
from Cordova just for this reason." Leonor's compensation was fairly substantial, given that one hundred ducats was the amount of many dowries that mid-
dling Sevillian women brought into marriage during this period. The governor
authorized the full payment, and the commissioners agreed that she should approach steward Diego del Postigo and have him disburse the money. But Leonor
de Morales returned on 6 April complaining that neither Diego del Postigo nor
the accountant Hernando de Porras would release payment in spite of the letter
of authorization. At this point the Count of Villar ordered a plague commissioner to collect the money and pay her.

Another woman who had worked at the Cinco Llagas Hospital, Juana de Es-
quivel, also petitioned for compensation. She asked to be paid sixteen ducats

for the time she had cared for plague-stricken women. Juana stated that she had worked for three and a half months for a promised six reales daily. The commissioners recommended that she should continue to "seek her justice," thus delaying any recompense Juana was entitled to.[2] The bills for medical care, as well as for guarding the numerous posts and many other services, were accumulating, and the city attempted to postpone payments as long as possible. Nevertheless, most people who were able to provide the necessary proof did get paid, though they might wait several months or longer.

Aside from trying to meet the escalating debts, the governor reshuffled assignments of some guards. On 27 March the Count of Villar ordered Diego de Toledo, who had served in Alcalá del Río for more than a month, to switch places with Bernaldino Ramírez, who had been stationed at Casaluenga. The alternating of posts was one way to ensure that officials did their jobs properly and did not establish close local ties, which might influence their conduct.

As Seville was attempting to keep out travelers and merchandise from places with known plague outbreaks, there were new complaints about the negligence of Triana's guards, because "many people pass through [Triana] and enter Seville without being asked for testimony and where they come from." The count took swift action and ordered Triana closed off to the outside, naming Triana vecino Cristóbal Romero to assist the guards at the one entrance that was to remain open, the street of Santo Domingo.[3] Romero, a wealthy seaman and the son-in-law of Triana jurado Juan Yáñez de Perea, was promised eight reales a day for his services. The governor instructed Romero to patrol, carrying the staff of justice, "day and night and not let or allow any people, cloths or other things" to enter from infected towns and to make sure that anyone who was allowed in "carries testimony that he is from a part and place that is healthy without plague." The governor had been warned by Jurado Sánchez de Soria, stationed at La Algaba, that "there is fraud in the passports," because the documents did not include a personal description or the type of clothing each person was wearing. Yet despite the shortcomings of the documentation, city officials relied on the only tool they knew to indicate that people entering Seville had not been in contact with the sickness.

In spite of all the efforts to contain the disease, more places were becoming infected, and fresh reports of suspicious deaths in Seville surfaced. The

2. AMS, sec. 13, siglo XVI, vol. 5 (26 March 1582).

3. Today's San Jacinto Street.

veinticuatro Luis del Alcázar informed the plague commission that he had learned from a courier who had passed through Lora del Río that there was plague there and that "the day before yesterday, Thursday, seven men died from the said sickness and yesterday, Friday, ten and today [30 March] in the morning there were six stricken by the disease and another six had died." There were also reports that people were perishing of the plague in Écija. Sevillian authorities immediately suspended all trade with Lora del Río and Écija. When the governor discovered the next day that Écija's regidor, García de Jerez, was in Seville buying wheat by the cartload for shipment to his town, he ordered him to leave, taking "his people and servants and clothing" with him, or face a fine of one thousand ducats. The constables located García de Jerez the following day, and after notifying him of the count's command, they escorted him outside the city walls and left him by the sanctuary of San Sebastián. That same day, guards at the Jerez Gate stopped muleteers from Écija with "a drove of animals carrying oil and other things" and ordered them to turn back.

By the second day of April the number of prohibited places Seville's town criers were proclaiming throughout the city was extensive: Constantina, Puebla de los Infantes, Castilblanco de los Arroyos, Jerez de los Caballeros, Segura de León, Lora del Río, Écija, Tarifa, Cartaya, Gibraleón, and La Redondela. At the same time, the authorities removed Cazalla de la Sierra from the list, no longer considering it a danger. Seville was now surrounded by plague-ridden communities in all directions, and as their number grew, so did the punishment for breaking the rules: people of "quality" were condemned to serve four years in the galleys without salary, while those of "low quality" received the same punishment and two hundred lashes. Any innkeeper who provided a room to a traveler from a proscribed town was threatened with one hundred lashes and a fine of one hundred thousand maravedís. The denouncer would be rewarded with a portion of the fine.[4]

4. AMS, sec. 13, siglo XVI, vol. 5. It is difficult to ascertain how often these punishments were actually carried out, but there are notices of thieves and of women who were illegally reselling meat or vegetables, for example, being whipped in the streets. Some thieves were even hanged. Hanging was a common punishment for murderers and homosexuals. See, for example, Francisco de Ariño, *Sucesos de Sevilla de 1592 a 1604*, ed. Antonio María Fabié (Seville: Ayuntamiento de Sevilla, 1993), 50–52, 57–58, 68–69, 80; or Pedro de León, *Grandeza y miseria en Andalucía: Testimonio de una encrucijada histórica (1578–1616)*, ed. Pedro Herrera Puga (Granada: Facultad de Teología, 1981), 411–28.

28

FLEEING DISEASE

Many people had left the town, fleeing the said disease.
—DIEGO ALONSO

T HE TOWN OF CASTILBLANCO de los Arroyos once again demanded attention from Sevillian authorities. On Saturday, the last day of March, Pedro Suárez de Venegas received orders to travel to Castilblanco and check on the number and status of the sick. The Count of Villar charged him with reporting on conditions in Constantina and Puebla de los Infantes as well. Jurado Suárez de Venegas, accompanied by the notary Martín de Castro, promptly left on his mission. The men spent the night in a small place called Burguillos, about two-thirds the distance between Seville and Castilblanco.

The following day, Sunday, after Mass, the jurado reached the outskirts of Castilblanco, where he was appalled to find thirty to forty huts "and in them many people who are dying of hunger." He immediately wrote the Count of Villar asking him to help these unfortunates, who had only "boiled weeds" to eat and had not tasted bread for a week. Their plight was exacerbated by being barred from nearby villages, and they desperately needed food and alms. Jurado Suárez de Venegas implored the governor to provide two or three cargas of bread, two cargas of fish, and one carga of olive oil "to distribute among all these wretches." The twelve friars living in the nearby Monastery of Santo Espiritus del Monte, who traditionally received their supplies from Castilblanco, were also without food. In closing, the jurado appealed to the count's Christian sentiments, reminding him that feeding these starving people would be of great service to God. The jurado's pleas reached Seville quickly. On 2 April the Count of Villar authorized shipment of one hundred fanegas of Sicilian wheat to Castilblanco. This was not a gift; the alhóndiga of Seville was to be reimbursed for the wheat on 1 August at the elevated rate of 26.5 reales (about

2.4 ducats) per fanega. The count ordered the town council of Castilblanco to distribute the grain primarily among the poor, and the most needy were to receive it first and foremost.

Jurado Suárez de Venegas and his notary did not enter Castilblanco; instead, they summoned the town's officials to the Fuente de la Gama, a place in the countryside about one league distant from the plague-stricken community. The jurado began his investigation by questioning one of the people living in the huts, farmer Diego Alonso. The farmer related that around the middle of February people started to sicken with "carbuncles and buboes." He stated that shortly before Lent he had left his home in Castilblanco "for the countryside where he is at present in a hut." Diego Alonso told the jurado that "many people had left the town, fleeing the said disease." He believed twenty to thirty people had perished in Castilblanco, though it seemed the situation was improving. The farmer thought that there were presently four sick being cared for by a physician sent from Seville and two local barbers. He claimed that no one had died for ten days and insisted that the principal problem now was lack of food among those who had fled to the countryside. They were reduced to eating weeds, he said, and he had "seen them cooking them in water without any other thing." The farmer was not as seriously affected by the food shortage and was able to "give to some of them the whey of his goats' milk."

The next witness, Castilblanco's magistrate Pedro Gutiérrez, provided similar testimony but with important variations in detail. He stated that of those who had perished, about half had died of causes other than the plague. He also pointed out that at present, the principal concern was hunger. Nevertheless, there were now thirty to thirty-two sick with the plague; about half of them were in the hospital, while the rest were being treated in their homes. The magistrate insisted that there had been no deaths for fifteen days, save an old woman who died because of her age and poverty. He praised the efforts of the physician, Licentiate Melchior de Rojas, who came from Seville at the beginning of March and had brought the much-needed plague remedies with him. He also mentioned the two local barbers. Pedro Gutiérrez bitterly complained that Castilblanco's council had no money, having spent all that they had available. The council's last resort was to sell tree bark from cork trees belonging to the town, but "the said bark cannot be sold." No buyers were coming because of the trade embargo and the fear of the plague.

Town officials were desperate to find wheat for their community. Gutiérrez admitted that the forty fanegas of wheat currently in the public granary, a meager quantity, he "took by force from some carters" who were transporting cartloads of wheat, though he did pay a hefty price for the grain: thirty-two reales a fanega, about triple the set price. The magistrate's testimony was echoed by the public notary, Alonso Rodríguez, who added that normally the town had two hundred fanegas of wheat on deposit. He lamented that the town could not pay the Sevillian physician or for the medicines needed to cure the sick. The notary emphasized the plight of the starving populace, noting that many "eat grass and mustard weeds," and some went to the countryside to kill goats "and eat them because of the great necessity." These men must have been relieved to learn that wheat was being sent from Seville, though the question of payment would have been troublesome.

The fear of the plague raging in Castilblanco spread to nearby communities. On 2 April, a man from Burguillos arrived in Alcalá del Río and informed Diego de Toledo that there was a rumor that a man who had come from Castilblanco had died from the plague. People feared that he had brought the disease to their village. Such information could not be ignored, and the jurado sent magistrate Antonio de Roa to Burguillos to investigate. The magistrate questioned Pedro Ruiz, the local barber surgeon who had treated the sick man. He could not shed much light on what caused the man's death, but he was quite certain that it was not the plague; he claimed to know the symptoms well. There was another sick man in Burguillos, Luis Martín de Cortegana, whom the barber had visited the day before, on 1 April. He found that he had "a tumor above the left groin and four pustules, one on the thigh and three on the tip of his buttocks." Not too pretty, but again the barber assured the magistrate that Luis Martín did not have the plague.

The barber surgeon returned that very day to check on his condition, but Martín was not at home. The man's wife told him that her husband had gone out to "collect firewood." Clearly, Luis Martín was feeling better, and there seemed to be no danger of contagion from him. The magistrate also questioned the local priest, who confirmed that there was no plague in Burguillos. Diego de Toledo sent the magistrate's report to the count and the plague commission in Seville.

In the meantime, Jurado Suárez de Venegas had left the outskirts of Castilblanco and traveled to Cazalla de la Sierra, where he arrived on Tuesday, 3 April. He assembled the same men who had testified several times already to ask them yet again about health conditions in Cazalla. The jurado questioned surgeon Andres Gutiérrez, physician Hernán Vázquez, and barber Francisco de Zamora as well as the local priests Luis Muñoz and Luis de Aguilar, and they all coincided in their testimony that the place was healthy.

While in Cazalla de la Sierra, Jurado Suárez de Venegas also secured testimony about conditions in Constantina in fulfillment of the count's instructions. He was able to question several vecinos of Constantina who happened to be in Cazalla. One was a millstone maker, Francisco Sánchez de Hojeda, who had just arrived. He told the jurado that approximately three and a half months earlier, for a period of about one month, three to four people were dying daily. But he insisted that this mortality had ended a month ago, and now Constantina was healthy.

Another traveler from Constantina, the sales tax collector Gaspar Fernández, concurred, though he put the earlier mortality at three to six people daily. He stated that Constantina's food shortage had been alleviated by a recent shipment of wheat. Fernández informed the jurado that the plague constable Francisco de Ocaña had finished his duties about twenty days earlier and in the past five days no one had died. He admitted that there were still about eight to ten patients convalescing in the hospital, cared for by the new surgeon, Bachiller Miguel Díaz, who had replaced the deceased Dr. Centurio.

This was encouraging testimony, and Jurado Suárez de Venegas decided to continue on to Constantina. He reached the Monastery of San Francisco, outside the town walls, and sent a messenger to gather certain witnesses he wanted to question: two magistrates and councilors, as well as Constantina's chief justice, the licentiate Francisco González Perellón, and the physician Miguel Díaz. They would join the jurado outside town the next day and give their depositions.

The first witness was surgeon Bachiller Díaz, who had arrived from Seville only four days earlier. His testimony was not nearly as optimistic as that of the two men the jurado had questioned in Cazalla. The twenty-six-year-old surgeon stated that while many of the sick had recovered, four people had died since his arrival in Constantina. There were presently two people, a couple, in the hospital suffering from the plague. The husband had a bubo and a carbuncle, and his wife had two buboes in the groin. The only other sick person was being treated at home. Miguel Díaz complained that the town council had not paid him, and he mentioned that he had spent six reales just yesterday to

buy "a hen and two loaves of bread for the sick." In addition he had given an-
other six reales to Garrido, the barber surgeon who lived in the hospital. He
knew that the town's money was kept in a special coffer at the Monastery of San
Francisco and complained that the officials refused to open it, something that
Constantina's chief justice had alluded to in his earlier letter to the Count of
Villar.

The next witness was Alonso Martín del Rincón, Constantina's magistrate,
one of the officials who had irritated Licentiate González Perellón because of
his unwillingness to release funds to pay the plague expenses. The magistrate
testified that since mid-January about fifty people had died of the plague, but
now there were only five patients in the hospital. The current physician seemed
effective, he reported, and there were plenty of medicines. Martín del Rincón
insisted that the town did not have the money to cover the costs, though he
thought that when the council collected the income from the town's properties,
the situation would improve. He contended that the city of Seville should help
pay the plague expenses, especially the salaries of the physician and barber. He
declared that the public granary had an adequate supply of wheat.

Next to testify were the two councilors, Juan Yáñez de Ureña and Juan
Hidalgo de Reina, about whom the chief justice had so bitterly complained to
the governor. Their testimony mirrored that of their colleague. Juan Hidalgo
denied any possibility of payment until perhaps the end of April, when the
town revenues were normally collected. Interestingly, Yáñez de Ureña acknowledged that there was money in the coffer at the Franciscan monastery and indicated that the council might be able to authorize some payment.

The next witness was the chief justice himself. Licentiate González Perellón stated that about eighty people, mostly poor, had died since the epidemic
began. He noted that he had written to the Count of Villar just yesterday, but
there was no courier to take the letter to Seville. González Perellón was exasperated because he had been writing to the governor regularly but had not received
a single response. He was not alone in complaining that the Count of Villar
was not replying to letters; others mentioned it also, usually at the beginning of
their missives to Seville. We know the communications arrived, and both the
count and the councilors read them and acted upon them. But it appears they
and the scribes were often too occupied to write back, or the responses were
both tardy and insufficient.

As in his letters, González Perellón had nothing but praise for the medical staff that he worked with, but he again complained about the town officials who refused to contribute any money to the plague fund. González Perellón, not to be defeated by the obstreperous councilors, had with the count's authority "embargoed all the propios and income of the council for food in the said hospital and the sick and the salaries of the physician, and barber surgeon." He had not touched any of the money deposited in the Franciscan monastery or the "sales taxes of His Majesty." The chief justice also disapproved of the town council's recent decision to sell wheat from the granary because the price was beginning to fall. He had argued against it, pointing out that it should be saved for a time of need, but to no avail. Nevertheless, in spite of the sale, some wheat was still available.

Having made the necessary inquiries in Constantina, Jurado Suárez de Venegas and the notary left the Franciscan monastery on Thursday morning, 5 April, in the direction of Puebla de los Infantes. Once again they stopped outside the town, about a half league away, in the Huerta de la Vera Cruz. From there they sent a man with orders to bring out local officials, the notary, and Licentiate Perea Durán, Seville's jurado overseeing the plague efforts in Puebla.

The first witness was farmer and town councilor Pedro López. He stated that since the end of December, in spite of the efforts of the two physicians sent from Seville, Pedro García Arroyal and later Licentiate Sosa de Sotomayor, about two hundred people had died. Most were adolescents, and only about fifteen adults had succumbed to the disease. There were still twenty patients in the hospital, about half of whom were improving. In the last week, "since it was cloudy . . . some . . . were stricken." Both the medicines and the pharmacist to dispense them also came from Seville, but there was no money left in Puebla to pay for them. Local authorities were buying bread for the poor, about one and a half fanegas a day, as well as hens and a ram. The town had left only the income from two tracts of pastureland that were not only grassy but had enough live-oak trees to produce substantial amounts of acorns. Unfortunately, there would not be any revenue "until the acorns come." The acorns, used to fatten pigs in the weeks leading up to slaughter, could not be harvested until the fall. But there still remained about fifty ducats and forty fanegas of wheat in the granary.

Jurado Suárez de Venegas then asked Pedro López whether the town would be able to store wheat brought from Seville and when the council would be able to pay for it. Storage was not a problem, there was a place nearby, but they could not pay anything until "the day of San Miguel [29 September] when the acorns would be sold." Even then, López was not certain that the council would be able to afford to buy the wheat, given the current high expenses and shortage of funds.

The next witness, Alonso García Velázquez, the steward of Puebla's cabildo, stated that there were presently about seventeen or eighteen patients in the hospital and twelve in their homes. He insisted that more people continued to be stricken. He knew Puebla's financial situation well and admitted that there was still the considerable amount of a thousand ducats in the coffers. The steward declared that the wheat was all gone and the town needed three hundred fanegas of it to survive until the new harvest. He recommended that it should be brought in carts from Seville and unloaded outside Puebla on land belonging to the Countess of Palma.

The testimony of Puebla's magistrate, Anton García Rebollar, was more optimistic. He suggested that the plague had been decreasing over the past twenty days and also blamed cloudiness for an increase in people stricken over the past week. He acknowledged that there were one thousand ducats in the treasury but insisted that the money was necessary to buy wheat for the poor and could not be used for hospital expenses. García Rebollar did not think that the town could cash in on the acorns any earlier than All Saints Day (November 1). He estimated that Puebla would need about eighty fanegas of wheat until new grain became available.

During his questioning the magistrate revealed that about two months before a man had appeared in town, a certain *Maese* (Master) Martín, who claimed to be a surgeon. Although the magistrate was impressed with the itinerant healer, who had successfully treated three people, Puebla's physician, Licentiate Sosa de Sotomayor, "did not want the said Maese Martín to cure because he did not have orders from the Señor governor." The physician had enlisted the help of Licentiate Perea Durán to drive the unlicensed practitioner out of town, and Maese Martín had confided in García Rebollar and another man that "he wanted to leave the said town because Licentiate Perea wanted to arrest him." In his testimony García Rebollar denounced the actions of Sosa de Sotomayor and Perea Durán, outsiders from Seville who had forced the healer to leave and had threatened the local council with a fine of thirty thousand maravedís if they allowed him to stay and treat the sick. García Rebollar defended Maese Martín, who "did his craft well and he told the poor that he would treat them for free."

It is unclear whether Licentiate Perea Durán testified, because although he had been summoned, there is no record of his testimony. Suárez de Venegas and his notary were able to finish their work on the outskirts of Puebla within hours, and by the afternoon they left in the southeastern direction. They reported, "we arrived to spend the night at the monastery of the Franciscan friars called San Luis, one league away from Palma [del Río]." The next morning the men continued to Palma del Río, where they negotiated with the Countess of Palma regarding Puebla's needs and to obtain permission to store wheat sent from Seville on her land. They left Palma in the afternoon, heading back in the direction of Seville, but they bypassed Lora del Río, where, according to what they heard in Palma, "every day six to seven people die of the plague." Instead, the jurado and his scribe spent the night at La Campana, east of Lora del Río, and the following morning they traveled back home, "and this day in the night we arrived in Seville." They claimed that they had spent a total of eight days on the road.[1]

1. AMS, sec. 13, siglo XVI, vol. 5.

29

POSTING GUARD

We will assign a very honorable man and of confidence.
—THE PLAGUE COMMISSION

WHEN THE COUNT OF VILLAR met with the plague commission on 2 April, he pointed out that now that Seville was surrounded by plague-stricken communities, greater care needed to be taken to protect it. He ordered jurados and constables to guard the city gates, and he set their salary at ten reales a day. Furthermore, he posted eight mounted constables to keep watch in the areas outside city walls. He charged the city's steward, Diego del Postigo, with selecting them and paying them the same daily stipend as those guarding the city gates. The councilors present at the meeting decided to make a list of all the veinticuatros and jurados currently in Seville who could inspect the city gates daily and at all hours. To ensure that the mounted constables were diligent in their patrols, they agreed to assign "a very honorable man and of confidence" to supervise the horsemen.

Of the thirteen entrances leading into the city, the councilors determined to keep only eight open. Extra guards were needed for the Slaughterhouse and Arenal Gates because they remained open at night. Two days later the assignments were made, to be effective for the next fifteen days:

Alonso de Avila, Macarena Gate
Pedro Ruíz de Santiago, Carmona Gate
Luis Alvarez de Soria, Slaughterhouse Gate
Juan Jara, Postigo del Carbón (Coal Gate)
Francisco de Alburquerque, Postigo del Aceite (Oil Gate)
Luis de Troya, Arenal Gate
Diego Gutiérrez Barba, Triana Gate
Alonso de Andrada Avendaño, Royal Gate

The next day, though, the governor modified the gate openings. The extramural Monastery of the Santísima Trinidad requested that the Sol Gate, the closest communication point with the city for the monks, be kept open. The Count of Villar obliged and assigned the jurado Juan Gómez Corona to guard it. At the same time the count ordered the Postigo del Carbón closed, though the Postigo del Aceite remained open because it was Lent, and the gate was near the fish market.

The governor had received the nominations for the eight mounted constables from Diego del Postigo, and on 6 April he officially assigned the men, each armed with a lance and a leather shield, to guard the immediate environs of the city. The count instructed the constables to work in pairs in four specific locations. From these locations, each guard would be responsible for a certain territory. For example, two horsemen were posted at the Monastery of San Isidoro del Campo to patrol the area on the "other bank of the Guadalquivir," beyond Triana. One constable was to guard the northwest area between the monastery and the towns of Santiponce and La Algaba, and the other the territory to the west of the monastery up to the village of Salteras.[1]

Three days after these assignments were issued, the plague commission met in the Count of Villar's quarters in the Alcázar to discuss the situation in the outlying communities. Jurado Suárez de Venegas, who had just returned to Seville, reported on conditions in Castilblanco, Constantina, Puebla de los Infantes, and Cazalla de la Sierra. After listening to the jurado, the plague commissioners agreed that the situation in Constantina was exacerbated by the fact that the sick were not properly treated for lack of funds. They ordered that anyone newly stricken should be taken to a hospital, and they advised Constantina's officials to use the town's sisa to cover plague expenses. If that was insufficient, there were always forced loans from wealthy residents. The central government in Seville placed the financial burden on the local council and reminded Constantina's officials that if they failed to provide the necessary treatment for their community's plague-stricken poor, they were entirely to blame for the consequences.

Jurado Suárez de Venegas informed the commission of the severe bread shortage in Puebla de los Infantes. The count and the plague deputies adopted a strategy similar to that applied in the case of Castilblanco. One hundred fane-

1. AMS, sec. 13, siglo XVI, vol. 5.

gas of Sicilian wheat from Seville's public granary would be transported to Puebla under the supervision of Jurado Suárez de Venegas. The town would reimburse Seville's alhóndiga at a rate of 2.5 ducats per fanega, and the 250 ducats were to be paid to Juan de Perea Durán, Seville's jurado stationed in Puebla. As in Castilblanco, the bread was earmarked for the most needy.

By mid-April it seemed that the worst was over in Castilblanco, and local officials wanted to let Seville know as quickly as possible of the improvements. On an auspicious day, 15 April, Easter Sunday, they compiled a report and sent it to the Count of Villar. The licentiate Melchior de Rojas, the surgeon who had been treating the sick since the beginning of March, testified that for the past eight days no one had been taken to the hospital. Juan Lozano, the town's plague constable, concurred that no one had been sick in the past ten days, and the hospital was empty. Gerónimo Díaz, the nurse who resided in Castilblanco's pesthouse helping the sick day and night, stated that for the past twelve days no one had been stricken, nor was there anyone currently being treated. Barber surgeon Francisco Díaz, who also resided in the hospital, declared that he had "bled and cured many sick" and that twelve people had died in the hospital during the outbreak, but that for the past fifteen days there were no patients and all was well. Two priests agreed, saying that for the past twenty days they had not attended or taken confession from anyone sick with the plague.

The Count of Villar received the report along with a letter from Juan Martínez on 17 April. Martínez declared on behalf of Castilblanco's town council that the community was healthy and requested permission for its residents and goods to enter Seville. The governor must have been convinced because he ordered that Melchior de Rojas be notified that his services were no longer needed and his salary for work in Castilblanco was ending. As in the case of other physicians returning to Seville after a tour of duty in plague towns, Licentiate Rojas was not allowed to enter the city immediately but was to await the count's authorization.[2] Even before the Count of Villar's order reached Castilblanco, the town's council had already dismissed Licentiate Rojas "because there was no one to cure," and the physician left town on Easter Sunday, shortly after he had testified. He did come back several days later attempting to collect his salary from Castilblanco's officials, and after a few days left again, though it is unclear where he went, since he could not yet return to Seville.[3]

2. Ibid.

3. AMS, sec. 13, siglo XVI, vol. 6.

At the same time that Castilblanco reported the restoration of healthy conditions, there was suspicion of the plague in Coria, a small town south of Seville. The count and the plague commissioners sent Diego de Toledo to make inquiries; he began his investigation on Monday, 16 April 1582. He questioned a local physician, the licentiate Miguel Cortés Altamirano, who testified that seventeen days earlier it was rumored that a sick man had come to an inn, the Mesón Blanco, from Sanlúcar de Barrameda. He was "sick with a fever" for two days and then died. Cortés Altamirano told Diego de Toledo that four days later he was called to the Mesón Blanco to see the innkeeper's son. He found him "with a fever, vomiting and swelling up, with many palpitations." The innkeeper's wife and daughters were lamenting "the day that they had received in their inn the sick man who died there and his clothing that he left behind, because the boy had taken it." The boy died within twenty-four hours.

But the sickness at the Mesón Blanco did not end there. Licentiate Cortés Altamirano was called back "to visit another, older boy at the inn." He found that the child was "humoral in the groin and having pressed it, he drew back in pain." The physician was not surprised to learn that the patient died three days later. Then, three days after that, Licentiate Cortés Altamirano was called to the inn yet again, this time to see another boy, twelve or thirteen years old, "with a tumor under his throat and a very high fever." The youth had been vomiting and "was so out of his senses" that even after the doctor "strongly pressed the tumor, he was quiet and did not show any palpitation." When the physician came out of the boy's room, "they showed him a nursing infant in the same inn" who was also sick and died that same day. Licentiate Cortés Altamirano concluded his testimony declaring that they all died within two days of becoming sick and that they were all infected by the man who had come to stay at the inn. But the physician insisted that these were isolated cases and that there was no other sickness in the area.

The following day, Tuesday, 17 April, Diego de Toledo wrote his report, stating that at the Mesón Blanco five people had died of the plague, the innkeeper's children and grandchildren who became infected by a sick man who stayed at the inn. The jurado added that he had also questioned the local priest and two barber surgeons, who all confirmed that there were no other cases of the disease. Diego de Toledo was a prudent man, and he instructed Coria's officials to keep careful watch on health conditions and to guard against the plague. He also ordered the innkeeper, his wife and remaining children, and his son-in-law to leave town and stay in the countryside. Food was to be provided to them, but there was to be no direct contact, nor could they return until receiving authorization from the Count of Villar. The Mesón Blanco was shut down.[4]

4. Ibid.

30

COVERED WITH BLACKISH SPOTS

She was covered with blackish spots and she was livid.
—MARÍA GONZÁLEZ

S SEVILLE FOUND ITSELF ever more tightly surrounded by infected communities, the situation in the city seemed to be deteriorating as well. On 5 April the plague commission learned that a candle maker who lived on Mar Street had died that day, and his wife and son were sick. The following day the deputies took down the testimony of Bachiller Rodrigo García de Flores, the physician who had treated the family. He stated that he had visited the candle maker, Juan Moreno, and found him in bed and delirious. The physician was able to ask him a few questions, and Moreno told him that the "day before his arm hurt and that he had an abscess underneath." He then examined the candle maker, "felt him under the said arm," but Moreno claimed that it did not hurt anymore because Dr. Juan Sánchez had prescribed an "unction of rose oil and it went away."

Indeed, Bachiller García de Flores did not find any lump, though he believed the candle maker "suffered from a poisonous disease and which carried malignancy because it had produced such a bad and pernicious transmutation that left him lethargic, and that is what he died from in two or three days." The physician added that he had gone back to the house that very afternoon to see Inés Alvarez, the candle maker's wife, who was "sick with a swelling in the groin," though he did not perceive any symptoms of malignancy. Her small son had a fever and was complaining of pain under his armpit, but when the physician examined him, he "did not find any bubo."

The apothecary Bartolomé de Barrientos, the candle maker's next-door neighbor, who knew the family well, was questioned the next day. He confirmed that "Doctor Flores" had treated Juan Moreno and his wife and son. It was Barrientos who prepared the medicines prescribed by the physician, and he believed that "they are for the said sickness of the plague." He had more news for the plague commission: the boy too had died.

The candle maker's brother, Gonzalo Martín, testified also. He said his brother had a "tumor above the heart and lethargy and the son had spots and he heard it said that he had a bubo." His sister-in-law, Inés Alvarez, had "a bubo," and she was in a bed with "two mattresses and two sheets and a blanket and two pillows." Her husband's and son's bedding had remained in the house after they died, but it was kept apart. As soon as the Count of Villar heard that the infected bedding was still in the house, he ordered it taken to the Arenal, where it was burned near the river. When a few days later, on 10 April, Inés died, her bedding was burned in the Arenal as well. If the governor and the plague commission feared that the family had died of the plague, their suspicions were confirmed on 16 April: Gonzalo Martín, who had testified only a few days earlier, had died "in the said house of the contagious disease within twenty-four hours." His bedding and linens met the same fate at the Arenal as that of his brother and family.[1]

The plague commission received other reports of sickness. On 6 April the deputies secured testimony from Dr. Pedro Gómez, who, along with Drs. Benito Carrero and Juan Rodríguez, had been charged by the commissioners with examining anyone in the city suspected of being sick. Dr. Gómez stated that four days ago he had gone to see two sisters of a fruit seller's widow who lived near the Royal Jail. They had fever, and each one had a lump, "one under the arm and the other beneath the throat," though the doctor believed that their symptoms were not as serious as was usual "in this contagious sickness." Furthermore, each one had menstruated, and they seemed to be improving. Therefore Dr. Gómez had not notified "His Lordship the Count in order not to disturb and agitate without reason." Dr. Gómez indicated that one of the women had been sick for five days and the other one for seven days now, and until fourteen days had passed "it cannot be said they are out of danger." Dr. Gómez's reference to menstruation was in keeping with traditional medical belief that in sickness the patient would experience a turning point, either for better or for worse, and this "crisis" was precipitated by a "sudden excretion of bad humors." Menstruation, vomiting, diarrhea, or heavy perspiration all signaled a turning point. In this case, one of the women "turned" from bad to worse, and she died on 11 April.[2]

1. AMS, sec. 13, siglo XVI, vol. 6.

2. Ibid. On prognosis and crisis, see Siraisi, *Medieval Medicine*, 134–35.

Reports of sickness in various parts of the city poured in. On 7 April Francisco Carrillo informed the plague commission that two girls had died three days earlier in the parish of Santa Lucía in the house of Bartolomé de Jerez. One girl had died of a "bubo," the other of typhus. The mothers of both girls as well as a barber surgeon were questioned. María de Herrera, Bartolomé de Jerez's wife, stated that her husband was a horse dealer and that their daughter Gerónima died of lethargy.[3] María Díaz, the mother of the other child, said that last Thursday her baby girl had been sick and died in her crib and that she "expelled skin from her mouth." Barber surgeon Andrés de Arjona had visited Gerónima the day she died. She had a very high fever, was delirious, and had "an abscess under her left arm." He believed that Gerónima's sickness was "pestilential" because of "the great degeneration that alters the spirits."

Sickness and death continued in the horse dealer's household. On 9 April the barber surgeon notified the cabildo about two new cases, "a boy and an old woman." For the past two days the boy had "a swelling in the groin and high fever" in addition to "fainting and vomiting." The old woman had the same symptoms, though less severe. The boy died the next day, and there was no follow-up on the woman's condition, though one wonders whether the dealer's house had been ordered locked. The count and the plague commission would have found sufficient reason to isolate everyone to prevent further spread of the contagion.

On 7 April came reports of people dying in another household, that of Juan de Céspedes, a hatmaker who lived "at the entrance to the Pajería," the prostitution district near the Triana Gate also known as the Mancebía. Barber surgeon Antonio de Solís had been called to the house and found three sick women there. One had a "bubo in the groin, a fever and was delirious"; she was dispirited and was vomiting and, not surprisingly, lacked appetite. The surgeon also observed typhus-like spots. She died five days after her symptoms first appeared. The second woman had a "carbuncle on her right calf," and she too had spots and fever and was unable to eat. She died on the seventh day of her sickness. The third woman was the hatmaker's mulatta slave, who had a fever and a "carbuncle on her right arm." She was still alive when the surgeon was giving his deposition but perished three days later.

The officials also questioned Juan de Céspedes. According to the hatmaker, one of the dead women was a beata, a holy woman, and he declared that she

---

3. The Spanish term is modorra, that is, encephalitis; see Chapter 27, n. 1, in this volume.

died of a chronic fever.[4] He indicated that she had a "pustule on her leg." The other woman suffered from "lethargy and spots," and what might have appeared as a carbuncle was instead "a swelling" that healed. When asked about the whereabouts of the bedding and linens, the hatmaker said that his "servant threw it out at the Laguna de la Mancebía" and that he "did not know who took it." The deputies went with Céspedes, found the articles, and burned them. By playing down the seriousness of the women's sickness, in stark contradiction to the barber surgeon's testimony, the hatmaker was hoping to dissuade authorities from locking his house and isolating the remaining residents. Given that the bedding was destroyed, it seems unlikely that he succeeded.[5]

Even at a time when the city was controlling all entrances by land, ships continued to arrive at Seville's port, merchandise was unloaded, and passengers and crew disembarked. Only when sickness actually appeared on board did authorities take notice. On 7 April the Count of Villar was informed that a ship from Brittany had anchored in the Guadalquivir River, and "they removed this morning two dead men and this afternoon they took out six sick men with two mattresses and other clothing." The governor ordered that no person or goods were to leave the ship, "under pain of death," and sent constable Alonso Rodríguez along with a notary to the port to make the pertinent inquiries.

When they arrived they discovered that the bedding that had been removed from the ship with the dead sailors had been burned in the Arenal. The constable questioned several people. First, Juan Ramos, customs duty guard, stated that he saw that morning two dead men taken off the Breton ship, *El Dragón*. They were carried "in a litter of La Caridad," the brotherhood founded to provide a Christian burial for the destitute, and the brothers of La Caridad took the bodies away. Then, between noon and one o'clock, Ramos observed two men loaded with two mattresses leaving the ship. Some time later four or five men left the ship, "staggering and it seemed they were sick," and went toward the Arenal Gate, but Ramos could not tell the constable where they went after that. The customs guard Alonso García de Almarea declared that the Breton ship carried wheat, which was being unloaded. He confirmed that there had been two dead on board and that five people were currently sick.

4. AMS, sec. 13, siglo XVI, vol. 6. The Spanish word is *ética,* defined in Covarrubias's *Tesoro* as "*calentura arraigada continua*" (continuous long-term fever). The modern equivalent is *fiebre hética* or *fiebre héctica,* and it is associated with extreme thinness and consumption, or tuberculosis.

5. AMS, sec. 13, siglo XVI, vol. 6.

The two subsequent witnesses were sailors. Nicolás Francés and Andrés Perra did not deny that two men had died on board and that others were ill, but their explanation for the malady was reassuring: overwork and too much wine. They testified that the men seen staggering from the ship had gone to a tavern in the Carretería, the neighborhood outside the Arenal Gate known to cater to sailor's needs, and became sick. Francés and Perra explained to the constable that their dead and sick companions "did not have nor have they any dangerous disease, rather it was the fatigue having worked to bring the said ship to this city, towing it, and having drunk a lot of wine." The two sailors insisted that it was this exertion coupled with the excess of wine that caused the men to have "fevers and stomach ache."

The two physicians who had visited the sick Breton mariners agreed. The licentiate Cristóbal Díaz del Prado and Bachiller García de Flores testified that they all had the same fevers "and complained about their stomachs." The doctors "examined their parts where pestilential abscesses tend to appear" and found none. Nevertheless, their fevers could be a portent of a serious ailment, and therefore the physicians advised that the sick sailors should return to the ship "and be treated there and they should be made to leave the city, being as it is fearful of outside sickness." Having heard the doctors' recommendation, the constable escorted the sailors back to the ship, and there, through interpreter Manuel de Voz, he admonished them not to leave the vessel, "on pain of death."

Reports of sickness streamed in. On Monday 9 April, María González, a fisherman's wife, testified about the death of her neighbor, Isabel de Medina. Last Thursday, "the Day of the Conversion of la Magdalena," the two women had gone together to "a sermon in Las Recogidas." María recalled that Isabel "had her menses" and returned to her house, where she "washed her legs with a small bucket of water from the well." She must have been thirsty, because she "drank a pitcher of water." In addition, Isabel "sent for half a loaf [of bread] from the depository and ate it soaked in vinegar," and María was convinced that "this caused her fever and vomiting." María González affirmed that this had happened five days before, and today Isabel died. She was there and "saw her dead and in the nude; she saw that she was covered with blackish spots and she was livid." Catalina González, who had also listened to the sermon at Las Recogidas, confirmed that Isabel was menstruating and added that "she perspired and became tired" during the sermon and therefore went home. Catalina's testimony regarding Isabel's activities after she returned to her house mirrored María González's deposition, except she noted that the bread was "warm." She too saw the corpse covered with spots.

In the following days, as reports of disease and death multiplied, the physicians employed by the municipality were busy visiting the sick and reporting to the plague commission. Dr. Pedro Verdugo had been called to examine Licentiate Fuentes de la Cerda. On Tuesday, 10 April, the physician testified that he had found Licentiate Cerda sick with "lethargy with its spots, the kind that normally appears every year at this time." The patient died, but Dr. Verdugo affirmed that "although this sickness is contagious, it does not compel the burning of the clothing nor taking the measures that are usually taken in the plague." The physician assured the authorities that in this case, "with washing and bleaching the clothes stay safe." The licentiate probably died of typhus, which according to Dr. Bartolomé Hidalgo "is such a common disease in Spain" and very deadly.[6]

That same Tuesday, Dr. Gómez informed city authorities that the previous day he had been to a house on Vírgenes Street, near the Triana Gate, where he saw three patients. First, he had examined a boy with "malignant pestilential fever" who had "a swelling behind the ear" and was "restless with nausea and vomiting." The boy succumbed that night, four days after becoming sick. Dr. Gómez also visited a seven or eight-year-old girl with a "swelling in the groin" and the same fever. The girl's mother also had a fever and "two carbuncles on her chest," and Monday night the physician was informed that her fever had risen and "a swelling appeared under her arm." These symptoms were a cause for concern, and the officials ordered the bedding in which the boy had died burned in the Arenal. The girl also perished, but her bedding had not been destroyed because her mother was using it. The mother did not long outlive her

6. Ibid.; Hidalgo de Agüero, *Thesoro*, fol. 286r. The Spanish word for typhus is *tabardillo* or *tabardete,* yet in the sixteenth century both words were also commonly used to describe a specific symptom, spots on the body, and such description could be applied to diseases other than typhus. The word *modorra*, which means lethargy, delirium, or encephalitis, was also used to denote a symptom, or it implied typhus, particularly in conjunction with the other symptom, tabardete. Dr. Hidalgo, in his short chapter on typhus (tabardillo), states that "in this fever delirium almost always comes (so much so, that even the common people combine them saying modorra and tabardete)," that is, lethargy and spots (*Thesoro*, fol. 288v). And not just the common people: Dr. Pedro Verdugo used precisely that terminology in the case of the Licentiate Fuentes de la Cerda: "*modorra con su tabardete*" (lethargy with its spots).

children; she died on 16 April, and this time all the bedding was incinerated in the Arenal.

Also on 10 April the plague commission learned that Gil de Aguilar, the priest of the Church of La Magdalena, had died suddenly. When the priest became sick, Dr. Gómez took him to his own house, where according to the physician he died of typhus. The doctor stated that the priest had a fever and was lethargic. He treated him for about a week and then on the eighth day, "he erupted with a few spots"; four to six hours later, he was dead. Dr. Gómez insisted that the priest did not have "the symptoms of contagious and pestilential fever, neither in the signs of the pulse nor urine." The physician did not think it necessary to do anything with the dead man's clothing or bedding other than to "wash it and bleach it." He argued that he let his own wife and children and servants remain in the house, which he would not have done had there been any fear of their contracting the plague.

Dr. Gómez reported on yet another case that same day, which did seem dangerous. He testified that the previous Friday afternoon he had visited a young woman, the daughter of a widow who lived near the river. According to the doctor, she had "a pestilential fever, having vomited green bile as is common to this disease." Furthermore, she had "a swelling in the groin" and died Sunday night, three days after becoming sick.

The reports of sickness continued the following day, Wednesday, 11 April. The plague commission learned that Alonso Vázquez, who had come from Cazalla de la Sierra, was sick in the neighborhood near the Convent of San Agustín, outside the Carmona Gate. He was immediately suspect "because he had come from the said town where there had been the plague." The deputies sent Dr. Benito Carrero to examine him. He found Vázquez "with a continuous fever and a weak pulse and a large lump in his left genitals." The patient told the physician that "he had fainted and vomited." He continued feeling faint and was vomiting while the physician was present, which led Dr. Carrero to "deduce that it is the plague that he has."

Dr. Pedro Verdugo had visited Alonso Vázquez earlier, and he testified that "he stopped treating him because it seemed to him that he had it." Presumably, the "it" referred to the plague. Dr. Verdugo's attitude seems unusual, considering that most doctors and even barbers used whatever medicines they thought appropriate to try to cure the plague victims.

In spite of the testimony of two physicians that Alonso Vázquez had the plague, the officials sent notary Cristóbal Pérez to question the sick man. Váz-quez was able to tell the notary that he had arrived six days earlier from Cazalla de la Sierra, accompanied by two Moriscos. He had entered the city through the Macarena Gate and went to Pedro de Ara's house in the Calería Vieja, the dis-trict where lime was produced. He was allowed in because he carried testimony from Cazalla that he was healthy. The previous Saturday he had begun "to feel sick." Normally when a deposition was taken, the person, if he or she knew how, would sign the document attesting to the truth of the statement. If the person was illiterate, then the notary would note it down and a witness, often another scribe, would sign instead. Although Alonso Vázquez knew how to write, the notary took certain precautions, noting that "I did not give it to him to sign, be-cause of the communicability of the paper and quill and to avoid that the said disease strikes me."[7]

Holy Week had begun on Palm Sunday, 8 April, and Maundy Thursday and Good Friday were reserved for religious processions and masses. Penitential confraternities wound their way through the narrow streets of Seville toward the cathedral, and, surely in time of plague, the penitents flagellated themselves with exceptional fervor. There were about twenty-six penitential confraterni-ties in Seville at this time, all devoted to the Passion of Christ.[8]

Holy Week provided a brief respite, for there were no reports of suspicious sickness until Saturday, 14 April. The plague commission learned then of the demise of shoemaker Diego Sánchez, on Mar Street, who had "two carbuncles and a bubo, from which he died." According to physician Juan Sánchez, the un-fortunate man had died of the plague, therefore his bedding was burned and the house sealed. The same day Dr. Bartolomé Hidalgo testified that he had visited a Morisco, García Herrero, who lived near the Macarena Gate with his daughter. Dr. Hidalgo stated that the Morisco had suffered from "a pestilential fever with great torment and choleric vomit," and he had "a bubo in the right groin." The man had died five or six days after he became sick, followed shortly by his daughter, who had developed the same affliction. The surgeon affirmed that both had "contagious diseases."

There were also reports of sickness in Triana, on Santo Domingo Street. The Count of Villar ordered constable Alonso Rodríguez to cross over to Triana and

7. AMS, sec. 13, siglo XVI, vol. 6.

8. Susan Verdi Webster, *Art and Ritual in Golden-Age Spain: Sevillian Confraternities and the Processional Sculpture of Holy Week* (Princeton, N.J.: Princeton University Press, 1998), 14–36.

investigate. The surgeon Pedro García Arroyal, who was once again back home and working for the city, filed his testimony on 14 April, stating that a woman baker in the Lucero Bakery "has carbuncles and a bubo and contagious symptoms." A young girl who lived above her was also sick, and she had "a bubo and two carbuncles on her thigh and pestilential symptoms." García Arroyal noted other cases, all on Santo Domingo Street. At the end of the street outside the guarded gate, "on the left hand side in a house of Moriscos," there was a woman with "a bubo and she had had pestilential symptoms," but according to the surgeon she was "out of danger." García Arroyal had treated a woman in a tavern next to a pastry maker on the street "with a bubo behind the ear," but she also had "a fever with spots." The woman had recovered "and at present is up and well," and her little boy "is also well and he had spots."[9] The recovery of these individuals, who probably suffered from the ubiquitous typhus, often deadly but not nearly as feared as the plague, was positive news for the plague commission.

The following day, Easter Sunday, the plague deputies heard from licentiate Gerónimo de Burgos. The physician testified that the day before he had been called to see "an old woman" in the Corral de Valverde in the parish of San Gil, near the city wall. She had "a continuous fever with chills and vomits and other pestilential symptoms and a pestilential bubón in the left armpit." Not a good prognosis, and when Licentiate Burgos returned this day, he found her dead. According to her relatives she died within three days of the onset of her illness. Not surprisingly, the physician recommended that all her bedding be burned, as indeed it soon was.

Also on 15 April there was news that coverlet maker (*colchero*) Andrés Sánchez Matamoros was sick, and the commissioners sent constable Alonso Rodríguez to inquire. He went to the house and found the coverlet maker's wife, but she refused to give her name. He also questioned a young man who swore that there was no one sick in the house, except for a woman who claimed she had "rheumatism." Two days later, a constable caught a man throwing out "two mattresses, two sheets, one blanket and one pillow," through the city wall into the Huerta de Colón. The items were quickly connected to the missing coverlet maker. The constable determined that he might learn more from Catalina de Breyza, Sánchez Matamoros' godmother, and he went to see her. She and her husband lived on Colcheros Street, near the Desamparados Hospital.

9. AMS, sec. 13, siglo XVI, vol. 6.

Catalina told the constable that "on Sunday night, already late," Andrés Sánchez Matamoros appeared at her doorstep muttering that "he was fleeing from justice, that they wanted to arrest him because of a bond." He seemed "somewhat indisposed," and when she asked him what was wrong he replied that "fleeing he had perspired and had caught a cold." They made him a bed where he remained until this morning, when they found him dead. Catalina declared that no physician had seen the coverlet maker and that she did not know what the cause of his death was, other than that "he died so suddenly." Catalina and her husband must have suspected something because she admitted that she gave a man four reales to remove Sánchez Matamoros's bedding to the nearby fields to burn it, though she was unsure whether he had done so. As noted earlier, he tried to dispose of it but was caught before he could finish the job.

Other notices of suspicious deaths reached city officials. Licentiate Salvatierra, the priest of San Gil Church, prepared a report on Sunday, 15 April, regarding four people who had died in his parish within the past two days, "suddenly, with signs of contagious and pestilential disease." Licentiate Salvatierra noted that "today, Sunday," Luisa Hernández, an old woman with "a bubo under her arm," had been buried; her sickness had lasted only two or three days. A thirteen or fourteen-year-old boy, a student, came down with a fever on Saturday night. Today, Sunday, "at noon a bubo appeared on the right side of his genitals, he erupted with spots, and at five o'clock he was dead, and he did not even last twenty-four hours."

Among the dead were two girls, one of them a twelve-year-old who had a "bubo on her genitals." The priest could not ascertain what the other girl, also twelve years old, died of, and he complained that "the problem with this business is that when [people] die of this disease, the others always conceal them and no one wants to say anything." The frustrated cleric commented that attempts to misrepresent the true cause of death "are sometimes at the cost of the one who does it, who pays with his life." He added that "they do not tell the truth even to us, who will administer the last rites, until after it becomes known." The priest's report was sent to the Count of Villar by a church official, who added that so far, those who succumbed were "poor people and badly nourished, but it is good to act so that if possible it does not spread."

On Monday, 16 April, the plague commission learned of the death of Luisa Gutiérrez, who lived alone on Vírgenes Street in the Cestería neighborhood outside the Triana Gate, in a room set apart. Her housekeeper testified that Luisa was stricken during Holy Week and "had something like a mump on her throat, fever and spots," but after the lump disappeared, Luisa died.[10] The same day there was news that a boy had died in a house on the Plaza of San Leandro. He was the son of a *bodegonero,* a proprietor of a peasant eatery, and Licentiate Francisco Cetina had visited the child.[11] The physician observed that he had "a bubo under his left arm, above the heart, pestilential fever and black typhus spots." Licentiate Cetina stressed that "the fever was extremely high and the said typhus spots were black, along with the great nausea and torment that he has." The physician returned the following day to find the boy had perished.

The next concentration of suspicious disease occurred in the prostitution district, where several cases were investigated on 17 April. Pedro García Arroyal left his house in Triana and crossed the pontoon bridge to visit a servant of constable Juan de Ribera in the Corral del Azufaifo in La Mancebía.[12] The surgeon examined him and found that he had a "bubo and pestilential fever." Moreover, there were other people sick in the rooming house, including a woman with "a bubo and a carbuncle."

Dr. Juan Sánchez provided further testimony about the neighborhood. The doctor had seen several patients and gave a detailed description of the symptoms of each. Dr. Sánchez visited an adolescent girl with "a carbuncle on her leg, a bubo on the thigh and another bubo under her arm and another on a thigh." In the same area, next to the Corral del Azufaifo, "a girl was dying with a bubo on her throat." In addition, her father "was in the same bed with two buboes in the groin." The girl died during the night, and her father the following day. In another house, the doctor saw a man with "a bubo" on his thigh, who later died. He also went to the nearby Corral de Barahona, where he treated a man with a "bubo on the thigh." In a house on Mar Street there were two young women with "two swellings on their thighs." Finally, in the Plazuela del Corral de Jerez in the house of the Genoese merchant Juan Bautista Spínola, which stood between the two small arches of the House of Trade, "a black man died this morning with a carbuncle on his chest and two buboes under his arms."

10. Ibid. The Spanish word was *papera,* a specific term referring to the type of swelling that appears during mumps, a common childhood disease. The housekeeper was describing the type of lump she had observed in a way that would have been familiar to anyone at the time, though this did not imply that Luisa died of mumps.

11. Sebastián de Covarrubias (*Tesoro*) did not leave a flattering picture of bodegoneros in his dictionary. He describes them, male or female, as people who "are normally dirty and greasy because of what they do, and they tend to be fat and lazy."

12. *Azufaifo* is the jujube tree.

Dr. Sánchez confirmed that all the people he had seen had "pestilential and poisonous symptoms according to the same order of last year."

On Thursday, 19 April, Dr. Diego de Tamayo testified that a woman he had visited in the parish of San Salvador died on Monday of "a pestilential fever and a bubo in the left armpit," and her brother also died of a "bubo." And this very Thursday, Dr. Tamayo examined a young man "near Santa Paula in the second house by the wall of the convent." He was close to death, "covered with black spots and [had] a bubo under his left arm and armpit."

On the same day, the Count of Villar learned that a female slave had become sick in the Royal Jail and was taken to the plague jail, outside the Macarena Gate. But the warden there refused to admit her, and "she wandered the countryside trying to enter this city," something that the councilors deemed of "great detriment to this republic." The plague commissioners agreed that they should find her a place to stay outside the city and that a physician should examine her. Licentiate Cristóbal de León saw the woman that Thursday afternoon and found that she had a fever and "a bubo on the top of her thigh." A constable took her to an inn outside the Macarena Gate, "the last one on the left-hand side," and the innkeeper, Catalina de Villafranca, put her in "a separate upstairs room," which she was not permitted to leave. The commissioners ordered Dr. Carrero to treat the sick slave, and they told the innkeeper to provide food and drink for her "guest."

Later in the day the governor and the commissioners determined that it was the deputy warden of the Royal Jail, Francisco González, who had ordered the woman's transfer to the plague jail. He was also the one responsible for letting her wander around when she had been refused admittance. The Count of Villar, displeased with such carelessness, gave orders to "arrest the deputy jail warden and put him in the prison of the Hermandad of this city," that is, the local militia's jail. The governor instructed that the deputy warden be interrogated regarding the slave's owner, the reason for her imprisonment, and why he transferred her from the Royal Jail.

The next day deputy warden González defended his actions. The woman's name was Gracia, and she was the slave of a cleric from Carmona. She was a runaway and was being incarcerated until her master came to claim her. González denied that he had released Gracia to the plague jail. He claimed it was the warden himself who, when he discovered she had developed a fever, "had ordered his mulatto slave to take her to the plague jail and indeed he took her." Later that morning the plague jail's warden came and complained that he "did not want to have the said black woman in his jail." Therefore the Royal Jail warden ordered his deputy to go to the plague jail and "remove the black woman and find her a house." Francisco González insisted that he had followed orders as best as he could under the circumstances, but he was unable to find any suitable place, "and for this reason and in order not to return her to the said jail he left the black woman in the countryside." The deputy warden later discovered that the Count of Villar had ordered her placed in an inn outside the gate.

Francisco González's justifications did not convince the count, who commanded the deputy warden to cover "at his expense the cure of the black woman and provide her with a physician and pharmaceuticals and the necessary sustenance." In addition, the governor ordered González to "pay for the house where she is and the woman who serves her until the black woman recovers or her master appears." Only if the deputy warden agreed to these terms would he be released from prison. When on 21 April Francisco González learned his sentence, he duly accepted the terms and was promptly freed.

On Thursday, 19 April, the governor received a petition on behalf of four orphans whose parents had recently perished. Francisco de Aguilar, the executor of the will of Alonso de Palencia and his wife, Juana Pérez, stated that the couple had died of "typhus and not the plague," and he noted that the Count of Villar, "for greater safety," had ordered their house shut. Aguilar contended that the deceased couple were seed sellers who left behind a sizable quantity of seeds and grain in their storehouse, including wheat. He argued on behalf of the four children that their father had died many days before, and the mother succumbed alone on "a very high floor," apart from everyone. Maintaining that "it is not just to detain the children" or the cereals in the storehouse, Francisco de Aguilar requested guardianship of the children, control of their possessions, and permission to lock up only the room where Juana had died.

Pedro García Arroyal testified on Aguilar's behalf. The surgeon stated that four days earlier he had seen Juana Pérez, the children's mother, on Alhóndiga Street, where the family lived. She was "covered with spots and had a bubo in the groin and burning fever." García Arroyal noted that other physicians had already "bled and purged her and did other remedies," apparently without success because when he saw Juana he believed that she would surely die, and indeed the next day she did. The surgeon confirmed that the sick woman was in a separate part of the house, "in an upstairs room above another upper room," and pronounced any clothing and goods downstairs to be safe for use by her heirs, that is her children.

Juana Pérez's symptoms illustrate vividly the dilemma facing early modern physicians attempting to diagnose disease and are indicative of the reasons why there were heated debates as to the severity of the health crisis. Juana had the spots (*tabardete*) characteristic of typhus, but at the same time she had a "bubo" (*seca*) in the groin, a sign of the plague. Pedro García Arroyal, an experienced surgeon who had seen many cases of both diseases, discounted the possibility that Juana died of the plague, but another physician might have argued differently. Given the descriptions of the symptoms of those stricken during the month of April and the diagnoses provided by the physicians, it appears that many had died of typhus rather than the plague.

Dr. Juan Gaitán de San Martín, then professor at the school of medicine of the University of Seville, suggested other less fearsome afflictions. He noted that the patients he had examined during the past eight days were suffering from "different sicknesses such as burning fevers and tertian fevers and lethargy and quinsy."[13] He had also seen "three or four, who appear to be sick with continuous fevers with tumors." The physician affirmed that none of these sicknesses had symptoms that "would obligate me to baptize the said diseases and tumors as pestilential because with moderate remedies they have diminished and improved and [the patients] are healthy." In closing, Dr. Gaitán de San Martín proclaimed that it was unnecessary to burn any of the clothing or bedding of the sick he had visited, because "none of them is a truly pestilential business."[14]

13. AMS, sec. 13, siglo XVI, vol. 6 ("*fiebres ardientes y tercianas y modorras y esquinancias*"). *Esquinancia* or quinsy is an acute inflammation of the tonsils, which become abscessed. Lethargy (modorra) refers to encephalitis. Matossian, *Poisons of the Past*, 14–18, suggests another possibility: food poisoning, called alimentary toxic aleikiia (ATA), caused by deadly mycotoxins in moldy cereals. The symptoms in severe cases include vomiting, fever, dark skin eruptions, including spots, possible "swelling of glands in the neck, armpits, and groin," and convulsions and delirium, among others. The author argues that people whose diets were based on cereals were especially susceptible and "that in the past ATA was often mistaken for an infectious and contagious disease." Given the severe food shortage, Seville's authorities were forced to procure grain from anywhere they could find it, and its quality and condition was questionable, as the many complaints of damp and smelly wheat indicate, and therefore a perfect breeding ground for the deadly toxins.

14. AMS, sec. 13, siglo XVI, vol. 6 (20 April 1582).

31

GRAVE CONSEQUENCES

From small beginnings very grave consequences would follow.
—DR. ALFONSO DAZA

IVEN THE CONFLICTING REPORTS regarding the sickness appearing among Seville's populace, the plague commission decided to turn to the city's physicians for advice on what steps to take. On 21 April the deputies asked the medical professionals to assess the cases they had treated in the past fifteen days and to declare these sicknesses as either pestilential or not. Because the pesthouses had been dismantled, the physicians were to give their opinion whether the situation warranted setting up temporary hospitals and convalescent houses. The deputies decided that it was not necessary to call a formal meeting of doctors and surgeons; instead, they should simply give sworn depositions.[1] Fourteen physicians and two pharmacists, including some of the city's best-regarded practitioners, gave detailed statements over the next two days.

Licentiate Martín de Busto, a thirty-seven-year-old surgeon from the San Pedro parish, stated that he had treated many sick in the past twenty days. He declared that some had "pestilential sicknesses and bad symptoms, vomit as well as spots, which are signs of poisonous humor." But the surgeon stressed that none of his patients had any buboes, and none of them died. He affirmed that "this sickness is common during this season," and he was certain that it was not the plague.

1. AMS, sec. 13, siglo XVI, vol. 6 (21 April 1582). Antonio Carreras Panchón, "Las epidemias de peste en la España del Renacimiento," *Asclepio* 29 (1977): 7–8, suggests that debates among physicians regarding whether a place was infected with the plague allowed the civic authorities to delay quarantine, which was costly and detrimental to local commerce, thus contributing to the spread of the disease. Only when mortality levels became high did city officials implement preventive plague measures.

The testimony of Licentiate Alonso López, a fifty-year-old surgeon from the Magdalena parish, was not as clear cut. He related having been called in to treat a woman and her son "who were stricken with the plague"; but when he arrived the woman had already been buried, and her son died soon thereafter. Licentiate López claimed that other people were sick with the plague as well. At the same time, the surgeon acknowledged that there were other sicknesses affecting the population, "lethargies and choleric fevers," but he predicted that the outbreak, which he qualified as "contagious and dangerous," would not last much longer, given that it was already approaching the end of April. Licentiate López's belief that the milder and dryer weather would reduce the likelihood of sickness was not uncommon among early modern physicians, who often attributed the rise in the number of sick to inclement weather.

Dr. Diego de Tamayo, a thirty-year-old surgeon from the San Salvador parish, stated that he had treated five people with the plague in the past fifteen days, "with their buboes in the groin and armpits," and three of them had died. Dr. Tamayo noted that he was currently treating a young woman "of the said disease of the plague" but had very little hope for her recovery, because this was "a very dangerous disease that comes with great fury." The young physician favored the founding of a hospital for the sick, to "prevent them from infecting each other." He commented that the people he had visited were poor and lacked means for a cure and that most of the sick in general were poor.

More physicians testified the next day, Sunday, 22 April, among them Dr. Bartolomé Hidalgo, who lived near the San Juan de la Palma Church. The famous surgeon concurred with some of his colleagues that several of the patients he had seen in the past fifteen days were "sick with the past sickness of the plague." Dr. Hidalgo, who worked in the Cardenal Hospital, had treated four people stricken with the plague; three of them had died. He had also seen three cases of the plague in San Gil parish and several others elsewhere in the city. But the physician pointed out that in addition to the plague, there were other diseases, such as "lethargies and typhus and tertian fevers and quinsy" and others, and they mostly occurred among common people. Nevertheless, the surgeon believed that "at the moment there is no need to set up a hospital, because there are no sick who would occupy it." Indeed, Dr. Hidalgo declared it would be detrimental to the community because even if the authorities stated that Seville was plague free, other places "would guard against this city and it would be of great disadvantage for the trade and dealings and provisions seeing that there is a hospital made for the said sickness."

The next physician, forty-year-old Dr. Benito Carrero of San Andrés parish, did not report any cases of the plague. He affirmed that in the past twenty days he had treated "two dozen" sick, most of them suffering from "fevers that physicians call malignant because they have bad symptoms." Indeed, Dr. Carrero's patients exhibited a variety of symptoms: "some had black and purple spots, others buboes on the genitals and throat and on the neck, and others carbuncles, and others all of these symptoms together and lethargies." Six of his patients had died, though the doctor emphasized that he did not treat any of them from the onset of their affliction and that most of them were poor. Dr. Carrero urged authorities to select at least two more doctors and surgeons and barbers, "learned and expert," to attend the sick poor, give them food, and care for them from the onset of their sickness, because that would halt the disease. He suggested that many could be cured in their own homes, "so that neither the city nor the district become aroused." They should follow the previous year's example and keep the sick confined in their houses, because otherwise they did not call a doctor until they are "on the brink of death." Priests could visit homes and, if they noted anyone ailing, report it to the doctors so that the sick could be treated, because those "who are given remedy from the beginning do not die."

Dr. Alonso Daza was more than fifty years old and an experienced surgeon, who lived on the Alameda de Hércules. He declared that he had not seen or visited "any person sick with the plague" this year or the year before. Nevertheless, Dr. Daza acknowledged that about four days before he had seen "two sick women" who were being treated by another physician, Juan Sánchez of Mar Street. He was curious and visited the women twice to see "for his own satisfaction whether it was the disease of the plague." According to Dr. Daza one of the women was "covered with carbuncles that are commonly called black spots." The other woman had "a carbuncle on her buttock." The doctor "took this to be a suspicious and dangerous business," but in spite of his initial curiosity he "did not return there again." Dr. Daza did not know of any plague cases, "other than having heard other physicians talk about it" after he questioned them "for his own satisfaction." After conversing with other physicians, he concluded that the problem was minimal, though he did not discount the possibility that it might be the beginning of a plague outbreak.

Dr. Daza stressed the importance of prevention. He recommended that the authorities "set up a comfortable place outside the city, so that poor and needy people could be cured and assisted in this said disease," and he warned that otherwise "from small beginnings very grave consequences would follow." Like some of his colleagues, he was concerned with keeping the populace calm. Since the current number of cases was still insignificant, there was no need to create "a scandal" by setting up a formal pesthouse. Dr. Daza concluded that a discreet house outside the city, with "a physician or surgeon" in charge who would treat the sick "in conformity with the good practice of medicine," should suffice for now.

Dr. Fernando de Valdés, at twenty-eight years of age, was the youngest man to testify. The surgeon lived on Sierpes Street and in the previous fifteen days had come across more than twenty people with "pestilential fever." Among the afflicted he saw some with "bad pustules and others with spots of typhus and others with none of these other than just pestilential fever, that might occur without anything coming from it." Dr. Valdés had seen patients in the Cinco Llagas and Amor de Dios Hospitals, and he had visited many in their houses and had witnessed this "pestilential disease." He believed that it was "necessary" to establish a special pesthouse because "there are at present many poor sick with this disease," and he pointed out that "being received in the ordinary hospitals . . . they suffer great necessity." Furthermore, Dr. Valdés noted that some of the poor who had come to these hospitals "have neither received the Sacraments nor been cured." In conclusion the young physician expressed his belief that the untreated poor "have already caused, are causing, and will cause much harm to the city transmitting the disease to others, also poor, in the corrales and rooming houses where they live." He urged the city to act without delay.

Forty-five-year-old Dr. Vidal Clavijo was convinced that there were cases of the plague in the city. He had seen six or seven people in the neighboring parishes of San Lorenzo and San Vicente "with burning fevers and vomit and nausea and tumors in the groin and armpits." Four of them had died. Dr. Clavijo had also visited a woman "sick with the said disease and with the characteristic symptoms." The surgeon admitted that he only saw the woman "one time" and left her to her own devices, "not wanting to continue the said cure because he learned that three slaves had died in the said house of the very disease." Dr. Clavijo noted that he distanced himself from treating this woman "because the house was small and ready for the other people to become infected and those who entered it." Nevertheless, he had learned that the woman had recovered, which raises the question what would have been her fate had the physician controlled his fear and bled and purged her and prescribed all the usual remedies. Yet he was not the only one who abandoned the premises: "the masters of the house have retreated to their hacienda" on the doctor's advice.

Dr. Clavijo thought that setting up a pesthouse would cause too much "scandal and harm" to the city. He advised the count and the jurados to make secret inquiries and if necessary call "a meeting of the most learned and expert physicians" to make recommendations on how to proceed. In closing, he warned against consulting physicians "who in order to gain notoriety with many more cases than they had seen inform the city secretly and publicly and cause fear among the residents and citizens for no reason."

Dr. Nicolás Monardes, who stated that he lived on Colcheros Street, had seen only one sick person, "a black woman in the house of Miguel de Jáuregui, with an inflammation in the throat of which she died."[2] Regarding the pesthouse, Dr. Monardes opposed it because of "the harm and scandal that might occur to the city and its residents, because there is no need for it."

Forty-two-year-old apothecary Rodrigo del Castillo, who lived on Francos Street, believed that there were only a few people in the city who might have the plague; he had dispensed many medicines but none for that disease. On the other hand, if "a place could be secretly designated where if someone were stricken with the plague he could be treated, it would be of great benefit to this city to separate the sick outside the walls." The pharmacist indicated that this would affect "primarily the poor who cannot be well cured in their homes." Rodrigo del Castillo stressed the importance of clearing away any clothing that a sick person, "dead or alive," might bring "because that is what tends to create much of this disease." The pharmacist urged the authorities to prevent anyone from entering who came from plague-stricken places and commented that "the other day they told him that there were many people from Écija spotted on the river," as well as from other towns that were infected. Seemingly unaware

2. AMS, sec. 13, siglo XVI, vol. 6. Unfortunately, Dr. Monardes's age became unintelligible when the manuscript was sewn together, but according to Rodríguez Marín (*Biografía*, 14, 20), Dr. Monardes was born in 1508, which would have made him seventy-four years old when he made his deposition. Francisco Guerra, *Monardes: Su vida*, 6, mistakenly took an older calculation for Monardes's birth date, 1493, which was effectively disproved by Rodríguez Marín in 1913.

of the governor's mandates, del Castillo admonished the count to make a list of places against which the city should guard. This was especially important since the "city was healthy and without any contagion because all of us are aided by the sunny weather and the winds that blow which tend to consume it."

Dr. Francisco Sánchez de Oropesa, a fifty-year-old physician from Carpintería Street, indicated that the cases of sickness he knew of "have signs of malignancy with dreadful symptoms, but they respond to the remedies," and those affected recover, something that would not occur with the plague. Dr. Sánchez de Oropesa had much experience and had talked with other physicians; most of the current cases, he stated, involved "burning malignant fevers with spots, lethargy, frenzy, sobs, shakes and a great appetite for food and these patients are treated and recover." He did not believe there was any plague and warned against "scandalizing and inflaming the city." The doctor was against setting up a pesthouse but advocated that "the city provide alms for the cure of the poor, and physicians and barbers to attend them," stressing that doing this with "rectitude and charity" would be the best course of action. He pointed out that with this charitable enterprise, "fear of the future would cease and at lower cost and without scandal."

Dr. García de Salzedo Coronel from the Santa Cruz parish concurred with most of the other physicians that he had not seen any plague cases, "nor is there up to now rumor in the street that frightens." To be sure, the forty-nine-year-old surgeon "had asked some of the modern physicians who cure this disease" whether they had encountered any cases of the plague and was told that there were none. Dr. Salzedo remarked that "few preventions would be necessary" and indicated that the most important measure in impeding the spread of any potential disease would be "to separate the sick from the healthy."

Fifty-nine-year-old surgeon Francisco de Castro of Francos Street declared that there was no plague at present, although about one month earlier he "saw a little bit of this disease, though very little, and in very few parts." The surgeon attributed the city's good fortune to God's giving "good weather." He commented that he spoke to a Father Pedro from the Church of Omnium Sanctorum in La Feria district, which had been particularly stricken by disease the previous year, and the priest told him "that for more than six days no Last Sacraments were given to any person." Francisco de Castro echoed most of his colleagues, maintaining that there was no need to establish a pesthouse because the few sick that there might be could easily be cured in their homes, and he warned that a hospital would "rouse this city and cause great fear and scandal among the residents."

Juan del Valle, a fifty-year-old apothecary and close associate of Dr. Nicolás Monardes, lived and dispensed medicines on Sierpes Street. He stated that some people came to his shop looking for medicines normally given in time of plague, but he only saw one person with the characteristic "tumor under the armpit." Juan del Valle had talked to his customers about the sickness, and some "were afraid having heard it said by other people that two or three have died from this disease of the plague." The pharmacist did not think it necessary to establish a pesthouse because "the weather is good and it would be a huge scandal and disturbance for this city." Juan del Valle, an astute businessman, admonished that setting up a hospital for plague victims would adversely affect commerce and "would result in lack of provisions which would cause great harm to the republic."

Licentiate Cristóbal de León, a fifty-five-year-old surgeon who lived near the Dominican Monastery of San Pablo, declared that he had not seen "one man touched by pestilence" in the past twenty days, except one on Colcheros Street, on Holy Wednesday (11 April), who had "two carbuncles on his right leg." The surgeon muttered that he only saw him once because the man "had resisted the remedies that he was providing," but he learned from another physician that he had died. Licentiate León advised against setting up a hospital and even spoke against a "meeting of physicians, because it would rouse the city and all the land too much." He stressed that there was hardly any sickness, and "the weather is good for withstanding the plague."

Dr. Pedro Verdugo lived on Alhóndiga Street, not far from the public granary. The forty-three-year-old surgeon affirmed that for the past eight days he had scoured the city, concerned with its state of health, and he had not "encountered one suspicious case of buboes." He conceded that there was an outbreak of typhus ("lethargies and spots") but added that "the city is now much improved." Dr. Verdugo reminded the officials that he had already advised that if "these diseases of lethargies and spots appear," they need to be treated "from the start," because then "almost all recover and are rid of them." He argued that a pesthouse was not necessary, nor would it be prudent "to create a scandal."

With five exceptions the city's medical practitioners agreed that Seville was free of the plague. They acknowledged that there was a deadly outbreak of typhus, a common disease of the spring season, and they stressed that if treated properly and, most important, on time, most patients recovered. Furthermore, they considered the mild late spring weather, with ample sunshine, an auspicious weapon against any contagion. Again, they found that the most affected were the poor. Given that the plague was not a threat, most of the physicians, particularly the older and experienced ones, opposed the creation of a pesthouse, which, they argued, would only cause unnecessary panic among the population and harm commerce. These men seemed more concerned with the city's reputation and the economic consequences of the stigma of the plague than with the health of its citizens, but to their credit, many did endorse some kind of charitable arrangement that would benefit the poor and provide them with medical treatment in their homes if they needed it.

When the plague commissioners and the Count of Villar met in his residence two days later to discuss the medical reports, they were clearly relieved. They agreed to send a letter to His Majesty, informing him that according to the physicians, "Blessed be Our Lord, Seville is healthy and free of the sickness of the plague." In spite of such a welcome finding, the plague deputies knew that their task to protect the city from the disease would only become more rigorous as they faced contagion in surrounding communities. They had recently shut four of the eight gates that had remained open to outside traffic. As of 22 April, only the Macarena, Triana, Arenal, and Carmona Gates allowed traffic, opening at five o'clock in the morning and closing at nine in the evening, and the key holders could only unlock the gates once the guards were in place. To underscore the seriousness of the city's intentions to keep undesirable people and goods out, a gallows was erected as a warning outside each gate as well as in Triana. The plague officials were still not entirely convinced that Cazalla de la Sierra was healthy, and they again included it in the list of places to guard against; at the same time they sent an emissary to the town to probe further. In addition to Cazalla, three more towns, on the southern coast, were now added to list: Cádiz, Arahal, and Conil.[3]

3. AMS, sec. 13, siglo XVI, vol. 6.

32

TRADE IS IMPEDED

We receive intolerable harm and injury
because our trade is impeded and shut down.
—SEVILLE'S MERCHANTS

THE COUNT OF VILLAR'S CAUTION before declaring Cazalla de la Sierra plague free proved to be warranted. On 25 April the governor received "very certain news" that Cazalla had "fallen back into sickness"; there were many sick and dead of the plague, including two prominent citizens, Don Cristóbal Moscoso and his wife, Doña María de Marchena. Almost at the same time that news of Cazalla's relapse reached Seville, Constantina's officials were attempting to prove that their town was now healthy. Three local physicians testified on 15 April to that effect. Juan Sánchez, a barber surgeon, stated that in the past he had "bled and treated the sick who had the disease of the plague," but now everyone was healthy. Francisco de Heredía, a physician who had worked in the pesthouse, affirmed that there were no more cases of "buboes." The surgeon Sebastián Garrido also declared the town to be healthy. Bachiller Miguel Díaz, the Sevillian physician who had replaced Dr. Centurio, reported on 24 April that for the past seven days there had been no new cases of the plague. He also mentioned to his superiors in Seville that Constantina's officials, who had been notoriously stingy in providing funds for the plague expenses, were planning to appeal his salary of forty reales because they thought it excessive. Considering the bad news from Cazalla de la Sierra, Seville's officials were in no hurry to act in the case of Constantina; the town would have to wait.

Conil, on the southern coast of Spain, was more successful in proving its healthfulness. Shortly after the Count of Villar added Conil to the list of plague towns, its resident physician, Licentiate Fernando Enríquez, sent a report to Seville affirming that the town was healthy and that he had not been called to visit anyone sick. He stated that he would know if anyone were stricken because he was "alone in my capacity in this town, with a salary that its council gives me annually of 138 ducats and one *cahíz* of wheat."[1] The local priest echoed the doctor's assertion regarding the town's health conditions. After the Count of Villar received these reports he sent Licentiate Gerónimo de Burgos to inspect Conil. When the physician reached the town, he accompanied Licentiate Enríquez in visiting three patients. According to Licentiate Burgos, one person had asthma and the other two suffered from continuous fevers. He vouched that there was no "plague or contagious disease" present and pronounced the town "very healthy." The count accepted this finding and on 12 May restored full communications with Conil. Local officials must have been relieved to have their town removed from the dreaded quarantine list.

The day after the stigma of plague was erased from Conil, the town of Carmona found itself on the list of places to guard against. On 13 May the Count of Villar was informed that people had come to the Carmona Gate of Seville warning that there was plague in Carmona "of which many people die." The governor took swift action. He questioned two guards of the Carmona Gate, who stated that three or four people had come from Carmona who revealed that the town "was guarding from its own outskirts because there was plague there." One of the travelers told them that there was plague also "inside the town and that many people were dying." As with other reports, the count ordered testimony to be taken, but without waiting for confirmation, he cut all communications with nearby town. Carmona's largesse in permitting the transit of merchandise from infected communities through the town en route to Seville cost them dearly.

Protecting Seville from deadly disease without harming the city's commercial interests seemed an impossible task. On 26 April 1582, the Count of Villar received an irate petition from a group of merchants. The men complained about the blocking of shipments of wine, vinegar, and textiles destined for the New Spain fleet, arguing that His Majesty would be defrauded of his rights if this merchandise did not proceed. They pointed out that "the said wines are much esteemed and valued in the Indies" and lamented, "we receive intolerable harm and injury because our trade is impeded and shut down." The merchants contended that "the wine and vinegar and skins in which it comes do not nor can they receive bad vapors, plague or contagion"; on the contrary, both wine

---

1. AMS, sec. 13, siglo XVI, vol. 6. A *cahíz* varied in size according to region; in Castile, it was equivalent to about 690 kilograms.

and vinegar were "a preservative and curative remedy against the plague." They went so far as to declare that "there could be nothing in the city more salubrious than the said wine and vinegar" and demanded that it be allowed to enter Seville freely.

The petitioners certainly would have had the medical profession on their side. Vinegar was the recommended antiseptic both for the body and for living quarters. Doctors stressed the importance of using water with vinegar to "sprinkle the dwelling." Dr. Hidalgo, for example, discouraged hot baths during a plague outbreak because "they relax the bodies and open the pores," thereby facilitating the entry of "pestilential air"; but "if those who in this time want to wash themselves for cleanliness, they should use vinegar and cold water and salt to invigorate the extremities."[2]

That same day, the Count of Villar received other petitions from individuals whose wine or vinegar shipments were en route to Seville or had just arrived at the outskirts of the city when the new and stricter regulations were announced. Mariana Pérez complained that she had ordered "four cargas of vinegar for the use of the peons who will reap my wheat from certain land that I have within the limits of this city." The muleteers bringing in the vinegar had just reached Seville as the new ban was proclaimed; Mariana lamented that this was unfair because it was too late to stop the shipment, and she asked permission to unload the vinegar, which the count granted.

The Sevillian wine merchant Pedro de Posada had a similar problem. Guards at the Macarena Gate stopped his shipment of 170 arrobas of wine from the Carthusian Monastery of Cazalla de la Sierra because the new ban had just taken effect. The governor authorized the merchant to bring in the wine. Luis Ponce de León had four hundred arrobas of wine shipped from Cazalla to Seville, directed to the royal shipyards. The wine was brought to the city to "be loaded on this fleet that is leaving now for New Spain." The Count of Villar allowed the muleteers to bring the carts with the wine to the shipyards, but as soon as the wine was transferred into barrels the animals and the wineskins were to be removed.

Wheat was a commodity sorely needed in the city, and the governor authorized entrance of most shipments. Juan Bautista Spínola, a wealthy Sevillian merchant of Genoese origins who lived near the House of Trade, announced

2. AMS, sec. 13, siglo XVI, vol. 6; Hidalgo de Agüero, *Thesoro*, fols. 279r, 280v. See also Mercado, *Naturaleza y modo de curar la peste*, fol. 67v.

on 30 April that a cargo of 2,810 fanegas of wheat was in the port. He assured the count that "the wheat that was taken in the Bay of Cádiz on the ships that brought it from Sicily, had not made a stop in any port or place." After the grain was inspected and testimony taken from various people, including sailors from the ships that had transported it from Cádiz to Seville, the Count of Villar allowed the wheat to be unloaded.

A Sevillian wood merchant, Pedro Alvarez de Castrillón, complained that plague guards had stopped his shipment of wood from Ribadeo, on Galicia's northern coast. He petitioned to be allowed to unload the wood and bring it into the city. Following the requisite report on the safety of the wood, the count granted permission to remove the cargo, but at the same time he sent a constable to supervise the activity and ensure that no other goods were taken from the ship.

Other merchandise was arriving in Seville, and after being duly stopped by the guards, the petitions streamed in. On 4 May Anibal del Cacha, a Florentine merchant residing in Seville, stated that he had merchandise from Italy sitting at the docks, including "paper, rice and cloths," and asked permission to unload it. The ship's master, a Frenchman named Alexandre Ferral, testified that he and his crew had learned about the restrictions while in Cartagena and therefore decided not to stop anywhere else until reaching Seville. He declared that everyone on board was healthy and produced a document to that effect issued in Cartagena on 31 March. The ship's notary, Honorat Brignole, testified that the *Santa María Buenaventura* had left Villafranca in the Duchy of Savoy, near Nice, and after stopping in Cartagena on Spain's Mediterranean coast, the ship proceeded directly to Seville. The Count of Villar ordered a medical report on 5 May, and three days later, Dr. Bartolomé Hidalgo, having inspected the men and cargo, pronounced that the goods were "safe from contagion, because if there were anything in them, the people on the ship would have been stricken, indeed they sleep on top of the said merchandise." With this evidence, the count authorized the commodities to be unloaded.[3]

When the plague commission met on 9 May in the Count of Villar's Alcázar quarters, one of the issues discussed was wine and vinegar from Cazalla de la Sierra. It was not in the city's interest to stop shipments of these goods, nor did the commissioners believe there was any need to ban wine and vinegar from entering, considering that these liquids could not harbor contagion. But the com-

3. AMS, sec. 13, siglo XVI, vol. 6.

missioners were concerned with how to unload them safely. One of the deputies proposed to have the carts with the wine or vinegar stop north of the city near the leper hospital of San Lázaro, or even further away from the city walls.[4] The merchandise would then be unloaded and the men and beasts who had transported it would return to Cazalla. After they left, men and animals from Seville would pick up the shipment and deliver it in the city.

Most of the commissioners agreed in principle, but there was some debate regarding details. Baltasar de Aguilar did not object to the procedure but recommended that "the carts should be washed there with vinegar in order to enter this city." Juan de Avendaño added that when the owners of the wine or vinegar go out to San Lázaro to retrieve the merchandise they should be allowed to read any letters that might have come from Cazalla, but as soon as they have read them, the missives should be burned. Gabriel de Perlin thought that it would be enough to simply unload the shipments "in the last houses of Seville, and if there were one in the countryside by itself," that would work also. He did not think it necessary to burn any letters coming from Cazalla, just "place them in vinegar two hours before they are given to the parties." At the end of the discussion, the Count of Villar remained ambivalent. He stated that the shipments should not be allowed to enter the city, but if they did permit it, then it should not jeopardize the health of its citizens. The governor preferred to decide each case separately; doing so would allow him to retain control of who brought in the merchandise and have the opportunity to have it inspected before granting permission.

There were other items on the agenda during this meeting. Seville's fruit sellers, who were in charge of collecting fruit tax revenue, were petitioning for permission to import cherries from Cazalla and Constantina. They declared that the first annual installment of the tax was paid from the income on cherries and other early fruits, and they complained that if these cherries did not come then they would be unable to pay it. They argued that "no bad vapors or contagion can come in cherries" and insisted that they were actually "a remedy against any kind of affliction and contagion."[5] Furthermore, the cherry or-

4. The leper hospital of San Lázaro, located near a principal road, had been used by other wine merchants to transfer or store wine coming from Cazalla de la Sierra. See Chapter 23 of this volume.

5. AMS, sec. 13, siglo XVI, vol. 6. Dr. Hidalgo recommended cherries during plague time, along with other "sour" or acidic fruit such as citrus, pomegranates, apples, pears, and quince. Luis de Mercado, on the other hand, discouraged eating any fruits or vegetables except lettuce or other leafy

chards were away from the towns "at least two or three leagues in the mountains and parts where there cannot be any sickness because they are cool and airy places." There was little discussion on this matter; most deputies opposed bringing the cherries into the city. Baltasar de Aguilar was willing to let them in but only if they were "put in vinegar for 10 days in some large containers" and stored at the inn of San Lázaro. But he was a lone dissenter, and when the vote was taken the fruit sellers' petition was denied.

Ships bearing merchandise from abroad continued to arrive. Given the difficulties and dangers facing ships trying to navigate the treacherous course of the Guadalquivir River in order to reach the inland port, many of the larger vessels chose to remain anchored in or near Sanlúcar de Barrameda, while smaller boats transported their merchandise and passengers to or from Seville. On 10 May the merchant Guillermo Stalenge reported that three ships arrived from England "loaded with merchandise" and were anchored about a league outside of Sanlúcar de Barrameda. He claimed that the ships bypassed both Cádiz and Sanlúcar and did not stop in either port. According to Stalenge, since the ships were "large and unable to go up the river, they were lightening their load," and part of the merchandise was being brought in on a boat, which had been stopped by the river guards. The merchant and the boat's crew wanted to bring it into the city and unload the shipment.

The Count of Villar ordered an investigation. The officials questioned two sailors, who confirmed that the ship had not stopped in either Cádiz or Sanlúcar. One of them gave the reason for not stopping: to avoid paying port dues, a lucky decision since both towns were on the governor's list of proscribed places. The count sent Dr. Juan Sánchez to inspect the vessel. The boat was moored near the Monastery of Los Remedios in Triana, and the physician found only three men aboard. He pronounced them to be healthy and the merchandise harmless. Dr. Sánchez recommended that the boat be allowed to enter the city, and the Count of Villar issued permission to unload the cargo.[6]

---

vegetables, "and these with vinegar and sugar, and fruits and drinks should be cooled with snow," that is ice. See Hidalgo de Agüero, *Thesoro*, fol. 280r, and Mercado, *Naturaleza y modo de curar la peste,* fol. 50v.

6. AMS, sec. 13, siglo XVI, vol. 6.

33

A PESTHOUSE FOR THE POOR

One cannot deal with all of them.
—DR. JUAN GAITÁN DE SAN MARTÍN

NCERTAINTY ABOUT THE PRESENCE of plague within Seville's walls soon resurfaced. Prodded by Dr. Rodrigo de León, the administrator of the Amor de Dios Hospital, the Count of Villar found it necessary once again to ask the city's physicians and pharmacists to state their opinions. On 15 May the governor called together a special committee to debate whether the disease was present and whether a hospital should be established to treat the poor. Some of the men had already testified three weeks earlier, when most of them concluded that there was no plague nor any need for a pesthouse. The present group included other physicians and pharmacists that the count had not heard from earlier.

The first to speak was Dr. Nicolás Monardes. He still maintained that "there are not many sick at present" and praised the measures employed by the Count of Villar as "enough and sufficient." He recommended that there should be a doctor, a surgeon, and a barber and that pharmaceuticals and monies necessary to cover the needs of the "destitute" should be provided. He urged secrecy and suggested that the poor sick "be taken under cover to a house," where they could be cared for by two women and a priest as they convalesced. Dr. Monardes again concluded that the current disease was not the plague, because "so few people sicken and die."

Dr. García de Salzedo offered a contrary opinion: given that there were some "buboes and carbuncles in the city, then it is the disease of the plague." He recommended that a place be set aside to treat the sick. Dr. Francisco Sánchez de Oropesa took his turn next. He stated that if the number of sick was too great to cure in their homes then the policy should be changed, and the city should establish a place where each person in need could have a bed. Nevertheless, Dr. Sánchez did not think enough people were dying to say that there was plague in the city.

Dr. Fernando Valdés also declared that there was sickness in the city and indicated that there were two hospitals in use for the afflicted. He had seen many patients with "pestilential fevers," which led him to believe that the present disease "can be called the plague." As he had argued earlier, Dr. Valdés recommended that to cure the poor there should be a "house or general hospital," because it was difficult to treat all the sick in their homes. Dr. León, who had advocated calling the meeting, also believed that the city "is not free from the disease of the plague." He too recommended the establishment of "a private house where the poor who have nothing to be cured with can be treated."

Dr. Juan Rodríguez reported that under the count's orders he had treated the "sickness that there was and is in Triana," and he stated that there were no new cases in the past three days. He believed that the disease could not be labeled "general plague" because fewer people were stricken by any kind of sickness than in other years. Therefore, Dr. Rodríguez did not see "the need to establish a house where the said sick can be gathered."

Dr. Juan Gaitán de San Martín, a professor of medicine at the University of Seville, had been charged by the governor with treating the poor in "one half of the city," and he did not encounter any cases of the plague, though "there are some diseases of pestilential fevers." Dr. Gaitán remarked that the problem with those who were "so destitute was that even though one takes as much care of them as had been done up to now, one cannot deal with all of them," and he favored the establishment of a special house to treat the poor.

Dr. Benito Carrero stated that the Count of Villar had ordered him to cure the poor in the other half of the city and that there was no plague there, although there were some "pestilential diseases." He added that in his part of the city there were "some sick with the said disease" and stressed that their number was "not small." The physician, who had before advocated early intervention as a way to combat disease, blamed the hot weather for the rise in the number of sick and noted that "more have died than had been dying before the heat came." Dr. Carrero changed his mind regarding the founding of a hospital; whereas earlier he believed it was inopportune because it might create panic in the city, now, three weeks later, he felt that it would benefit the "poor and destitute stricken by this disease" to have a separate place where they could be treated.

The count had assigned Dr. Pedro Gómez to cure the sick in the extramural neighborhoods of "Carretería and Cestería and Humeros." Dr. Gómez believed that given the condition of the sick, the disease "can be called the plague." He urged the city to establish "very quickly a house where they can be collected and cured" and warned that otherwise the city could face problems. In his 22 April deposition, Dr. Diego de Tamayo had affirmed that he had treated several cases of the plague. Since then he had been charged with curing some of Dr. Carrero's patients, and given what he had seen he did not believe that "what there is can at present be called the plague." Nevertheless, the physician warned that it could be "the great beginning to having it" and argued that "if no urgent remedy is made it could very quickly expand." Dr. Tamayo again recommended that "in order to prevent this," it would be wise to establish a separate house to treat the poor.

Licentiate Pedro Suárez de Venegas was more to the point. He had no doubt that the current sickness in Seville "can be called the plague and be given the name of plague." Convinced that the city was facing an outbreak of the dreaded disease, he urged a hospital for the poor be established "to prevent the harm that could occur if it increases." Dr. Fernando Alemán disagreed, declaring that "it cannot be called the plague nor can it be given its name . . . nor is it the plague, because the air is not corrupt." Nonetheless, Dr. Alemán supported the establishment of a house in which to cure the "poor destitute sick."[1]

Present also were several apothecaries, who primarily reported on the amounts of medicine they had been dispensing. Juan del Valle stated that in the past four days there were not "as many sick as before" and noted that he had fewer customers coming in with prescriptions. Francisco Ribera, an apothecary dispensing medicines in the Carretería, Cestería, and Humeros, said that in the past four to five days "less had been prescribed in his pharmacy than before." Juan Jiménez affirmed that in the past four days he had dispensed "medicines for four or five sick" and that in the previous days even fewer. Rodrigo del Castillo claimed that in his shop he had given out in the previous four days "a larger amount [of medicines] than in the past days," and he declared that "yesterday

---

1. AMS, sec. 13, siglo XVI, vol. 6. Dr. Fernando Alemán belonged to an important converso family, and he was the father of Mateo Alemán, the author of *Guzmán de Alfarache,* a popular picaresque novel first published in 1599. See Pike, *Aristocrats and Traders,* 83, 88; Gil, *Los conversos y la Inquisición,* 3:215–16; and Alexandra Parma Cook and Noble David Cook, *Good Faith and Truthful Ignorance: A Case of Transatlantic Bigamy* (Durham, N.C.: Duke University Press, 1991), 174.

and the day before twelve or thirteen were dispensed and today seven or eight." Gerónimo Ortiz, in charge of supplying medicine for "the half of the city on the right-hand side that Dr. Carrero had under his charge," noted that the "said disease had grown in the past eight days." He had provided more medicine in the past four days than earlier.

The last pharmacist to speak was Juan Martínez, a resident of the Santa Catalina parish. He was in charge of dispensing medications in the part of the city administered by Dr. Gaitán de San Martín and "the barrio of San Bernardo and San Agustín and outside the Macarena Gate," which was in the care of the surgeon Francisco de Castro "and in his absence, Licentiate Padilla." Indeed, Licentiate Juan Tomás de Padilla had taken over for Francisco de Castro on Monday, 7 May, because the surgeon became ill, and he continued to substitute for him until 17 May. Licentiate Padilla requested payment of ten ducats from the Count of Villar, the same salary the stricken surgeon had been earning, and was actually paid five hundred maravedís daily for the ten days that he had covered for his colleague. In his deposition, boticario Juan Martínez affirmed that in the past three days he had given out less medicine than previously, and he remarked that on this day he had filled only one new prescription.

At the end of the meeting, after "all the said physicians had given their opinion," the count asked to have "their sayings and declarations" put in order. When officials compared all the statements, they concluded that "the majority appear to have said and declared that there is not the said sickness of the plague in this city." The governor, however, took note that most of the physicians had recommended the establishment of a special hospital for the poor sick. Thus, in spite of declaring the city plague free, the count ordered the plague commission to find "houses where the sick can be gathered." He directed the deputies to set salaries for those involved and to charge the expenses to the plague account. The governor was a prudent man, keeping in mind that the physicians were not unanimous in their verdict. For the purposes of trade and the economic well-being of the city it was imperative to announce to the outside world that there was no plague in Seville, but at the same time it was wise to tend to the poor sick, who if left to their own devices could ignite a more serious disease outbreak.

The following week, on 21 May, the plague commission met in the Count of Villar's residence to finalize the establishment of a pesthouse. They all agreed to once again "open the Cinco Llagas Hospital" for the poor sick with the plague and charged Dr. Rodrigo de León with its administration. The commission-ers authorized the hiring of the necessary physicians and barbers as well as the procurement of appropriate medicine, food, and bedding for the patients. They also authorized establishment of a convalescent house, using the same format as the previous year. To cover the expected costs, the deputies decided to request a loan of twelve thousand ducats.

The consensus among Seville's physicians that the city was plague free brought some relief to the authorities, though they continued to wrestle with the question of the presence of the plague in surrounding communities. The recurrence of the plague in Cazalla de la Sierra troubled Seville's officials, and they sent yet another inspector, Licentiate Ramírez de Sierra, to ascertain the gravity of the outbreak. Like his predecessors, he interviewed physicians, phar-macists, and priests, all of whom agreed that yes, people had perished from the plague in April, but now, in May, the situation was improving; many witnesses, however, indicated that Cazalla was far from being entirely healthy.[2]

2. AMS, sec. 13, siglo XVI, vol. 6.

34

CONFLICT WITH TOWN OFFICIALS

They have imprisoned him in shackles.

— DOÑA MARÍA DE BUSTO

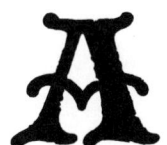 T ABOUT THE SAME TIME that Licentiate Ramírez de Sierra was conducting his inspection in Cazalla de la Sierra, there was trouble in nearby Constantina. When the Count of Villar sent Bachiller Miguel Díaz there, on 20 March, to replace the deceased Dr. Centurio, he had stipulated his salary at forty reales a day, including travel time. The new physician arrived in Constantina around 1 April and began to treat the sick. The governor had charged the local council with paying the surgeon from the town's own treasury, but Díaz complained repeatedly that he had not been paid and that the officials wanted to reduce his salary.

About a month and a half after the surgeon arrived in Constantina, his wife, Doña María de Busto, petitioned the count on her husband's behalf. She claimed on 15 May that since her husband had been away he had not collected anything for his services from the town of Constantina. "They have imprisoned him in shackles," she lamented, "and are otherwise mistreating him, trying to kill him at all costs." Doña María charged that the officials were intimidating her husband so that he would stop asking for payment, and she begged the governor to send a constable to Constantina to exercise justice and ensure that her husband was properly paid.

Doña María included a petition to the count that her husband had penned in Constantina on 8 May. Miguel Díaz complained that he was not receiving his daily salary, and he accused the officials of "planning to forcefully drive me out of the said town, all with the end to be able to say that I had left for a better place without curing the sick." The Count of Villar responded by ordering Constantina's officials to pay the surgeon immediately, and he also mandated the town's chief justice, Licentiate Francisco González Perellón, to set free the beleaguered physician.

The count's order reached Constantina on 18 May and elicited an immediate response. Constantina's officials defended themselves, stating that the accusations were false and insisting that they had not mistreated or imprisoned the surgeon. They counterattacked, alleging that Miguel Díaz had committed "crimes" in the town and that he intimidated his poor patients. They accused the physician of blackmailing the plague-stricken poor, "threatening them that if they do not pay him, regardless that he is collecting the salary, he would have to take them to the hospital." Furthermore, they claimed, he told these defenseless patients that he would "expose and display them before a notary so that they would be taken to the said hospital." The pesthouses, set up by municipal officials with the best of intentions to cure the poor sick, struck terror in the popular mind, and the threat of being removed to them could apparently be used to coerce people. These hospitals were often overcrowded, dirty, and smelly places where many patients died after being subjected to painful remedies.

The following day Constantina's officials claimed that they had paid the surgeon the six hundred reales (about fifty-five ducats) he was owed and that indeed he had collected more than two hundred ducats, "which they have been forced to allow for," and they insisted that they should not have to pay him anything else. As soon as Miguel Díaz learned of the accusations against him, he went to see the chief justice, Licentiate González Perellón. The surgeon stated that the claim that he had received a payment of two hundred ducats was untrue, and he stressed that he had cured the poor "without any profit, instead if they wanted to give it to me, I did not take it." "I do not remember what the rich gave me," he added, though he conceded that he might have received "just two or three baby goats," but he insisted that they gave them to him "of their own will without me asking for them." Miguel Díaz felt so certain in his righteousness that he demanded a public proclamation in the principal plaza of Constantina on Sunday, asking anyone who had been sick and had paid the surgeon to step forward and denounce him. The chief justice accepted the challenge: there was a public announcement in the town square on 21 May, and again three days later, yet no one came forth to accuse the surgeon of any misconduct.

Much of Miguel Díaz's conflict with local authorities stemmed from a disagreement over where and how the plague sick should be treated. The surgeon had ordered the sick removed from their houses and taken to the hospital, but the officials refused to comply, believing that the patients could be better cared for in their homes. In addition, according to the surgeon's denunciation of 20 May, Constantina's authorities permitted people purporting to be physicians to effect cures, although they lacked medical knowledge, and "because of them many people have died and are dying of the said contagion." Miguel Díaz demanded that "the men who say they are curing the disease of the plague, neither see nor visit any of the sick." He charged that "they do not cure them, nor do they know the remedies for this said disease," and the surgeon went so far as to accuse them of stealing prescriptions "that I have given in the pharmacy." He alleged that town officials failed to provide him with assistance to search out the sick who were in hiding and blamed them for the increase in the spread of the disease. In conclusion, Miguel Díaz complained that the chief justice, González Perellón, was not only unhelpful but had been interfering with the proper treatment of the plague.

That same day, enlisting Constantina's notary Anton del Castillo and invoking his commission by the Count of Villar to cure the sick, Miguel Díaz duly challenged the chief justice, requiring him to remove the sick from their homes and take them to the hospital. Francisco González Perellón was not amused as he replied sarcastically, "Pretty rubbish you are telling me, having decreed that the sick should be cured in their homes and now you ask that they be taken to the hospital!" Indeed, the outraged chief justice called the surgeon "fool," to which Miguel Díaz sniffed in reply, "you are the magistrate and you can say it, but you are well aware that you know who I am outside of here." According to the notary who witnessed the verbal sparring, the two men "were angrily disputing" until the Señor Licentiate González Perellón had had enough and took the surgeon to jail, exclaiming that he was an "offensive, ill-mannered, dirty rogue." As he was dragged away, the surgeon asked notary Anton del Castillo to take down certified testimony about his mistreatment and imprisonment. At some point the surgeon managed to escape and fled to a nearby church. As was customary, the notary complied with Díaz's request and "remained writing the said notification by the entrance of the chief justice's house." When the document was finished, "I went down the street and I found the said Miguel Díaz in the cemetery of Our Lady of la Encarnación of this town and he asked me for testimony of how I saw him there taking sanctuary."[1]

1. AMS, sec. 13, siglo XVI, vol. 6. The documents were witnessed by two local citizens, a scribe, Cristóbal de Haro, and Gonzalo Infante.

The chief justice did not wait long before countering the surgeon's allegations. On 22 May he fired a stern reply. He protested being blamed for the increase in the number of sick and accused Miguel Díaz of "great malice." González Perellón insisted that local physicians had recommended that those stricken with the plague should be cured in their own houses whenever possible because "experience has taught them that more sick recover in their homes than in the hospital." The chief justice also complained about the Sevillian surgeon's contempt for local physicians and indicated how wrong it was for Miguel Díaz to ask that they be barred from treating the sick. Indeed, "most of those who are stricken call for the said physicians because they are generally considered correct in the cures." González Perellón also defended the use of the same prescriptions for the plague, since after all they all knew the common remedies for the disease. Furthermore, the poor were treated and fed in the hospital, and "God be praised" there were only four patients there at present, and health conditions in general were improving. The chief justice also pointed out that Miguel Díaz's commission in Constantina was limited and claimed there was no indication of when or how his salary was to be paid. In closing, González Perellón reiterated that the surgeon was acting out of malice and accused him of making formal demands, attempting to make González Perellón angry to the point where he "let loose some words for which he could be reprimanded."

Miguel Díaz responded the following day. He insisted that the local surgeons were taking advantage of his own prescriptions because they were not learned physicians "and they know nothing." What was more, as the chief justice was surely aware, "none of them knows how to read and write," which was why he was preparing a report to the Count of Villar. As far as there being only four patients in the hospital, Miguel Díaz blamed it on "misdeed and negligence because for the past eight days there are more than thirty men stricken by the said contagion in this town." He stressed that he did not even take into account those who had died because "the said surgeons do not know how to apply the necessary medicines" and refused to send the sick to the hospital. Hence "every day more become infected," and he lamented that because his orders had been contradicted, many would die. Miguel Díaz reminded the chief justice that he had been sent by the count from Seville with ample authority to effect the cure of the plague and that he was a "meritorious person," who did not deserve the mistreatment he had been subjected to.

The ensemble of charges and countercharges was completed in Constantina on 28 May and sent to Seville for a decision. The Count of Villar reviewed the documents and on 4 June ordered Constantina's officials to pay the salary due to Miguel Díaz. At the same time the governor requested a full report on the town's health conditions, while reminding local authorities to ensure that infected clothing and bedding was burned.[2]

It is difficult to assess which of the men to believe. Certainly, the chief justice had worked well with Dr. Centurio, and the two men repeatedly professed mutual respect. Miguel Díaz seems to have antagonized local authorities from the beginning and never cooperated with González Perellón in the way his predecessor had. It is possible that the locals saw him as a haughty physician from the capital who refused to take into account anything suggested by the town's medical practitioners. At the same time, the chief justice, who had his own troubles with Constantina's town council and could have been the physician's ally, found any challenge to his honor and authority intolerable.

Eventually the plague ended in Constantina and Cazalla de la Sierra, as well as the rest of the region, but the fiscal repercussions were felt for a long time afterward. The plague epidemic of the 1580s became part of Constantina's popular lore. According to a local legend, while the town was suffering from the deadly plague, a young shepherd named Melchor, who lived outside of Constantina with his mother, went to the Robledal Valley while tending his flocks. There in the late afternoon the Virgin appeared to the boy, ordering him to convince the townspeople to come in a procession to the spot where she had revealed herself. Only then would the epidemic end. Melchor told his mother what had happened to him, and the next day she reported it to the parish priest of Constantina. After receiving what he believed was a sign affirming the authenticity of the vision, the priest was convinced; and following the pilgrimage, the town's health was restored. The Virgin of Robledo continues to be venerated to this day.[3]

Measures to prevent contagious disease during the early modern period were for the most part ineffective, and whatever success there was depended largely on luck and the virulence of a given episode. Sometimes, as in the case of Seville in the early 1580s, the remedies and fortune seemed to have worked together, and the outbreaks would be relatively mild. At other times, though

2. AMS, sec. 13, siglo XVI, vol. 6.

3. See Antonio Grados Fernández, *Melchor y la Señora del Robledo* (Constantina, Spain: Imprenta Gamo, 1984).

the same actions and preventive measures were implemented, the results were markedly different. Seville's next serious encounter with the plague came in 1599, and the city's steps to stop its spread were almost identical to those employed twenty years earlier. But this time, thousands of people died, and when in 1649 the plague again visited Seville, it swept away almost half its people and contributed to the city's general decline.[4]

4. AMS, sec. 3, vol. 7, doc. 17. Regarding Seville's decline, see Antonio Domínguez Ortiz, *Orto y ocaso de Sevilla* (Seville: Universidad de Sevilla, 1981).

EPILOGUE

GENTLEMAN OF PRUDENCE

A gentleman of great prudence, truthfulness, and Christianity.
—RODRIGO DE CASTRO, ARCHBISHOP OF SEVILLE

S EVILLE'S PHYSICIANS HAD DECLARED the city plague free, and on
22 June 1582 a solemn procession wound its way through the streets,
bearing the images of Santa Justa and Santa Rufina as well as San
Roque and San Sebastián, "through whose sovereign assistance the
disease had some temperance."[1] The cabildo and the Count of Villar, though relieved that the deadly disease had diminished its grip, continued to face other
crises and, after a few months, a recurrence of sickness. The governor's tenure
at the city's helm was nearing its end, and the Count of Villar began looking
for new postings.

As was customary with royal officials, the count's "job performance" would
be evaluated. The residencia was a long-established administrative inquiry
undertaken at the end of an official's tenure and designed to prevent graft and
malfeasance in office. A judge (*juez de residencia*) conducted the investigation,
following public announcement of the process. Potential complainants were
given thirty days to press charges, both public and secret, and the judge then reviewed the evidence. If any faults were found the official under review could be
fined, exiled, or barred from new appointments. There were problems with the
review system, and charges could be petty, sometimes resulting from person-
ality conflicts. But in general the *residencia* kept royal officials in check.

The Count of Villar, in various letters to the king and the royal council, provided detailed reports of his accomplishments as Seville's governor, boasting
of his successes. He intended the documents to be favorably reviewed in order

1. Ortiz de Zúñiga, *Anales eclesiásticos,* 4:115.

to secure future employment and reward. The normal period of service as governor of Seville was three years, and the Count of Villar was considering his future as early as the spring of 1582. In a subsequent letter to the king he complained about his health and the expenses incurred in office that far exceeded his stipend of 1,860 ducats. Furthermore, as he had indicated elsewhere, he had come often to the king's and the city's financial rescue, using his own money, during his tenure in Seville. Now he claimed he was financially strapped and blamed his "poverty" for his inability to provide sufficient dowry for one of his daughters, who consequently remained unmarried. He had many children, several of whom had died either in battle or from disease. The Count of Villar lamented the loss of four sons "in the naval war of the Lord Don Juan and in Flanders" and the sickness and death, from what he believed to be the plague, of two of his younger children after he arrived in Seville.[2] He claimed that the years during which he had served the city had been exceptionally difficult, and he pointed out that he had stayed beyond the normal term because it would have been inopportune to have left at the height of the plague epidemic. He related to the king that he himself had been struck twice by the contagious disease, and although "Our Lord was served to deliver me from the said sickness," the stress and general ailment that he had been suffering from while serving the city were endangering his life, according to his physicians. Indeed, his doctors recommended that he leave Seville as soon as possible. The count indicated that his "house and property have necessity of my intervention," and he was ready to return to his estates to recuperate his health and wealth. He asked the king for "pensions for two of my sons for their studies." In closing, the count requested an audience with the king or with his confessor, Friar Diego de Chaves, as soon as possible, because he preferred to discuss certain issues in person rather than commit them to paper.[3]

The Count of Villar's departure from Seville and the relinquishing of his

2. The Battle of Lepanto (1571) against the Turkish fleet was won by the Spanish forces led by Don Juan of Austria, Philip II's half brother.

3. BL, Mss. Add. 28343, fols. 345r–46v; BL, Mss. Add. 28344, fols. 213r–19r; regarding the count's salary, see Domínguez Ortiz, "Salarios y atribuciones," 209. For the political influence wielded by royal confessors, whose access to the monarch was not limited to spiritual matters, see Magdalena S. Sánchez, *The Empress, the Queen, and the Nun: Women and Power at the Court of Philip III of Spain* (Baltimore: Johns Hopkins University Press, 1998), 18–22.

duties at the city's helm were delayed for almost another year. Furthermore, the rejoicing in the summer of 1582 that the plague had ended was premature. In May of 1583 the count wrote that people were still being stricken, and although the plague raged mostly in the surrounding countryside, Seville was also affected. Again the count's health suffered, and from February to early May he was "sick in bed and in great danger of dying."[4]

About three weeks later (4 June 1583) the count wrote to the king's secretary, Mateo Vázquez, reporting on fiscal issues. He concluded the letter with a detailed commentary pointing out that he had "served with all my strength," but he added that his energy "is waning because of lack of health." Moreover, although the judge in charge of conducting his residencia was already in the city, he could not proceed because the new governor, Don Juan Hurtado de Mendoza, the Count of Orgaz, had not yet arrived. Hence the Count of Villar continued to govern Seville and its extensive territory while impatiently waiting to be relieved. At the same time he assured Mateo Vázquez that he did not wish to appear to complain and was only interested in serving His Majesty.[5]

In a long report on 11 August 1583 he repeated a request for authorization to travel to Court as soon as possible after the completion of the residencia. In the same missive, before detailing his achievements, he asked the king for recompense for his service and pressed for a lifetime appointment as head of the Royal Mint of Seville, a prestigious as well as lucrative position. He stressed that he had served in Seville approaching five years "without doing a thing regarding my estate and businesses which resulted in many losses for me."

The count argued that he needed some form of recompense "because although I do not owe a real, or anything else, nor have I been in debt, I have nothing." He again emphasized that the period of his governorship was one of the most calamitous in memory. One crisis followed after another, and the count pointed out how well he had dealt with them. He highlighted the persistent drought and serious crop failure and the consequent food shortages, and he reminded the king that he had organized the purchase and distribution of grain to alleviate the scarcity. He pointed to his intervention over a three-year period to help wipe out a locust infestation that threatened harvests. By imple-

4. BL, Mss. Add. 28369, fols. 105r–108v.
5. BL, Mss. Add. 28369 (4 June 1583).

menting effective measures, the count boasted, he had led the city and its district through serious epidemics of influenza, typhus, and plague. He noted that the measures included the founding of new hospitals and the creation of a cordon sanitaire to block the passage of infection into the city. He had made efforts to ascertain the city was clean and had ample fresh drinking water.

He had ensured the quick rebuilding of the gunpowder factory after the disastrous explosion and fire that destroyed parts of Triana. He helped the city raise and house local troops for the Portuguese campaign. He had overseen the billeting and health care of ill local and foreign troops in Seville. The Count took credit for supervising the embargo of Portuguese goods during the annexation, helping to direct the strengthening of fortifications along the border, and improving the coastal guard against foreign ships. He had tried to maintain order and protect the city, including from the unruly men on the Sicily galleys that had entered the port. He had blocked a potentially dangerous uprising of Moriscos in the city and surrounding countryside. He had secured substantial tax revenues, loans, and outright "gifts" from the parsimonious Sevillians for King Philip's military needs, which were enormous and rising in the 1580s. He had been in charge of numerous items that were outside the jurisdiction of the municipal government yet were important for administration. He had directed the embargo of the gold and silver arriving on the treasure fleet returning from the Indies, following the king's orders. He had assisted in the transfer of three hundred thousand ducats to Flanders, again as the king had ordered.

The count admitted that his relations with officials of the Inquisition, and the Royal Audiencia, were often strained, but he insisted that he had always acted in the service of God and His Majesty. He recalled that in spite of the fact that the archbishop and regent had been entrusted with the task, it was he, the count, who had taken over and with care and diligence executed the transfer of San Fernando and the other corpses to their resting place in the new Royal Chapel in Seville's cathedral. Don Fernando concluded by saying that he believed he had done his work well and had served His Majesty with "the highest care, liberty and honesty." The count again mentioned the loss of his children to the plague and in battles, as well as his own bouts with the disease, underscoring the direct and profound impact the plague had had on him and his family. In closing, he declared that it seemed that such sacrifices and services "deserve remuneration" and pledged to continue to serve His Majesty "until death."[6]

By late August 1583 the administrative review of the Count of Villar was finally completed. On 26 August the count informed the king that "Licentiate Varela who was sent to this city to conduct my residencia, was here for seventy days before the Count of Orgaz came and I could retire from office." The review process took the necessary thirty days, and the Licentiate Lope García Varela interviewed "a great number of witnesses and of different estates and conditions" regarding the Count of Villar's conduct and his government. They all agreed that the count "had served with great Christianity and integrity"; based on such laudatory testimony the judge pronounced a very favorable formal sentence on 23 August praising the governor's devoted service to the Crown. He called the count a "great gentleman," and recommended to the king that "he should be given ample reward and that it be public because for him it will be an incentive and for others an example."[7] Such unanimous approbation of an official was not common and reflects well on the count's tenure in Seville.

The accolades for the outgoing governor came not only from formal testimony presented to Judge Varela but from the highest religious authority as well, and most significantly, it was unsolicited. On 9 September 1583 Seville's archbishop Don Rodrigo de Castro penned in his own hand a confidential letter to the monarch stating that "the Count of Villar, who was this city's governor, has now completed his post, which he fulfilled as well as was expected given his manner of conduct. He is a gentleman of great prudence, truthfulness, and Christianity." The archbishop stressed that neither the count nor anyone else knew that he was writing this letter, confessing to being moved only by his desire to bring to His Majesty's notice someone that the king could have full con-

6. There is a rather extensive report of the count's administration of Seville summarizing his most important accomplishments. That undated report, "Relación de las cosas en que el Conde del Villar, asistente que fue de Sevilla, servio a Su Magestad en cinco años o casi que tubo el oficio," 1579–1583, is found in the Biblioteca Nacional, Madrid (BNM), mss. 9372, fols. 160–61. In the British Library is a related document, Mss. Add. 28344, fols. 213r–19r, dated 11 August 1583; at the end of this document there is a final letter signed by the Count of Villar. In these papers we see the relationship between the materials in the Archivo General de Indias, the Biblioteca Nacional in Madrid, and the British Library. The set at the British Library not only does much to clarify when the letter and report were made but also sheds important light on the personal life of the count.

7. Archivo General de Indias (AGI), Indiferente general 740, ramo 174.

fidence in. The archbishop vouched that the count would continue to serve the Crown loyally and well "in any important business."[8]

The count's many years of service to the Crown had left him rich in experience but, according to his frequent complaints, financially poor. He now had two principal options: return to his estates in Jaén or secure a higher and more profitable office, perhaps even in the overseas colonies. Given his advanced age and ill health many must have expected his career to be over when he left Seville. For several months after his tenure as governor had ended, the Count of Villar seemed content to remain in Andalusia. He hoped to regain his health and to improve his economic standing. He also was willing to travel. Long before he had retired from his post, the count had repeatedly asked permission to go to Court to inform the king personally of his activities as Seville's governor.

The count's sacrifices and loyalty did not remain unrewarded The king was looking for a new viceroy to govern Peru, and on 27 August 1583 the council in Madrid was charged to add the count's name to a list of potential candidates for the Andean viceroyalty. Not long thereafter, on 3 September, the king issued a royal order designating the Count of Villar as viceroy of Peru.[9] Owing to unforeseen circumstances and delays the count almost lost the position, but in the end he was able to set sail from Sanlúcar de Barrameda for the Indies on 30 November 1584, "Saint Andrew's day."[10] His wife remained behind hindered by poor health, but he was accompanied by his eighteen-year-old son, Gerónimo de Torres y Portugal, and his nephew, Don Diego de Portugal (not to be confused with the veinticuatro of Seville active in the city government while the count was governor), who eventually became judge and president of the Royal Audiencia of Charcas. The transatlantic crossing and the long trip south from Panama exhausted the new viceroy, and his frail health caused new delays. He did not reach the colonial capital of Lima until the end of November 1585.

8. BL, Mss. Add. 28344, fols. 245r–46v.

9. AGI, Indiferente general 740, ramos 171 and 293.

10. According to Pierson, *Commander of the Armada*, 53, the Duke of Medina Sidonia had complained to the king's secretary, Mateo Vázquez, about widespread corruption involving Seville, Mexico, and Peru, and he also included the outgoing governor of Seville, the Count of Villar. The duke tried unsuccessfully to block the Count of Villar's appointment as viceroy of Peru and suggested instead his uncle, the Marquis of Villamanrique, one of Seville's chief justices, who subsequently became the viceroy of New Spain in 1585.

The training the count had received as royal governor of Seville provided important experience, but nothing could lay the foundations needed to prepare him for what he faced in Peru as viceroy of a territory covering half a continent. There was the threat and reality of foreign attack on shipping along the western coast of South America in what had been Spain's own sea, the Pacific Ocean. That his tenure coincided with the time of the Spanish Armada certainly complicated matters. Never good in normal times, communications between the colonies and the motherland broke down for months during the conflict with England. The viceroy spent much time protecting various sources of the Crown's revenue, including the royal fifth due from precious metals taken from Potosí and other mines, as fleets attempted to transport the treasure to Spain. There were natural disasters, such as a major earthquake that destroyed much of the city of Lima and damaged surrounding countryside. The Creole aristocracy were even more of a challenge to rule than Seville's had been. The Count of Villar's relationship with the local branch of the Holy Office of the Inquisition became so explosive that he was excommunicated. And the most disastrous epidemics to sweep Spanish South America decimated the Amerindian population during his term. When the Count of Villar left Peru in 1590 his residencia was still incomplete, and the results, which were delayed until 1593, and after the count's death, were very different from those in Seville a decade before. The inspector levied 128 charges against him and his government, including bribery and nepotism, and it took years before his heirs were able to sort out the mess.[11]

In Andean America, the Count of Villar's attempt to deal with a deadly outbreak of smallpox and measles mixed with influenza and typhus was destined to fail, in spite of good intentions and strenuous efforts. Certainly, his experience with contagious disease was invaluable, and he tried to implement measures of prevention and cure similar to those he had ordered in Seville. But in the Indies the circumstances were very different. The devastating epidemics spread rapidly, killing mostly Amerindians. When colonial officials became aware that a deadly epidemic was quickly moving south from the Quito region, passing from village to village, the count turned to the medical profession for help, as he had done in Seville years earlier. On 21 March 1589 he convened a meeting of several doctors in Lima. The viceroy asked if any cases had been

11. AGI, Indiferente general 740, ramo 271; AGI, Patronato 190, ramo 43, fol. 3; AGI, Justicia 485.

reported in the city yet and what cures they recommended for those stricken. The physicians agreed that there were no cases of the diseases at present in the capital. As to cures for the sick in the hinterland, they recommended that the *encomenderos* (those who held Indian grants) should "go to the affected villages and take gifts of sugar, raisins and oil and preserves and barley." In addition they should provide honey and oil for medicines. The doctors stressed that once the disease made its appearance, "above all the Indians should be exempt from work and household service." They should be kept out of the sun and shielded from the wind, bled, and isolated from the rest of the village. The doctors advised that the sick should be placed in hospitals; if there were none, then churches or any public buildings could serve to separate the sick, provide care for them, and prevent others from becoming infected. The Count of Villar agreed and ordered the Indian governors and encomenderos of any town or village where infectious disease was rampant to "do and carry out" all that the physicians had recommended.[12]

Whether these orders were fulfilled is unclear, but given the nature of the colonial system and its insatiable demand for Indian labor, it seems unlikely that many encomenderos, whose livelihood depended on the tribute they collected from their charges, would have kept anyone from working merely to prevent sickness. Indeed, the viceroyalty comprised such a vast territory that close supervision was virtually impossible. In the end, a series of epidemics— smallpox, measles, influenza, and typhus—swept the entire western half of South America, devastating the Amerindian population. The count's efforts were in vain. Given the high susceptibility and mortality among the Amerindians, it is unlikely that the impact of the combination of diseases could have been lessened, even if the recommended measures had been followed.

Although the Count of Villar's replacement arrived in Lima's port of Callao on 28 November 1589, he was unable to depart Peru until 2 May of the following year, on the annual treasure fleet heading for Panama. Disembarking in the Pacific seaport, the count and his contingent, including his son Don Gerónimo, escorted the Crown's silver across the isthmus to the Caribbean port of Nombre de Dios. From there they sailed to Cartagena de Indias, where they arrived on 2 July 1590, and transferred the silver to the homeward bound fleet of Pedro

12. BNM, 3043, fols. 422–25. For locating and transcribing this document, we want to thank Miguel Costa, whose Ph.D. dissertation, "Patronage and Bribery," sheds much light on the administration of the Count of Villar as Peru's viceroy.

Menéndez Márquez.[13] By the time his ships were ready to sail for Havana and on to Spain, the count had fallen too ill to continue. He remained in Cartagena for more than a year before he recuperated enough to embark for Havana and continue home. He finally sailed from Havana sometime after 20 November 1591 and reached Spain on 18 January 1592, a return journey that lasted two years.[14]

After arriving in Spain, the Count of Villar was planning to stay in Seville until retiring to his estate in Jaén.[15] Unfortunately, his health began to fail again, and he died shortly before midnight on 12 October 1592 in the Alcázar, where he had lived as Seville's governor a decade earlier. The day he died the count summoned a notary to compose his will, which was to supersede all his prior testaments. His shaky signature indicates the gravity of his condition. He was just as detailed in the disposition of his estate as he had been in administering Seville and, later, Peru. The Count of Villar was married twice and had many children: thirteen with his first wife and twelve with his second wife, Doña María Carrillo de Córdoba. Most of his children had predeceased him, many in infancy, but there were two younger sons from his first marriage and four from his second marriage still alive and ready to battle one another over their father's estate. The oldest son with Doña María, Don Gerónimo, who had traveled with him to Peru, was named along with his mother as one of the executors of the will. Doña María was to assume the guardianship of their minor children. Three days after the Count of Villar's death the notary opened and read his will in the presence of his son Don Gerónimo, the magistrate of the Royal Audiencia, and the current governor of Seville, Don Francisco de Carvajal, as well as other witnesses.

Like other sixteenth-century Spaniards of his class, he was concerned about his legacy, and in his will he left detailed instructions to ensure his memory would be perpetual. In addition to the standard religious proscriptions, the masses for his soul in various churches and convents, he made certain that his family tomb in the cathedral of Jaén was a fitting memorial and that the seat

---

13. Roberto Levillier, ed., *Gobernantes del Perú, cartas y papeles, siglo XVI* (Madrid: Juan Pueyo, 1925), 11:306–17.

14. Ibid., 11:322–26. AHPS, Protocolos notariales, leg. 17720. The information comes from the Count of Villar's will, which is sewn between folios 428r and 435r in the notary's bundle. The numeration of this insert is folio 33r–v.

15. AHPS, Protocolos notariales, leg. 7291, fols. 759r–v. The count was in Seville on 10 July 1592.

of the mayorazgo (estate), the Condado del Villardompardo, would be a solid and permanent reminder of his life and that of his forefathers. In his will he gave careful instructions to his grandson Don Juan de Torres y Portugal, the new Count of Villar, on how to maintain the business and family fortune. He left him a virtual blueprint on how the family castle in Villardompardo was to be rebuilt, bearing a marble plaque with the family coat of arms and an inscription on its exterior wall. The count also described his vision for the family chapel in the cathedral of Jaén, including the paintings of the large retable, the placement of the family coat of arms, and the iron gate with its inscriptions and images.[16]

Following the count's death, his body, dressed in the habit of the Order of Santiago, was placed in a lead box and put inside a wooden coffin; it was then moved from the Alcázar to the Monastery of San Diego, outside the Jerez Gate. A royal *cédula* (decree) of 19 July 1589, inserted with the will, had provided for the transport of the count's body to Jaén. A few days after the Count of Villar's death, the current governor of Seville authorized money for the guides, carts, and beasts of burden and appointed constable Francisco de Herrera to oversee the trip. The count's last journey was about to commence.[17]

16. AHPS, Protocolos notariales, leg. 17720. The original agreement regarding the chapel had been worked out with Bishop Don Diego Tavera in Jaén on 8 March 1557 by notary Pedro Ochoa, and a copy was placed "in the Archive of my papers that I have in the Fortress of the said my town of Villar," along with other papers.

17. AHPS, Protocolos notariales, leg. 17720, fols. 419v–27v.

GLOSSARY

aceite: Oil

alcabala: Sales tax

alcalde mayor: Chief justice, appellate judge

alférez mayor: Chief standard-bearer

alguacil mayor: Chief constable

alguacil de la peste: Plague constable

alhóndiga: Public granary

almud: Dry measure of about 27.75 liters. Two *almudes* equal a *fanega.*

almojarifazgo: Customs duty

arenal: Sandy ground

arrendador: Tax farmer

arroba: Liquid measure of about 12.5 liters

asistente: Royal governor in Seville and some other cities

atarazanas: Shipyard

Audiencia: Royal appellate court of justice

bachiller: Bachelor, the lowest university title

barbero: Barber

barbero cirujano: Barber surgeon

beata: Holy woman

bodegonero: Proprietor of a peasant eatery

botica: Pharmacy

boticario: Pharmacist

bubón: Large bubo

caballero: Knight

caballero veinticuatro: Alderman

cabildo: City council

cahíz: Measure equivalent to about 690 kilograms

cañas: Javelin jousting

caños: Water pipes

carbón: Charcoal

carga: Dry measure, approximately four *fanegas.*

caridad: Charity

carne: Meat

carnero: Ram

cédula: Decree

Casa de la Contratación: House of Trade

colchero: Coverlet maker

Contaduría: Accounting office

converso: Jewish convert to Christianity

corral: Rooming house with a central patio; courtyard

corregidor: Royal governor

corrida de toros: Bullfight

cuadrilla: Squadron, team

cuadrillero: Squadron or team leader

curandero: Healer

ducat: Gold coin worth 375 *maravedís* or 11 *reales*

encabezamiento: Tax assessment

encomendero: Holder of an Indian grant

enfermero: Male nurse

fanega: Dry measure, approximately a bushel, or 55.5 liters

fiel ejecutor: Inspector of weights and measures

fuente: Spring, source

fuero: Royal charter, privilege, granted to a town

fulano: So-and-so

hidalgo: A member of the lower nobility

honras fúnebres: Devotional service for the deceased

hospitalera: Female hospital worker

huerta: Plot of land, field

infante: Prince

juego de cañas: Jousting games

juez: Judge

jurado: Councilman

league: Measure of distance, about 5.57 kilometers

letrado: Person skilled in the law

lugar: Place

maese: Master

maestre: Shipmaster

maravedí: Basic unit of currency

marismas: Alluvial floodplain

matadero: Slaughterhouse

mayordomo: Steward, treasurer

mayorazgo: Entailed estate

mesonero: Innkeeper

modorra: Lethargy, encephalitis

Morisco: Muslim convert to Christianity

paz: Peace

postigo: Small city gate

procurador mayor: Chief representative or solicitor

propios: Income-producing municipal properties

Protomedicato: Tribunal that examined and licensed medical professionals

real: Silver coin worth thirty-four *maravedís*

reconquista: Reconquest

regidor: Alderman

rejón: Short spear

residencia: Review of an official's administration at its conclusion

sanbenito: Penitential garment worn by those condemned by the Inquisition

sangre: Blood

seca: Bubo, swelling

sisa: Excise tax

sol: Sun

solicitador del almojarifazgo: Customs agent

tabardete: Spots on skin, associated with typhus or other contagious diseases

tabardillo: Typhus

vara: Measure equal to approximately 835 millimeters or slightly
    less than a yard

vecino: Head of household, citizen, neighbor

veinticuatro: Alderman

venta: Countryside inn

MEDICAL TERMS

In translating Spanish terms of the most common symptoms discussed by the contemporaries, we have attempted to be consistent. Here is the list of the English words and their Spanish equivalents:

abscess: *Apostema*

bubo: *Landre, seca*

carbuncle: *Carbunco*

lump: *Bulto*

pimple: *Grano*

pustule: *Nacido*

spots: *Tabardete*

swelling: *Seca*

tumor: *Nacencia* (rarely, *nacido*)

BIBLIOGRAPHY

PRINTED PRIMARY SOURCES

Amelang, James S., trans. and ed. *A Journal of the Plague Year: The Diary of the Barcelona Tanner Miquel Parents, 1651.* Oxford: Oxford University Press, 1991.

Ariño, Francisco de. *Sucesos de Sevilla de 1592 a 1604.* Edited by Antonio María Fabié. Seville: Ayuntamiento de Sevilla, 1993.

Caro, Rodrigo. *Antigvedades, y principado de la ilvstrissima civdad de Sevilla. Y chorographia de sv convento ivridico, o antigva chancilleria* [1634]. Seville: Ediciones Alfar, 1998.

Cervantes, Miguel de. "Novela de Rinconete y Cortadillo." In *Novelas ejemplares,* edited by Harry Sieber, 1:189–240. Madrid: Cátedra, 1990.

Chaves, Cristóbal de. *Relación de la cárcel de Sevilla.* Madrid: Clásicos El Arbol, 1983.

Covarrubias Orozco, Sebastián de. *Tesoro de la lengua castellana o española* [1611]. Edited by Felipe C. R. Maldonado and Manuel Camarero. Madrid: Editorial Castalia, 1994.

Enríquez, Enrique Jorge. *Retrato del perfeto médico.* Salamanca: Casa de Iuan y Andres Renau, 1595.

Hidalgo de Agüero, Bartolomé. *Thesoro de la verdadera cirugía y la via particular contra la común.* Seville: Francisco Pérez, 1604.

León, Pedro de. *Grandeza y miseria en Andalucía. Testimonio de una encrucijada histórica (1578–1616).* Edited by Pedro Herrera Puga. Granada: Facultad de Teología, 1981.

Levillier, Roberto, ed. *Gobernantes del Perú, cartas y papeles, siglo XVI.* 14 vols. Madrid: Juan Pueyo, 1925.

Mercado, Luis de. *Libro en que se trata con claridad la naturaleza . . . y modo de curar la enfermedad vulgar, y peste. . . .* Madrid: Imprenta del Licenciado Castro, 1599.

Monardes, Nicolás. *Historia medicinal de las cosas que se traen de nuestras Indias occidentales que sirven en medicina. . . .* [1574]. Seville: Padilla Libros, 1988.

Morales Padrón, Francisco, ed. *Memorias de Sevilla (Noticias sobre el siglo XVII).* Cordova: Monte de Piedad, 1981.

Morgado, Alonso de. *Historia de Sevilla* [1587]. Seville: J. M. Ariza, 1887.

Ortiz de Zúñiga, Diego. *Anales eclesiásticos y seculares de la muy noble y muy leal ciudad de Sevilla* [1796]. 5 vols. Seville: Guadalquivir, 1988.

Pacheco, Francisco. *Libro de descripción de verdaderos retratos de ilustres y memorables varones* [1599]. Edited and with an introduction by Pedro M. Piñero and Rogelio Reyes Cano. Seville: Diputación Provincial de Sevilla, 1985.

SECONDARY SOURCES

Aberth, John. *From the Brink of the Apocalypse: Confronting Famine, War, Plague, and Death in the Later Middle Ages.* New York: Routledge Press, 2000.

Albardonedo Freire, Antonio José. *El urbanismo de Sevilla durante el reinado de Felipe II.* Seville: Ediciones Guadalquivir, 2002.

Arrizabalaga, Jon, John Henderson, and Roger French. *The Great Pox: The French Disease in Renaissance Europe.* New Haven, Conn.: Yale University Press, 1997.

Betrán, José Luis. *La peste en la Barcelona de los Austrias.* Lleida, Spain: Milenio, 1996.

Bilinkoff, Jodi. *The Avila of Saint Teresa: Religious Reform in a Sixteenth-Century City.* Ithaca, N.Y.: Cornell University Press, 1989.

Biraben, Jean-Noël. *Les hommes et la peste en France et dans les pays européens et mediterranéens.* 2 vols. Paris: Mouton, 1975–76.

Brockliss, Laurence, and Colin Jones. *The Medical World of Early Modern France.* Oxford: Oxford University Press, 1997.

Calvi, Giulia. *Histories of a Plague Year: The Social and the Imaginary in Baroque Florence.* Berkeley and Los Angeles: University of California Press, 1989.

Campbell, Anna Montgomery. *The Black Death and the Men of Learning.* New York: Columbia University Press, 1931.

Campos Díez, María Soledad. *El Real Tribunal del Protomedicato castellano (siglos XIV–XIX).* Cuenca, Spain: Universidad de Castilla-La Mancha, 1999.

Carmichael, Ann G. "Bubonic Plague." In *The Cambridge World History of Human Disease,* edited by Kenneth F. Kiple, 628–31. Cambridge: Cambridge University Press, 1993.

———. "Diseases of the Renaissance and Early Modern Europe." In *The Cambridge World History of Human Disease,* edited by Kenneth F. Kiple, 279–87. Cambridge: Cambridge University Press, 1993.

———. *Plague and the Poor in Renaissance Florence.* Cambridge: Cambridge University Press, 1986.

Carmona García, Juan Ignacio. *Crónica urbana del malvivir (s. XIV–XVII): Insalubridad, desamparo y hambre en Sevilla.* Seville: Universidad de Sevilla, 2000.

———. *El extenso mundo de la pobreza: La otra cara de la Sevilla imperial.* Seville: Ayuntamiento de Sevilla, 1993.

———. *La peste en Sevilla.* Seville: Ayuntamiento de Sevilla, 2004.

———. *El sistema de la hospitalidad pública en la Sevilla del antiguo régimen.* Seville: Diputación Provincial, 1979.

Carreras Panchón, Antonio. "Las epidemias de peste en la España del Renacimiento." *Asclepio* 29 (1977): 5–15.

Christian, William A., Jr. *Local Religion in Sixteenth-Century Spain.* Princeton, N.J.: Princeton University Press, 1989.

Chueca Goitia, Fernando, Antonio Domínguez Ortiz, Antonio Hermosilla Molina, and others. *Los hospitales de Sevilla.* Seville: Real Academia Sevillana de Buenas Letras, 1989.

Cipolla, Carlo M. *Cristofano and the Plague: A Study of the History of Public Health in the Age of Galileo.* London: Collins, 1973.

———. *Fighting the Plague in Seventeenth-Century Italy.* Madison: University of Wisconsin Press, 1981.

Coleman, David. *Creating Christian Granada: Society and Religious Culture in an Old-World Frontier City, 1492–1600.* Ithaca, N.Y.: Cornell University Press, 2003.

Cook, Alexandra Parma, and Noble David Cook. *Good Faith and Truthful Ignorance: A Case of Transatlantic Bigamy.* Durham, N.C.: Duke University Press, 1991.

Cook, Noble David, and José Hernández Palomo. "Epidemias en Triana (Sevilla, 1660–1865)." *Annali della Facoltà di Economia e Commercio della Università di Bari,* n.s., 31 (1992): 53–81.

Costa, Luis Miguel. "Patronage and Bribery in Sixteenth-Century Colonial Peru: The Government of Viceroy Conde del Villar and the Visita of Licentiate Alonso Fernández de Bonilla." Ph.D. diss., Florida International University, 2005.

Defourneaux, Marcelin. *Daily Life in Spain in the Golden Age.* Translated by Newton Branch. Stanford, Calif.: Stanford University Press, 1979.

Domínguez Ortiz, Antonio. *Autos de la Inquisición de Sevilla (siglo XVII).* Seville: Biblioteca de Temas Sevillanos, 1994.

———. *Orto y ocaso de Sevilla.* Seville: Universidad de Sevilla, 1981.

———. "Salarios y atribuciones de los asistentes de Sevilla." *Archivo hispalense* 7, no. 20 (1946): 207–13.

———. *La Sevilla del siglo XVII.* Seville: Universidad de Sevilla, 1986.

———. *La sociedad española en el siglo XVII.* Madrid: Consejo Superior de Investigaciones Científicas, 1964.

Domínguez Ortiz, Antonio, and Bernard Vincent. *Historia de los moriscos: Vida y tragedia de una minoría.* Madrid: Alianza Universidad, 1997.

Domínguez-Rodiño y Domínguez-Adame, Eloy. "El Hospital de las Cinco Llagas." In *Los hospitales de Sevilla,* by Fernando Chueca Goitia, Antonio Domínguez Ortiz, Antonio Hermosilla Molina, et al., 89–117. Seville: Real Academia Sevillana de Buenas Letras, 1989.

Eire, Carlos M. N. *From Madrid to Purgatory: The Art and Craft of Dying in Sixteenth-Century Spain.* Cambridge: Cambridge University Press, 1995.

Fernández-Carrión, Mercedes, and José Luis Valverde. *Farmacia y sociedad en Sevilla en el siglo XVI.* Seville: Biblioteca de Temas Sevillanos, 1985.

Fortea Pérez, José Ignacio. "Sevilla y las Cortes de Castilla en el reinado de Felipe II." In *Sevilla, Felipe II y la Monarquía Hispánica,* edited by Carlos Alberto González Sánchez, 49–80. Seville: Ayuntamiento de Sevilla, 1999.

Fraga Iribarne, María Luisa. *Conventos femeninos desaparecidos: Sevilla—siglo XIX.* Seville: Ediciones Guadalquivir, 1993.

Friedman, Ellen G. *Spanish Captives in North Africa in the Early Modern Age.* Madison: University of Wisconsin Press, 1983.

Gil, Juan. *Los conversos y la Inquisición sevillana.* 5 vols. Seville: Universidad de Sevilla, 2000–2001.

González Díaz, Antonio Manuel. *Poder urbano y asistencia social: El Hospital de San Hermenegildo de Sevilla (1453–1837).* Seville: Diputación de Sevilla, 1997.

González Sánchez, Carlos Alberto, ed. *Sevilla, Felipe II y la Monarquía Hispánica.* Seville: Ayuntamiento de Sevilla, 1999.

Grados Fernández, Antonio. *Melchor y la Señora del Robledo.* Constantina, Spain: Imprenta Gamo, 1984.

Granjel, Luis S. *La medicina española renacentista.* Salamanca, Spain: Universidad de Salamanca, 1980.

———. *Médicos españoles.* Salamanca, Spain: Universidad de Salamanca, 1967.

———. "Vida y obra de Sorapán de Rieros." *Asclepio* 24 (1972): 63–75.

Guerra, Francisco. *Epidemiología americana y filipina, 1492–1898.* Madrid: Ministerio de Sanidad y Consumo, 1999.

———. *Historia de la medicina.* 2 vols. Madrid: Ediciones Norma, 1982–89.

———. *Nicolás Bautista Monardes: Su vida y su obra (ca. 1493–1588).* Mexico City: Compañía Fundidora de Fierro y Acero de Monterrey, S.A., 1961.

Herlihy, David. *The Black Death and the Transformation of the West.* Cambridge, Mass.: Harvard University Press, 1997.

Hermosilla Molina, Antonio. *Cien años de la medicina Sevillana.* Seville: Diputación Provincial, 1970.

Herrera Puga, Pedro. *Sociedad y delincuencia en el Siglo de Oro.* Madrid: Biblioteca de Autores Cristianos, 1974.

Hess, Andrew C. "The Moriscos: An Ottoman Fifth Column in Sixteenth-Century Spain." *American Historical Review* 74, no. 1 (1968): 1–25.

Hiltpold, Paul. "The Price, Production, and Transportation of Grain in Early Modern Castile." *Agricultural History* 63, no. 1 (1989): 73–91.

Horrox, Rosemary, trans. and ed. *The Black Death.* Manchester, U.K.: Manchester University Press, 1994.

Kagan, Richard L. *Lawsuits and Litigants in Castile, 1500–1700.* Chapel Hill: University of North Carolina Press, 1981.

———, ed. *Spanish Cities of the Golden Age: The Views of Anton van den Wyngaerde.* Berkeley and Los Angeles: University of California Press, 1989.

Kamen, Henry. *Philip of Spain.* New Haven, Conn.: Yale University Press, 1997.

Kiple, Kenneth F., ed. *The Cambridge World History of Human Disease.* Cambridge: Cambridge University Press, 1993.

Livi-Bacci, Massimo. *Population and Nutrition: An Essay on European Demographic History.* Cambridge: Cambridge University Press, 1991.

López Alonso, Carmen. *Locura y sociedad en Sevilla: Historia del Hospital de los Inocentes (1436?–1840).* Seville: Diputación Provincial, 1988.

Lunenfeld, Marvin. *Keepers of the City: The Corregidores of Isabella I of Castile, 1474–1504.* Cambridge: Cambridge University Press, 1987.

Lynch, John. *Spain under the Habsburgs.* Vol. 1, *Empire and Absolutism, 1516–1598.* New York: Oxford University Press, 1965.

Mate, Mavis E. *Daughters, Wives, and Widows after the Black Death: Women in Sussex, 1350–1535.* Woodbridge, U.K.: Boydell and Brewer, 1998.

Matossian, Mary Kilbourne. *Poisons of the Past: Molds, Epidemics, and History.* New Haven, Conn.: Yale University Press, 1989.

Mena, José María de. *Las calles de Sevilla.* Seville: Editorial Castillejo, 1994.

Molina Martínez, Miguel. "Los Torres y Portugal: Del señorío de Jaén al virreinato peruano." In *Andalucía y América en el siglo XVI: Actas de las II jornadas de Andalucía y América,* edited by Bibiano Torres Ramírez and José Hernández Palomo, 2:35–66. Seville: Escuela de Estudios Hispano-Americanos, 1983.

Mollat, Michel. *The Poor in the Middle Ages: An Essay in Social History.* Translated by Arthur Goldhammer. New Haven, Conn.: Yale University Press, 1986.

Montero de Espinosa, D. J. M. *Antigüedades del convento casa grande de San Agustín de Sevilla, y noticias del Santo Crucifixo que en él se venera* [1817]. Seville: Imprenta Municipal, 1995.

Moraleja Pinilla, Gerardo. *Historia de Medina del Campo.* Medina del Campo, Spain: Mateo Alaguero, 1971.

Morales Padrón, Francisco. *Los corrales de vecinos de Sevilla.* Seville: Universidad de Sevilla, 1997.

———. *Historia de Sevilla: La ciudad del quinientos.* Seville: Universidad de Sevilla, 1983.

Nader, Helen. *Liberty in Absolutist Spain: The Habsburg Sale of Towns, 1516–1700.* Baltimore: Johns Hopkins University Press, 1990.

Pérez Moreda, Vicente. *Las crisis de mortalidad en la España interior, siglos XVI–XIX.* Madrid: Siglo XXI, 1980.

Pérez Murillo, María Dolores, Jesús María de la Casa Rivas, Antonio Dueñas Olmo, and Angeles López Díaz. "Aspectos urbanísticos y sociales del Arenal de Sevilla en el siglo XVI." In *Andalucía y América en el siglo XVI: Actas de las II jornadas de Andalucía y América,* edited by Bibiano Torres Ramírez and José Hernández Palomo, 2:273–302. Seville: Escuela de Estudios Hispano-Americanos, 1983.

Pérez-Mallaína, Pablo E. *Spain's Men of the Sea: Daily Life in the Indies Fleets in the Sixteenth Century.* Translated by Carla Rahn Phillips. Baltimore: Johns Hopkins University Press, 1998.

Perry, Mary Elizabeth. *Crime and Society in Early Modern Seville.* Hanover, N.H.: University Press of New England, 1980.

———. *Gender and Disorder in Early Modern Seville.* Princeton, N.J.: Princeton University Press, 1990.

Phillips, Carla Rahn, and William D. Phillips. *Spain's Golden Fleece: Wool Production and the Wool Trade from the Middle Ages to the Nineteenth Century.* Baltimore: Johns Hopkins University Press, 1997.

Pierson, Peter. *Commander of the Armada: The Seventh Duke of Medina Sidonia.* New Haven, Conn.: Yale University Press, 1989.

Pike, Ruth. *Aristocrats and Traders: Sevillian Society in the Sixteenth Century.* Ithaca, N.Y.: Cornell University Press, 1972.

———. "The Converso Family of Baltasar del Alcázar." *Kentucky Romance Quarterly* 14 (1967): 349–65.

———. *Enterprise and Adventure: The Genoese in Seville and the Opening of the New World.* Ithaca, N.Y.: Cornell University Press, 1966.

———. *Linajudos and Conversos in Seville: Greed and Prejudice in Sixteenth- and Seventeenth-Century Spain.* New York: Peter Lang, 2000.

———. "An Urban Minority: The Moriscos of Seville." *International Journal of Middle East Studies* 2, no. 4 (1971): 368–77.

Rodríguez Marín, Francisco. *La verdadera biografía del doctor Nicolás Monardes* [1913]. Seville: Padilla Libros, 1988.

Rojo Vega, Anastasio. *Enfermos y sanadores en la Castilla del siglo XVI.* Valladolid, Spain: Universidad de Valladolid, 1993.

Sánchez, Magdalena S. *The Empress, the Queen, and the Nun: Women and Power at the Court of Philip III of Spain.* Baltimore: Johns Hopkins University Press, 1998.

Sánchez-Arjona, José. *Anales del teatro en Sevilla desde Lope de Rueda hasta finales de siglo XVII* [1898]. Seville: Ayuntamiento de Sevilla, 1994.

Schwarz, Klaus. *Die Pest in Bremen: Epidemien und freier Handel in einer deutschen Hafenstadt, 1350–1713.* Bremen, Germany: Selbstverlag des Staatsarchivs Bremen, 1996.

Siraisi, Nancy G. *Medieval and Early Renaissance Medicine: An Introduction to Knowledge and Practice.* Chicago: University of Chicago Press, 1990.

Slack, Paul. *The Impact of Plague in Tudor and Stuart England.* Oxford: Oxford University Press, 1990.

———. "The Response to Plague in Early Modern England: Public Policies and Their Consequences." In *Famine, Disease, and the Social Order in Early Modern Society,* edited by John Walter and Roger Schofield, 167–87. Cambridge: Cambridge University Press, 1991.

Torres Ramírez, Bibiano, and José Hernández Palomo, eds. *Andalucía y América en el siglo XVI: Actas de las II jornadas de Andalucía y América.* 2 vols. Seville: Escuela de Estudios Hispano-Americanos, 1983.

Trexler, Richard C. *Public Life in Renaissance Florence.* Ithaca, N.Y.: Cornell University Press, 1991.

Vázquez García, Francisco, and Andrés Moreno Mengíbar. *Poder y prostitución en Sevilla.* Seville: Universidad de Sevilla, 1995.

Velázquez y Sánchez, José. *Anales epidémicos: Reseña histórica de las enfermedades contagiosas en Sevilla desde la reconquista cristiana hasta nuestros días (1866).* Seville: Colección Clásicos Sevillanos, Ayuntamiento de Sevilla, 1996.

Vioque Cubero, Rafael, Isabel M. Vera Rodríguez, and Nerea López López. *Apuntes sobre el origen y evolución morfológica de las plazas del casco histórico de Sevilla.* Seville: Ayuntamiento de Sevilla, 1987.

Walter, John, and Roger Schofield, eds. *Famine, Disease, and the Social Order in Early Modern Society.* Cambridge: Cambridge University Press, 1991.

Webster, Susan Verdi. *Art and Ritual in Golden-Age Spain: Sevillian Confraternities and the Processional Sculpture of Holy Week.* Princeton, N.J.: Princeton University Press, 1998.

Wilson Bowers, Kristy Sue. "Plague, Politics, and Municipal Relations in Sixteenth-Century Seville." Ph.D. diss., Indiana University, 2001.

INDEX